A Colour Atlas of Demonstrations in Surgical Pathology

Royal College of Surgeons of Edinburgh

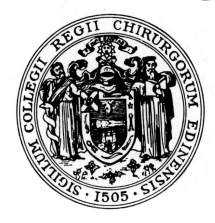

Volume 2

Head and Neck
Endocrine System
Breast
Skin

Wolfe Medical Publications Ltd

Contents

Foreword

The quality of the clinical practice of surgery, the art of teaching and the development of research are unquestionably dependent upon sure foundations in the basic sciences of anatomy, physiology and biochemistry and the ability to apply them. The understanding of surgical disease and its pattern of evolution depends upon this fundamental knowledge together with a full appreciation of pathology, including dynamic or 'living' pathology as Moynihan called it. This new series on Surgical Pathology is based on the unique collection of specimens from the Museum of the Royal College of Surgeons of Edinburgh which houses one of the largest and most historic collections of surgical pathological specimens in the United Kingdom. This material is now presented in a synoptic and illustrative form which makes understanding and learning easy. It has evolved from the development of a series of demonstration boards which have been on permanent display singly or in groups in the hall over the past few years. This method of presentation was originally devised in the Wellcome Museum for Tropical Diseases in London and adapted to our needs by the then Conservator, Professor D.E.C. Mekie, and his colleagues. They have met with considerable acceptance from postgraduate students and other visitors and it was this that inspired their publication. I am proud to be associated with this important publication which has been authorised by the College.

John Gillingham C.B.E.

Acknowledgements

The Editors have been aided in their task of co-ordinating the contributions received and arranging the layout of the material. This has been achieved with the aid of a team to whom tribute is paid for their great contribution and advice.

Dr W.A. Copland has scrutinised and provided much of the radiographic material. Dr N. MacLean has again prepared the histopathological illustrations. He has also undertaken the preparation of the captions with careful emphasis on the essential features necessary for interpretation. Dr M.O. Wright has advised on the content required for the proper understanding of essential physiology and has been responsible for the contribution in this field in the part of this volume dealing with the endocrine system.

The Editors must express their gratitude to Mr A.I.S. Macpherson for scrutiny and preparation of text and to Mr J.A. Ross for advice and reading of proofs. The photography has again been undertaken by Mr M. McKenzie the College photographic technician who has maintained his high standards of excellence. Much of the onerous work has been undertaken by Mrs Violet Tansey exhibiting her high skill in the preparation of the manuscript for publication.

6

Contributors

Mr U. Chetty	*Edinburgh*
Mr J. Cook	*Edinburgh*
Sir James Fraser Bt	*Edinburgh*
Mr A.D.B. Harrower	*Airdrie*
Professor J.A.A. Hunter	*Edinburgh*
Mr I.S. Kirkland	*Edinburgh*
Dr N. Maclean	*Edinburgh*
Dr K.M. McLaren	*Edinburgh*
Mr A.I.S. Macpherson	*Edinburgh*
Dr J.A.M. Murray	*Edinburgh*
Professor K. Shanmugaratnum	*Singapore*
Professor J.C. Southam	*Edinburgh*
Miss A.B. Sutherland	*Edinburgh*
Mr A.C.H. Watson	*Edinburgh*
Professor D.H. Wright	*Southampton*
Dr M.O. Wright	*Edinburgh*

Introduction

An essential requirement for the surgeon is a knowledge of the pathology of lesions encountered in practice to the point where the individual tissue changes can be visualised, and an ability to recognise with accuracy the nature and character of lesions when exposed at operation. Such knowledge may be partly achieved from textbooks but a full visual concept can only be adequately acquired by the study of specimens whether as seen fresh in the operating room, exposed at post mortem examination or as found in museums. The Museum of the Royal College of Surgeons of Edinburgh was commenced in 1807 for this very purpose and has continued to grow and evolve to meet new concepts. It is now chiefly used by postgraduate students preparing for the Fellowship examinations and research workers.

It is essential as well as convenient that these two methods of approach should be conducted simultaneously. In recent years, therefore, the College Museum collection has been supplemented by a series of demonstrations on which photographs together with histological, radiological and clinical illustrations and diagrams are associated with an appropriate text. The text has been in synoptic form and arranged schematically to indicate logical lines of learning. The text covered essential related embryology, anatomy and physiology together with an account of the aetiology and nature of the lesion as would be found in larger textbooks. The demonstrations have thus integrated the visual advantages of the study of specimens with the systematic approach of the textbooks.

This work is based on these demonstrations which have been revised and expanded to meet the needs of postgraduate students preparing for Fellowship examinations or for more advanced higher diplomas. This revision has been undertaken by individual contributors who possess expertise in the different fields. The demonstrations are identified by the alpha-numeric index of the museum catalogue.

Part I – Head and Neck

Acquired Lesions

The acquired lesions including inflammatory, metabolic and neoplastic, occurring in the head and neck are numerous, diverse in character and frequently the site is incidental. Many are of minor significance and receive only minimal mention to assist in the differential diagnosis. In a majority of instances the lesions are described according to their anatomical site but lesions of similar pathology are grouped together according to the site most commonly affected.

Of the many congenital deformities of the head and neck some are ill defined in embryological terms, and may form part of a generalised congenital syndrome sometimes associated with chromosomal abnormalities. Others are well defined and can be directly related to the development of the craniofacial complex and the branchial arches.

1

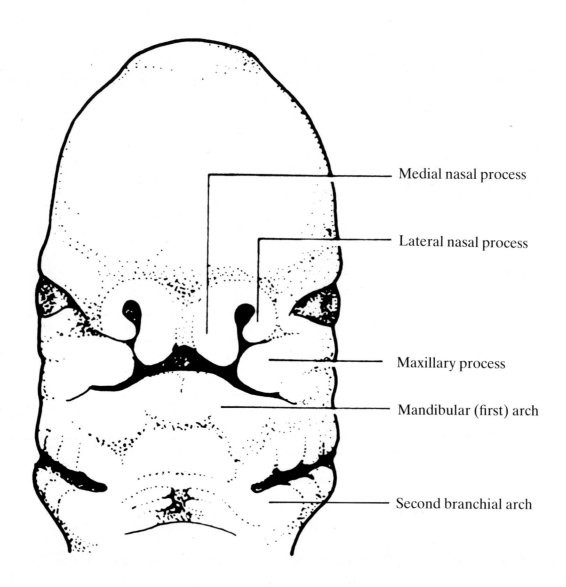

Medial nasal process

Lateral nasal process

Maxillary process

Mandibular (first) arch

Second branchial arch

1   Development of skull and face – 6 week embryo.

Major craniofacial anomalies

Since the pioneering work of Tessier (1967) these have become amenable to surgical correction. Those most important surgically are considered below.

Ocular hypertelorism

Hypertelorism was fully described by D. M. Greig in 1924 and is characterised by an increase in distance between the orbits. Clinically it can be distinguished from telecanthus (increased distance between the medial canthi) by measurement of the interpupillary distance. There is still argument about the classification of hypertelorism but it is no longer considered to be an entity in itself. It is found in association with a number of different syndromes (e.g. craniofacial dysostosis, acrocephalosyndactyly) and with frontal encephalocoele or meningocoele. It is the most important feature of the median cleft face syndrome (frontonasal dysplasia) where it is associated with a broad, bifid or cleft nose.

The skull abnormalities include hypoplasia of the sphenoid and an increased width of the ethmoid. Intelligence is frequently normal. The illustrations are those of the original case studied by Greig. The patient died aged 22 years of pulmonary tuberculosis.

2

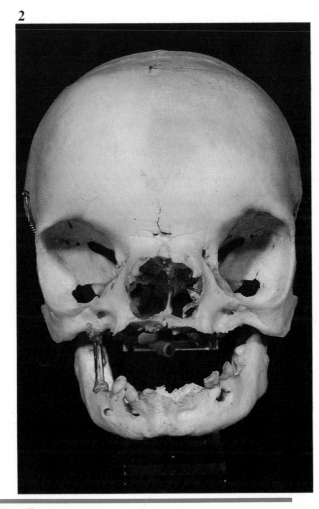

2a

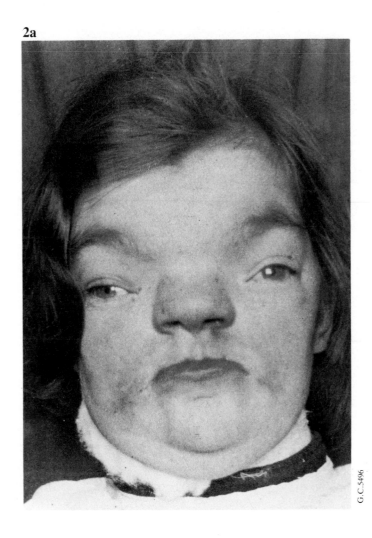

G.C.5496

Reference

GREIG, D. M. (1924) *Edinburgh Medical Journal* n.s. xxxi. **560**.
TESSIER, P. (1967) *Entretiens sur la Chirurgerie orbito-Cranienne*. Paris.

Major craniofacial anomalies *(Continued)*

Craniofacial dysostosis

This condition is also known as Crouzon's syndrome. It is characterised by premature cranial synostosis and maxillary hypoplasia causing:

(a) bilateral exophthalmos and hypertelorism
(b) parrot beak nose
(c) relative mandibular prognathism
(d) cranial deformity – brachycephaly – in which the skull shows a short A – P, and a wide transverse diameter.

The condition usually results from an autosomal dominant inheritance but some sporadic cases have been reported.

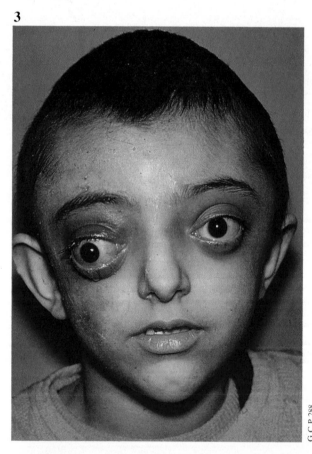

3 Craniofacial dysostosis. A 7-year-old boy showing hypertelorism and exophthalmos which is particularly severe on the right.

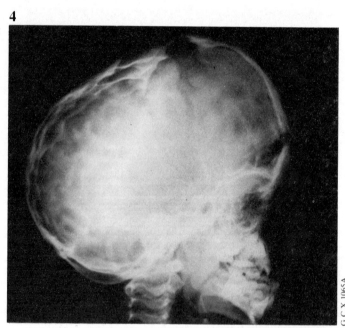

4 A similar case. Lateral radiograph showing craniofacial deformity with widening of the coronal sutures and premature synostosis of the other sutures.

Acrocephalosyndactyly

The condition is also known as Apert's syndrome.
  (a) There is a craniofacial deformity similar to Crouzon's syndrome with hypoplastic maxilla and exophthalmos. The cranium is acrocephalic or brachycephalic with a high, steep forehead.
  (b) In addition there is syndactyly of all fingers and toes with short, broad thumbs and big toes. Most cases are sporadic.

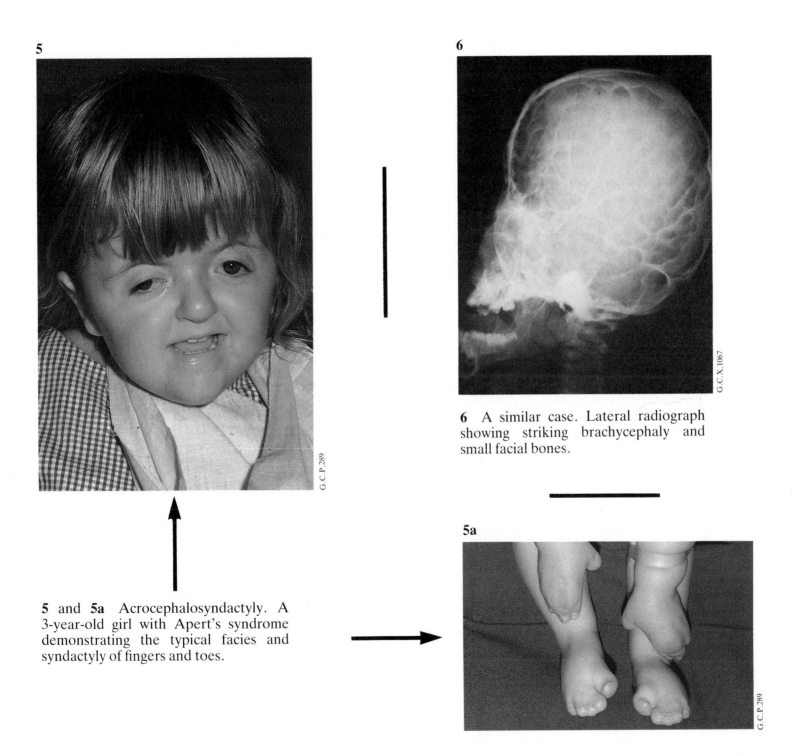

6 A similar case. Lateral radiograph showing striking brachycephaly and small facial bones.

5 and **5a** Acrocephalosyndactyly. A 3-year-old girl with Apert's syndrome demonstrating the typical facies and syndactyly of fingers and toes.

Major craniofacial anomalies *(Continued)*

Cranium

Anomalies of the cranium fall into two groups:

1 Those in which there is a primary skull defect due to faulty development and in which neurological features may occur secondarily. Many of these skull lesions result from premature fusion of the sutures.

   The neurological features result from compression and distortion of the brain. In certain instances surgical intervention by division of the fused sutures in the young baby may be helpful.

Examples

Acrocephaly (turricephaly, oxycephaly)

All sutures fused. This gives a tall pointed skull.

Scaphocephaly (Dolichocephaly)

Sagittal suture fused. Resulting in a long narrow skull.

Brachycephaly

Coronal and lambdoidal sutures fused. Leading to a broad short skull.

Plagiocephaly

Asymmetrical fusion of sutures. Giving an asymmetrical skull.

2 In the second group of lesions the primary defect is faulty development of the brain with distortion of the young developing skull, e.g. hydrocephalus.

These anomalies are considered as primary neurological disturbances and are dealt with in a later volume.

Acrocephaly

7

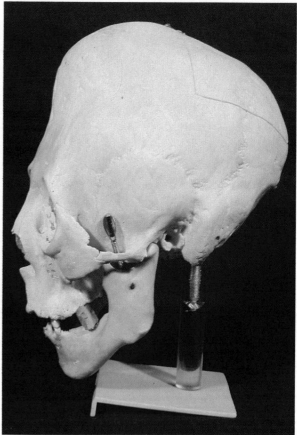

G.C.9644

7 Note fusion of all sutures.

14

Scaphocephaly

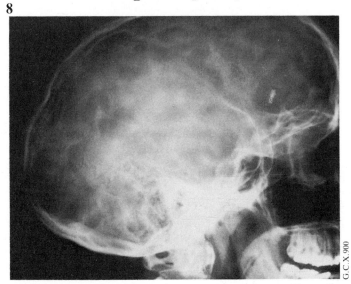

8 The coronal sutures are prematurely fused.

Brachycephaly

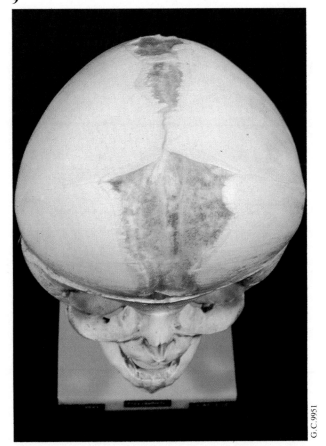

9 Note fused coronal suture and widely open fontanelles.

Plagiocephaly

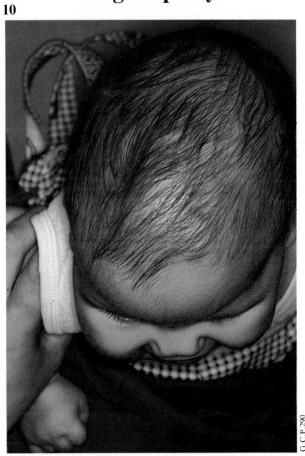

10 There is asymmetry of the vault due to premature fusion of the right coronal suture. Note also the bifid nose.

First and second branchial arches

11

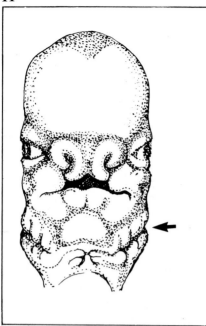

11 The first and second branchial arches and the first groove which lies between them give rise to the upper and lower jaws, muscles of mastication and facial expression, the external and middle ears and the eustachian tubes. In the embryo the maxillary and stapedial arteries supply the first and second arches respectively. Any failure of development of these embryonic structures will lead to defects of the tissues and organs that arise from them.

Mandibulofacial dysostosis

12 This syndrome is also known as the Treacher Collins syndrome or the Franceschetti–Klein syndrome. The condition is transmitted as an autosomal dominant anomaly with incomplete penetrance and variable expressivity. There is inhibition of growth at about the seventh week of embryonic life affecting the mesenchyme related to the neural crest which should migrate to the first and second branchial arches. The essential features are:

1 Hypoplasia of maxillae, zygomatic arches and mandible.
2 Antimongoloid slant of palpebral fissures.
3 Colobomas of lower eyelids.
4 Ear deformities.

The deformities are always symmetrical (cf. hemifacial microsomia).

12

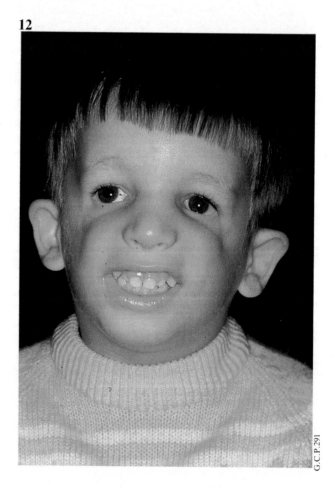

G.C.P.291

Hemifacial microsomia

This is known also as '1st branchial arch syndrome' or '1st and 2nd branchial arch syndrome'. The condition is occasionally inherited but most instances are sporadic. Other causal factors may be noted, e.g. thalidomide. It is due to hypoplasia of structures supplied by the stapedial artery during development and may be caused by a haematoma at the origin of this artery in the embryo. It presents with some or all of the following:

1 Hypoplasia of hemimandible and maxilla.
2 Hypoplasia of soft tissues of the cheek including muscles, parotid gland and facial nerve.
3 Macrostoma.
4 Ear anomalies, from accessory auricles to microtia. If severe, the middle ear is always involved.

The deformity may be bilateral but is never symmetrical. Asymmetry increases with growth in severe cases.

13

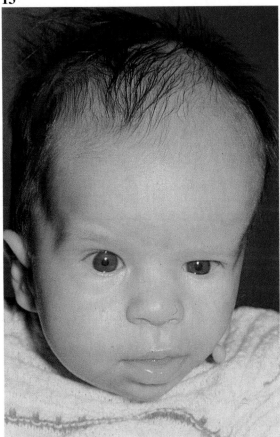

G.C.P.292

13a

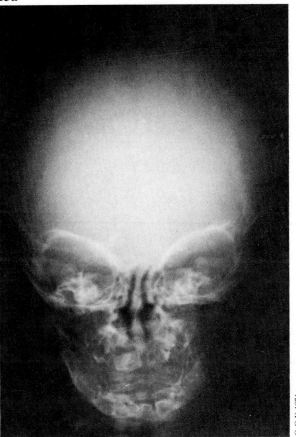

G.C.X.1074

13 This patient has left sided hemifacial microsomia. Note the hypoplasia of the maxilla, mandible and related soft tissues. The ear deformities are dealt with overleaf.

13a A.P. view of skull and face of the same child. Note the absence of the vertical ramus of the left mandible and hypoplasia of the other bones of the left side of the face. As a result, what should be the mid-line forms a curve, concave to the left.

First and second branchial arches *(Continued)*

External and middle ear – Microtia

Hypoplasia of the external ear or pinna (complete absence is termed anotia). The degree of the deformity varies greatly. When it is severe the middle ear is also hypoplastic. Examples are shown below.

14

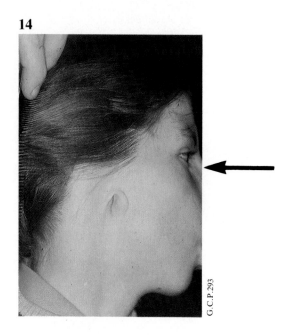

G.C.P.293

14 Here due to thalidomide. Note the absence of the external ear and its replacement by a low set blind cleft passing upwards and medially, surrounded by a rudimentary bar of cartilage. Relate this to the primitive ear in the six-week-old embryo.

15

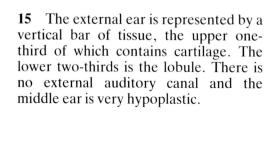

G.C.P.294

15 The external ear is represented by a vertical bar of tissue, the upper one-third of which contains cartilage. The lower two-thirds is the lobule. There is no external auditory canal and the middle ear is very hypoplastic.

16

G.C.P.292

16 A bar of tissue representing the lobule lies at a lower level than normal. On the cheek anterior to it, is an accessory auricle. This child also has hemifacial microsomia illustrated in (**13**).

17

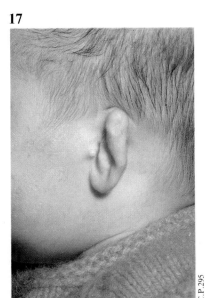

18

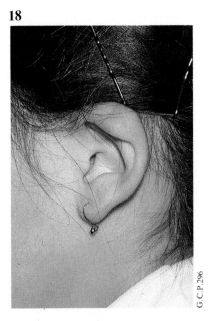

17 The pinna is partly formed and there is a slit-like external meatus but no tympanic membrane and a hypoplastic middle ear.

18 The ear is almost normal but the upper part of the pinna is folded forward in a 'cup ear' deformity. Its circumference is reduced confirming hypoplasia. The meatus and middle ear are normal.

Macrostoma

19

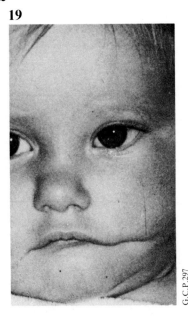

19 Lateral facial cleft. An example of a left sided cleft extending from the angle of the mouth towards the ear, and a mild hypoplasia of mandible, maxilla and associated soft tissues.

Other developmental lesions

Facial clefts

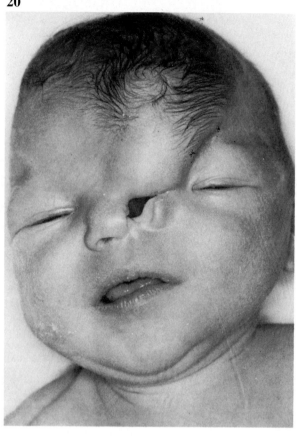

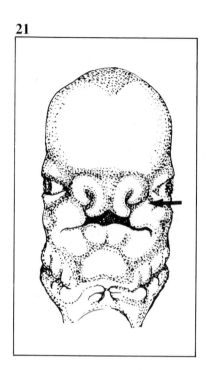

20 and **21**   Many other rare clefts have been described and have been variously classified. An example is seen here of an oblique facial cleft due to persistence of the naso-optic furrow.

External angular dermoid cyst

22   A cyst lined by squamous epithelium situated on the outer end of the supra-orbital ridge due to defective closure of the groove between the maxilla and the frontal process. There is a corresponding underlying bony depression.

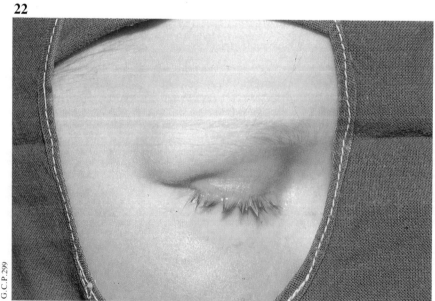

Dermoid cyst of nose

23

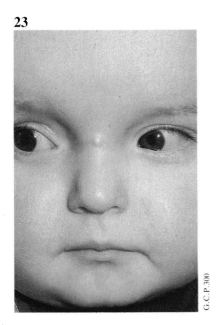

24

24a

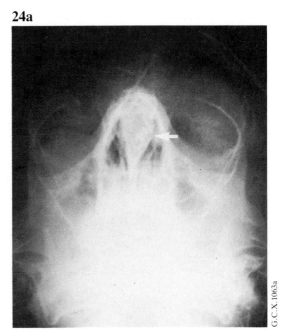

23 The illustration shows a child who presented with a recurrently infected mid-line swelling of the nose. This was a dermoid cyst due to partial failure of fusion of the medial nasal processes.

24 and **24a** An apparently superficial cyst may communicate deeply and even intracranially. The X-rays show a cyst lying in the septum. Note the tooth in the cyst which may also contain hair.

Mid-line scalp defect

Bifid nose

25

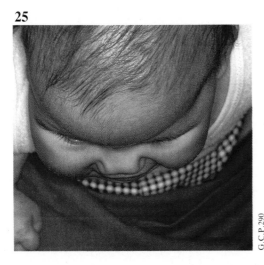

26

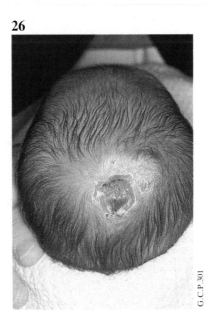

25 Another example of defective mid-line mesodermal penetration. *See also* **(10)**

26 The scalp may also be affected by a failure of mesodermal penetration. This is a mild example and healed spontaneously.

A. C. H. Watson

Cleft lip and palate

Clefts of the lip and palate produce disfigurement and disturbances in feeding, hearing and speech. From birth the feeding of the infant requires skilled management and in later life, especially after operative intervention, speech training is essential. These anomalies present the greatest challenge to the surgeon both in regards to timing of intervention and the technique of repair of the defects. For an understanding of these complex congenital deformities it is necessary to study the normal development of the face and jaws and the variations of anomalies which occur.

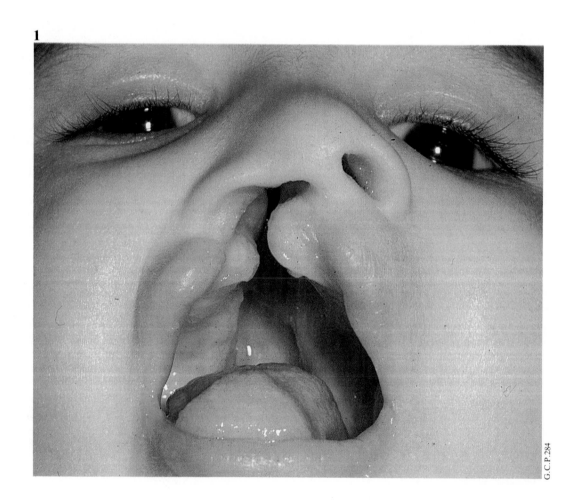

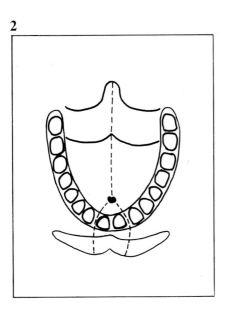

2   Lip and palate – human.

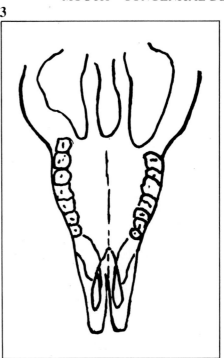

3   Palate – sheep.

The formation of the palate and the tooth bearing ridges which form the alveoli has in the course of evolution undergone many changes and a study of comparative anatomy of skulls reveals this. It illustrates too that while the major part of the palate lying posteriorly is formed by two palatal shelves arising from the maxillae, the premaxilla is a separate bone attached to the anterior edge of the vomer and bearing a small alveolar segment in which develop the incisor teeth. In the herbivorous animals, e.g. the sheep and horse, very clearly seen is the marked forward placement of the premaxilla and the intervening gap between the incisor teeth and the molars located posteriorly. In many animals including man, however, the palate is a single united plate with a single continuous alveolar margin.

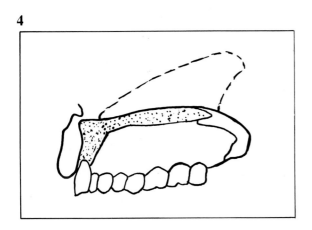

4   Premaxilla and vomer – human.

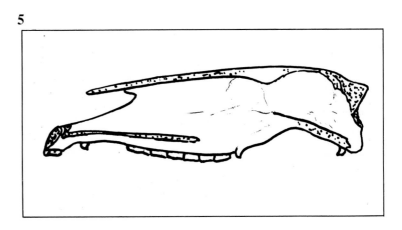

5   Premaxilla and vomer – horse.

Cleft lip and palate *(Continued)*

Embryology

There are two component elements in the formation of the lip and palate:
1 The fronto-nasal process.
2 The maxillary processes.
It is convenient to trace the early stages of the development of these separately.

Fronto-nasal process

The fronto-nasal process develops in the mid-line at the upper margin of the stomatodaeum. Covered by epithelium it increases in size by the growth of underlying mesothelial elements. The process is subdivided on its free anterior extremity into four sub-processes. These are the right and left medial and lateral nasal processes. The olfactory pits lie between the medial and lateral nasal processes on each side.

The approximation and merging of the medial nasal processes during the fifth and sixth weeks give rise to the intermaxillary segment which represents the anterior (cephalic) end of the palato-pterygo quadrate bar. This is situated in the mid-line of the vault of the stomatodaeum. Posterior to the intermaxillary segment the nasal septum develops. The intermaxillary segment develops into:
1 Part of the upper lip (prolabium).
2 The underlying premaxilla bearing the incisor teeth.
3 A small triangle of palate immediately behind the premaxilla which will lie anterior to the incisive foramen.
These constitute the 'primary palate'.

6

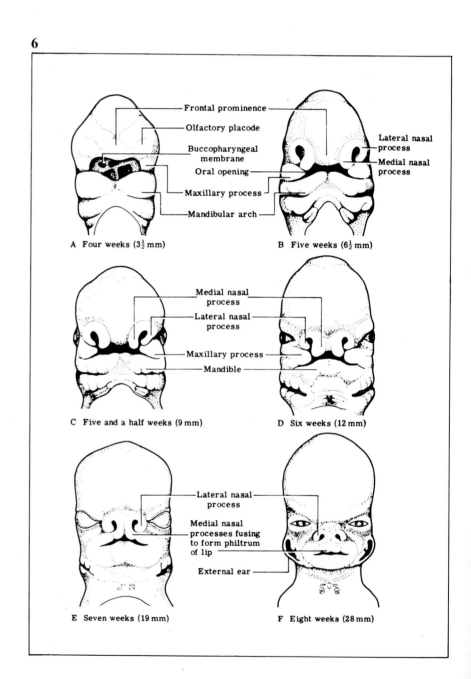

A Four weeks ($3\frac{1}{2}$ mm) B Five weeks ($6\frac{1}{2}$ mm)
C Five and a half weeks (9 mm) D Six weeks (12 mm)
E Seven weeks (19 mm) F Eight weeks (28 mm)

Maxillary processes

Very early in embryonic development a series of branchial arches develop in the lateral wall of the primitive pharynx (*see* (**6**)**A**). The arches do not project freely across a gap but are elevations above the surface of the embryo caused by the development of underlying mesenchymal growth centres. The grooves between them become obliterated as growth proceeds and the centres coalesce.

At four weeks the primitive mouth (stomatodaeum) is bounded below and at the sides by the first or mandibular arches. Each arch is described as having developed into two processes, the lower or mandibular process and the upper or maxillary process. The maxillary processes lie below the projecting forebrain forming the upper and lateral boundaries of the stomatodaeum (*see* (**6**)).

By six weeks the maxillary processes have now increased and there develops along their inner surfaces a rounded ridge extending along the whole length from before backwards. In front, this ridge is close to but separated from the primary palate and forms the palatal shelf.

7

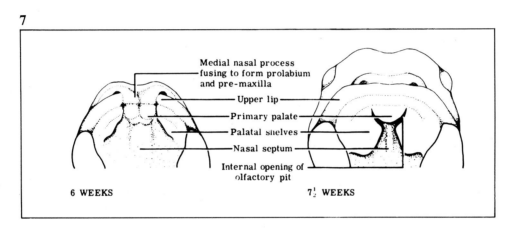

6 WEEKS   7½ WEEKS

7 Synchronously with these changes is the further development of the nasal septum. It forms a vertical partition to the upper part of the stomatodaeum. Commencing anteriorly it extends backwards as far as the posterior ends of the palatal shelves of the maxillae.

8

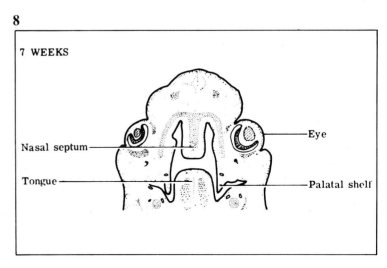

7 WEEKS

8 By the seventh week the palatal shelves are well defined. The tongue, which develops from the second arch extends upwards and occupies the whole of the stomatodaeum. The palatal shelves are therefore separated by the tongue and moulded downwards by the pressure which it exerts. During this period there is an upward and forward development of the third arch. Later this process expands into the palate and is concerned with the development of the palatal muscles and constitutes the posterior pillars of the fauces.

Cleft lip and palate *(Continued)*

Development of the nose and lip

The development of the nose is intimately related to the changes previously described. The olfactory pits are initially separated from the stomatodaeum by a membrane which breaks down to form the nostrils. The two medial nasal processes fuse. These fused processes are the site of the formation of the columella of the nose and central part of the upper lip (prolabium). From the lateral nasal processes the alae are formed. Synchronously the development of the upper lip and alveolus is taking place. During the sixth week of embryonic life mesoderm continues to flow into the maxillary processes and the medial nasal processes filling the grooves between them and creating the complete upper lip and alveolus. Note that the prolabium does not contribute materially to the musculature of the upper lip and in operative reconstruction, especially of the bilateral cleft, it is important to bring into apposition the muscle tissue derived from the maxillary processes.

Fusion of palate

9 From the eighth week, fusion of the premaxilla and the palatal shelves occurs. Fusion commences anteriorly where the tongue is less massive. More posteriorly the palatal shelves are still separated by the tongue but, by the growth of the mandible and extension of the neck, the tongue descends and moves backwards. The palatal shelves of the maxilla come to lie above the tongue and assume a horizontal plane.

9

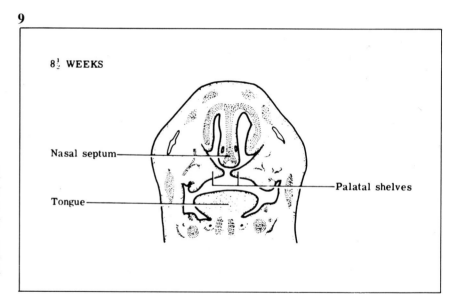

8½ WEEKS

Nasal septum

Tongue

Palatal shelves

10

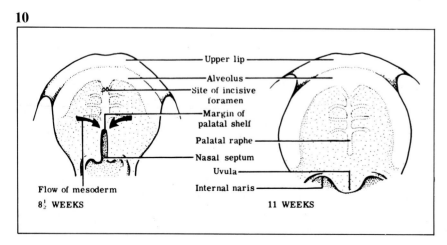

Upper lip

Alveolus

Site of incisive foramen

Margin of palatal shelf

Palatal raphe

Nasal septum

Uvula

Internal naris

Flow of mesoderm

8½ WEEKS

11 WEEKS

10 As the shelves grow, their edges approximate. Fusion now occurs from before backwards from the incisive foramen. Above, the palatal shelves are in contact with and later fuse with the nasal septum. That part of the palate which is attached to the septum is the future hard palate while the portion not attached becomes the soft palate.

Developmental anomalies

The complex process of development and fusion inherent in the formation of the lip and palate may be arrested at any point. The resulting malformation varies greatly in character from the complete cleft which represents total failure of the process, to notching of the lip or bifid uvula which represent minimal lesions.

Genetic factors

The families of 'cleft' patients have an increased susceptibility to the deformity. There are two epidemiologically distinct groups:

	1 Clefts of Lip± Cleft Palate	2 Clefts of Palate alone
Sex ratio	More common in males	More common in females
Incidence	0.8 – 1.6/1000 births	0.36 – 0.49/1000 births
Familial incidence	4% chance of similar cleft in siblings and children of patient when parents unaffected.	2% chance of similar cleft in siblings and 6% in children of patient.

If one parent and one child are affected the chance of a cleft in another child rises to almost 14%.

Teratogens

Clefts have been attributed to the effect of drugs and certain teratogens have been incriminated. Many are known to cause clefts in animals, e.g. cortisone and hypervitaminosis A. Rubella virus and the drugs Thalidomide and Aminopterin have been proved to cause clefts in man.

Classification

The degree of failure of fusion varies widely and the resulting clefts are of different degree and form. It is convenient to classify them on an embryological basis. Clefts affecting lip, alveolus and the line of fusion between the premaxilla and the palatal shelves, i.e. clefts anterior to the incisive foramen, are collectively termed 'clefts of the primary palate'. Clefts posterior to the incisive foramen which result from failure of the palatal processes are described as 'clefts of the secondary palate'.

Cleft lip and palate *(Continued)*

Complete cleft

Bilateral

Bilateral cleft lip extending into the nostril on each side and associated with a 'Y' cleft of the hard and soft palate is the most gross form of anomaly. It represents total failure of the process of fusion. The unrestrained premaxilla projects far forwards in front of the palatal shelves. The gap between the two segments of the hard palate may be wide, partly because of deficiency of tissue and partly because of distorted muscle action. Through this gap can be seen the inferior border of the nasal septum. There has been a failure or delay of mesodermal migration, the grooves between the medial nasal process and maxillary process have broken down giving rise to a cleft of the lip and alveolus. Similarly the palatal shelves have failed to fuse and a cleft of the secondary palate has resulted. These features are illustrated in the accompanying diagram and clinical photograph.

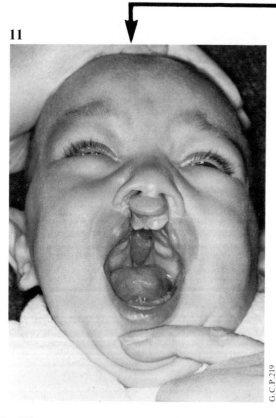

11

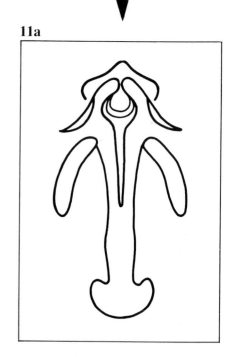

11a

A one-week-old girl with a complete bilateral cleft of lip and palate. Note the premaxilla and prolabium suspended from the anterior end of the nasal septum. The columella is absent with resulting gross deformity of the tip of the nose.

11 The protrusion of the premaxilla can be a major problem in treatment. The tension of the orbicularis muscle created by repair of the lip restrains the forward growth of the premaxilla and the lateral elements of the maxillary arch grow forward to form a more normal relationship as growth proceeds.

11a The construction of the normal muscle relationships in repair of the soft palate acts in a similar way. The muscles in a cleft palate lack a central anchorage and therefore act as distractors of the margins of the gap of both the soft and hard palate. Early repair of the muscles will result in a restoration of muscle function and some degree of narrowing of the gap.

Unilateral

The cleft may be unilateral, fusion having taken place between the premaxilla and the palatal shelf on one side. As a result the premaxilla and nasal septum will show deviation.

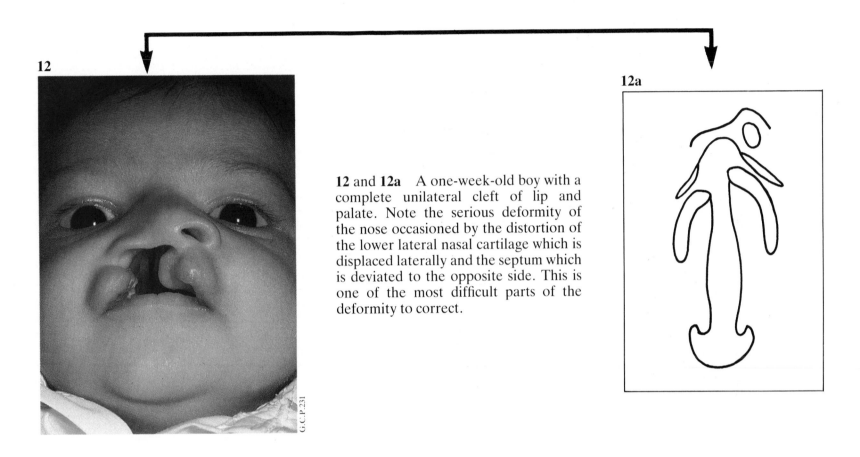

12

12a

12 and **12a** A one-week-old boy with a complete unilateral cleft of lip and palate. Note the serious deformity of the nose occasioned by the distortion of the lower lateral nasal cartilage which is displaced laterally and the septum which is deviated to the opposite side. This is one of the most difficult parts of the deformity to correct.

Incomplete clefts

Where failure of fusion has been partial the resulting clefts may affect elements arising from either the primary or secondary palate. These are described separately.
1 Cleft lip – those mainly affecting the lip and nostril (primary palate).
2 Cleft palate – those in which the major defect is of the palate (secondary palate).

Cleft lip and palate *(Continued)*

Cleft lip

Failure of fusion of the maxillary and fronto-nasal processes, completely or incompletely, results in a cleft involving the parts derived from the primary palate. The simplest form is represented by a notching of the lip – failure of closure of the lower end of the cleft between the medial nasal process and maxillary process. The most extreme form is where the cleft of the lip extends into the floor of the nostril and is associated with a cleft of the alveolus. The cleft may be unilateral or bilateral.

13a
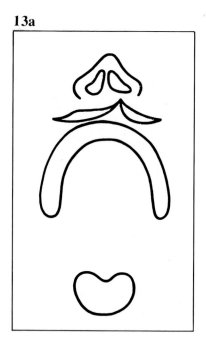

13b
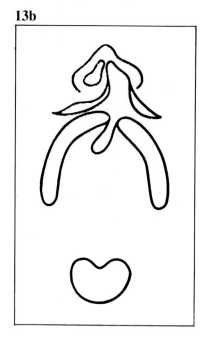

13c
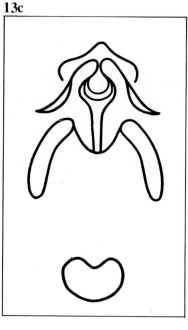

13a Incomplete cleft of lip.

13b Complete unilateral cleft of lip and primary palate.

13c Complete bilateral cleft of lip and primary palate.

13
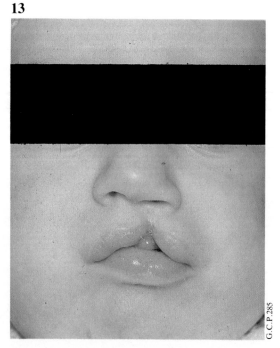

13 Boy with incomplete unilateral cleft of lip alone. Note the minimal nasal deformity.

Nasal deformity

The deformities of the nose are significant and disfiguring. The ala is flattened and expanded laterally. The anterior septum is deviated towards the side of the deformity and the columella is shortened so that the tip of the nose is drawn downwards and backwards.

Cleft palate

Clefts involving only the secondary palate range in severity from those which involve both the hard and soft palate from the incisive foramen to those limited to the soft palate or uvula. The septum may be wholly unattached or attached to one or other palatal shelf. The defect has been ascribed to:

1 Failure of development of palatal shelf growth centres.
2 Failure of descent of the tongue.
3 Failure of shelves to swing horizontally.
4 Failure of fusion of apposed epithelium.

14

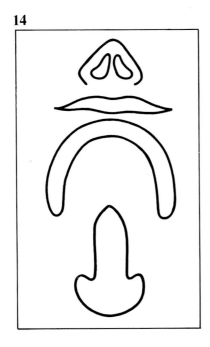

14a

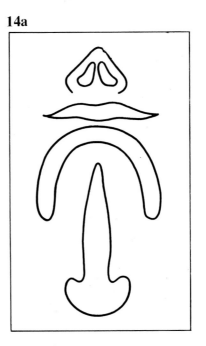

14 Cleft of the soft palate alone.

14a Cleft of the whole secondary palate.

Submucous cleft palate

15

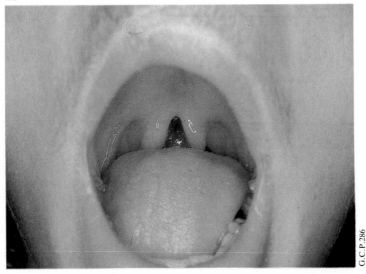

This minimal malformation of the palate is often missed until speech problems arise. Oral and nasal mucosa of the palate are intact, but there is no muscle union. It can be recognised by: bifid uvula, a groove in mid-line of soft palate and by a notch in posterior border of hard palate. Many people with submucous clefts speak normally.

15 Boy aged 10 years with 'cleft palate' speech.

G.C.P.286

31

Cleft palate (*Continued*)

Normal soft palate function

The soft palate (velum) consists of two layers of mucosa with muscle and aponeurosis in between. The muscles form two slings which pull the palate upwards and backwards to separate the nasal and oral cavities during speech and swallowing. The superior constrictor muscle sends fibres into the soft palate and contributes a sphincteric element to closure. This is particularly important in swallowing but is also significant in some normal speech.

Muscles of palate

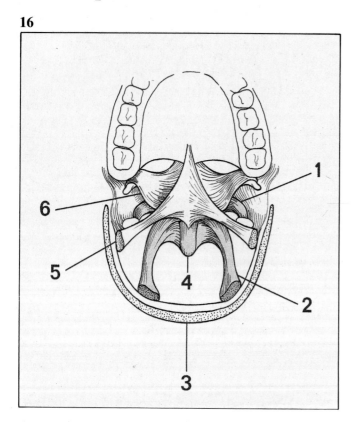

16 Muscles of soft palate from below.

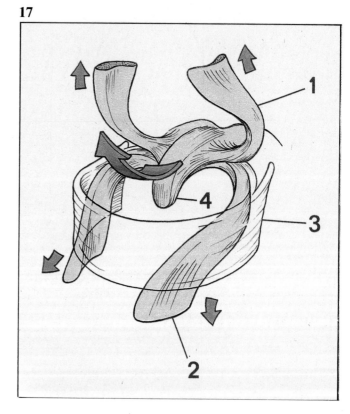

17 Posterior oblique view of normal soft palate showing directions of muscle pull.

Key

1 Levator palati	**2** Palato-pharyngeus	**3** Superior constrictor
4 Musculus uvulae	**5** Palato-glossus	**6** Tensor palati

Radiological studies

At rest, the nasopharyngeal airway is open.

During phonation of the sound 'ss' the soft palate moves upwards and backwards to close off the nasal cavity from the pharynx.

18

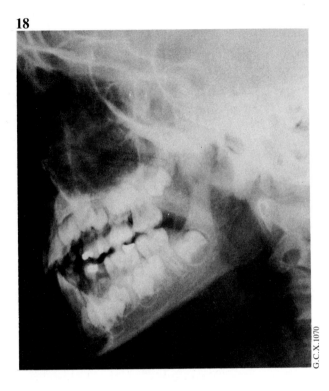

G.C.X.1070

19

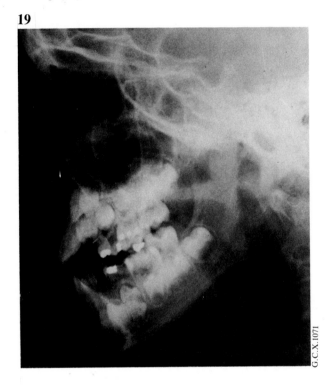

G.C.X.1071

18a

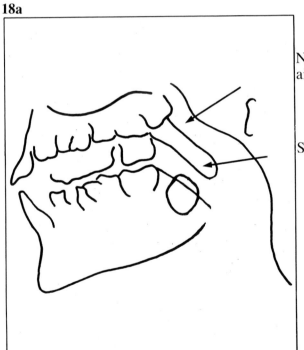

Nasopharyngeal airway

Soft palate

19a

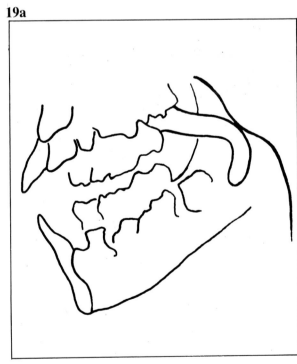

Cleft palate *(Continued)*

Defective soft palate function

20

In the cleft palate the slings do not exist. The muscles of the palate are inserted into the posterior margins of the hard palate and the sides of the cleft. Therefore, on contraction they may widen the cleft.

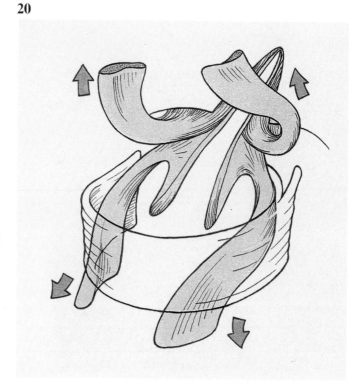

20 Cleft palate – posterior oblique view demonstrating distortion of palatal muscle slings.

Anteroposterior shortening of the soft palate which is an important factor in causing inability to close the nasopharynx is a component of the deformity of cleft palate. This can be difficult to correct at operation if there is tissue deficiency and may persist even if the cleft has been closed.

When the palate is short the patient can often effect closure with the help of the superior constrictor which produces an inward movement of the side walls of the pharynx and sometimes forward movement of the posterior wall – the so-called Passavant's ridge. This leads to a sphincteric type of closure.

Occasionally even when the palate is short it will achieve contact with the posterior pharyngeal wall when there is hypertrophy of adenoid tissue thus giving occlusion of the nasopharynx. Removal of the adenoids in such cases can cause nasal speech.

The levator and tensor palati muscles arise in part from the eustachian tube and its function is disturbed when there is a cleft. This may lead to retention of secretions in the middle ear causing deafness. Imperfect closure of the lower end of the tube may also occur and infection may pass upward from the nasopharynx.

Radiological studies

X-rays from a patient in whom the cleft palate has been repaired. At rest, the position of the palate is demonstrated but observe that it is attenuated.

During phonation of the sound 'ss' there is a persisting gap between soft palate and posterior pharyngeal wall which allows nasal escape of air during speech.

21

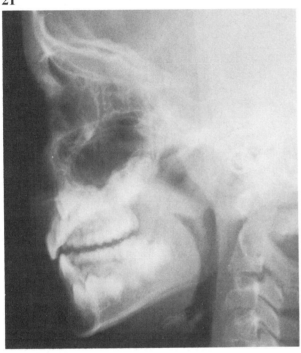

21a

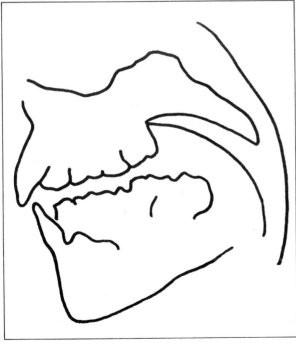

22

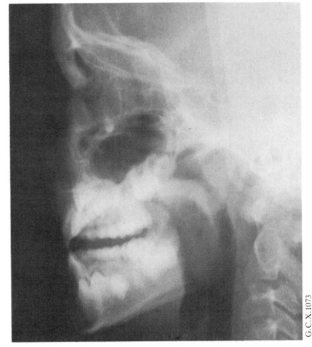

22a

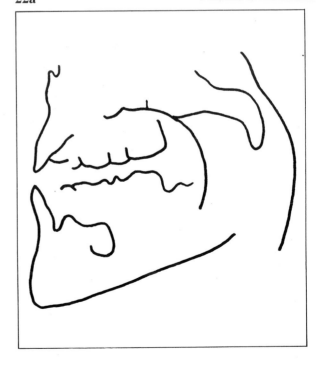

Cleft palate *(Continued)*

Blood supply

The blood supply of the palate is of great surgical significance. The operative closure of a cleft palate involves raising mucoperiosteal flaps based on the greater palatine arteries. Success depends upon maintenance of the blood supply both during the incision defining, and in elevation of the flaps. Damage to the blood supply during operation may lead to failure of closure of the cleft.

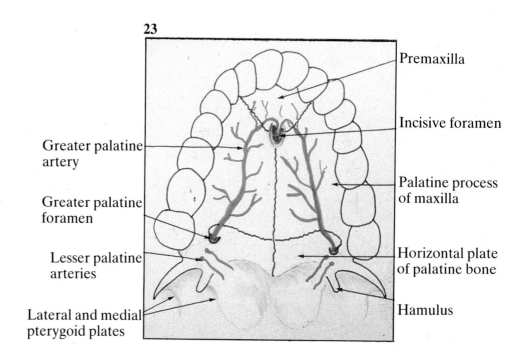

Combined lesions

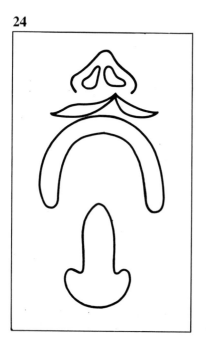

This term covers the many examples where incomplete clefts of the lip and palate are associated and represents a partial failure of fusion at both extremities of the embryonic cleft.

24   Incomplete cleft of lip and palate.

Median cleft lip

25

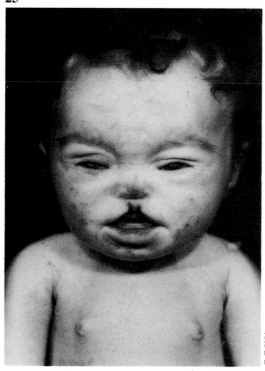

Median clefts of the upper lip are rare anomalies. The example illustrated shows gross hypoplasia of structures arising from the intermaxillary segment. They may also occur in association with hypertelorism and bifid nose in the 'median cleft face' syndrome.

Pierre Robin syndrome

(Robin Anomalad)

26

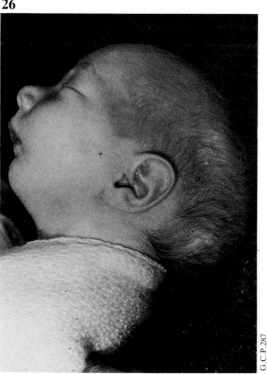

A small, retrodisplaced mandible, glossoptosis and neonatal respiratory distress, often associated with cleft palate. The small mandible may be due to hyperflexion of the neck secondary to oligohydramnios. The tongue has no room to descend and the palatal shelves cannot come together and fuse. The mandible develops after birth and may reach normal size.

26a

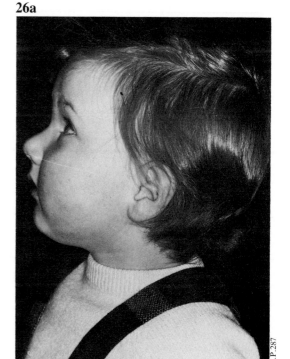

A. C. H. Watson

Thyroglossal duct

Thyroid anlage appears in the 2 − 2.5mm embryo. From its point of origin between the first and second branchial arches the thyroglossal duct passes downwards and forwards in the midline to reach a point anterior to the body of the hyoid.

It curves upwards behind the bone lying between the hyoid and the thyrohyoid membrane. It then passes downwards in front of the thyroid cartilage and the upper rings of the trachea.

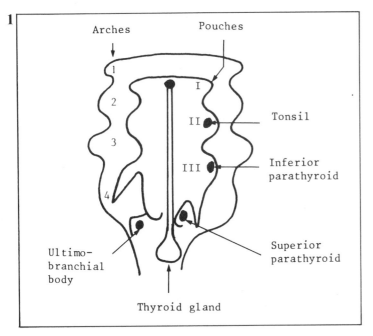

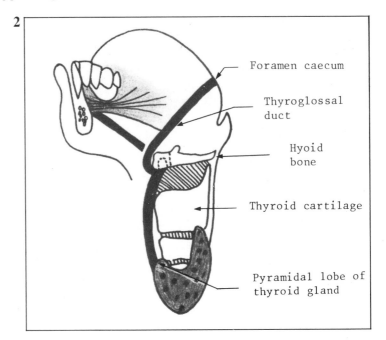

1 and **2** The isthmus of the thyroid gland lies opposite the second and third rings of the trachea. The two lateral lobes extend above and below these rings. The lower part of the tract above the isthmus may also be the site of thyroid glandular elements and forms the so-called pyramidal lobe. The point of origin of the tract is represented in the adult by the foramen caecum at the junction of the anterior two thirds and posterior third of the tongue.

The thyroglossal tract is lined by pseudo-stratified and ciliated columnar cells. Mucous glands and occasionally a squamous lining may be present.

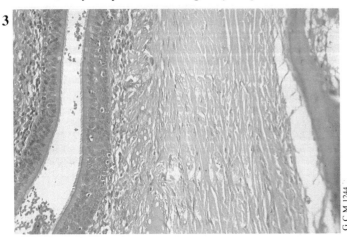

3 Thyroglossal duct. The duct (left) is lined by columnar ciliated epithelium. It is attached to the hyoid bone (right) by a broad band of hyaline fibrous tissue. (*H&E × 125*)

Thyroglossal cyst – fistula

The connection between the cervical thyroid and its point of origin normally disappears. Remnants of the connection may persist as:

1   a thyroglossal cyst

2   a fistula opening at the foramen caecum

Infection is common and may lead to a cutaneous sinus.

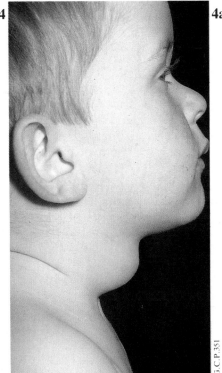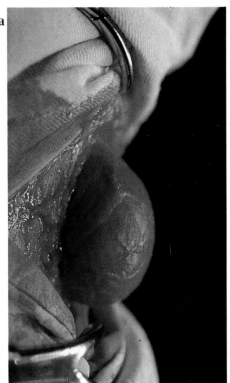

4 and **4a**   Thyroglossal cyst clinically and at operation.

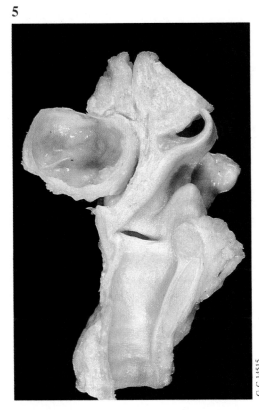

5   Thyroglossal cyst. The specimen was an incidental finding at necropsy on an elderly woman. The cyst which has tilted the epiglottis backwards has a thick fibrous wall. It was filled with mucin and has a shining epithelial lining.

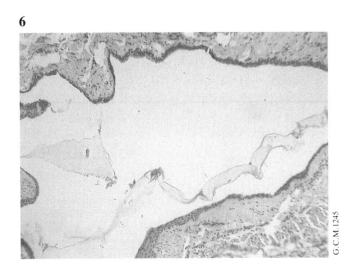

6   Thyroglossal cyst. This portion of the cyst is lined partly by columnar epithelium (top) and partly by squamous epithelium (bottom). (*H&E × 90*)

Ectopic thyroid tissue can occur at any level of the tract including the tongue (lingual thyroid). (See p. 213)

Malignant change may occur in the lining of cysts and the majority of these tumours are papillary carcinomas.

Branchial cyst – fistula

Branchial cysts lie medial to the upper third of the sternomastoid muscle. They originate from the branchial pouches, usually the second or fourth. The first and second branchial arches grow more rapidly than the others and cover them, forming the cervical sinus. Usually this disappears entirely. If the ectoderm between the second and fourth arches fuses before the cervical sinus disappears it gives rise to a branchial cyst. If the second arch fails to fuse and the sinus persists a branchial fistula occurs. Branchial fistula opens externally at the anterior border of the sternomastoid at the junction of the upper two-thirds and lower third. Its upper end is in or near the tonsillar cleft. The track of the fistula (or sinus if there is only an external opening) passes between the VII and XII nerves superficially and the IX nerve deeply on the side wall of the pharynx and between the internal and external carotid arteries i.e. between the nerves and arteries of the second and third branchial arches.

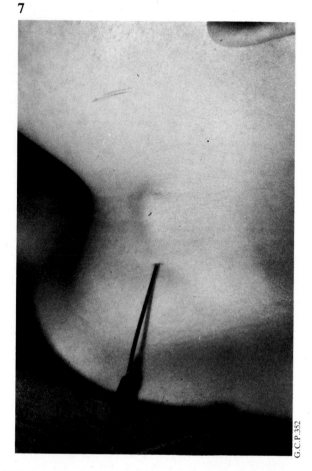

G.C.P.352

7 The lower end of a branchial tract which discharged pus intermittently. (Probe in fistula.)

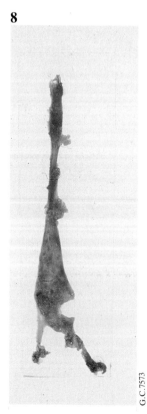

G.C.7573

8 Branchial sinus. From a boy aged 5 years who had an intermittent discharge from a minute opening at the junction of the middle and distal thirds of the anterior border of the left sternomastoid muscle. The sinus track was about 7cm long. The lowest portion was V-shaped. The trumpet shaped portion above it passed deep to the cervical fascia and on to the carotid sheath. The elongated part ran upwards to the supratonsillar fossa and was separated from the pharynx by only the thin pharyngeal mucous membrane.

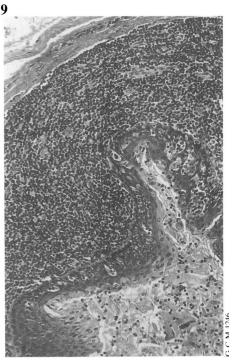

The lining is with non-keratinised squamous epithelium closely resembling that of the pharynx, or occasionally by stratified columnar epithelium with surface cilia. A feature is the presence of a large amount of subepithelial lymphoid tissue.

The connective tissue of the wall is dense and fibrous or loose and areolar. There may be mesodermal remnants in the wall e.g. cartilage.

9 Branchial cyst in an adult. This small part of the wall is lined by squamous epithelium. Exfoliated cells lie in the lumen mixed with lymphocytes. Hyperplastic lymphoid tissue forms most of the thickness of the wall and is enclosed by a fibrous capsule. (*H&E × 160*)

In childhood branchial cysts cause 20% of lateral neck masses.

Infection is common if there is an opening to the pharynx or skin, staphylococcus being the usual infecting organism but coliform organisms may be present.

Branchial carcinoma

Arising from persistent remnants of the branchial cleft or a cyst carcinomatous change may occur. This complication usually occurs after the age of 40 years. The tumours may be cystic or solid and are generally globular. Invasion of adjacent tissues and lymph nodes may be early or late. The tumour becomes fixed.

The structure is that of an epidermoid carcinoma containing flat squamous cells. Kerato-hyaline granules may often be present. The younger cells of such tumours tend to lose their adult flat appearance and infiltrate the tissues. The squamous cells may become more and more atypical producing cellular carcinomas of many types. (See p. 90)

Pre-auricular sinus

Pre-auricular sinuses are rare. They occur anterior to the tragus either as a small pit or a track leading backwards and upwards. These originate from the first branchial cleft.

Torticollis

The essential feature of this deformity is a contraction of the sternomastoid muscle leading to a lateral deviation of the head associated with torsion to the opposite side.

Aetiology

The aetiology is unknown. There are several theories:

1   Congenital, the cervical deformity being associated with other anomalies.

2   Ischaemia of sternomastoid. This muscle is segmental. Each segment has an individual blood supply and it has been held that there is limited vascular communication between the segments. The upper third of the muscle is supplied by a branch from the occipital artery, the middle third by a branch of the superior thyroid artery and the lower third from the inferior thyroid artery. The artery to the middle third is apparently particularly vulnerable. The ischaemia leads to muscle death and fibrotic replacement.

3   Trauma during labour leading to acute kinking and thrombosis of the artery and associated vein.

Pathology

The initial clinical manifestation is the development of an ovoid 'tumour' in the sternomastoid during the first six weeks of life. This swelling is attributable to degenerative changes in the muscle fibres with an associated oedema. The tumour disappears slowly. During this phase there is fibrous replacement of the damaged muscle and evidence of contraction increases.

Associated changes

Usually become evident about the first year of life:

10

1   Soft tissue contracture
— scalene muscles
— carotid arteries
— fascial layers of neck including the carotid fascia

2   Skeleton
— face
— skull

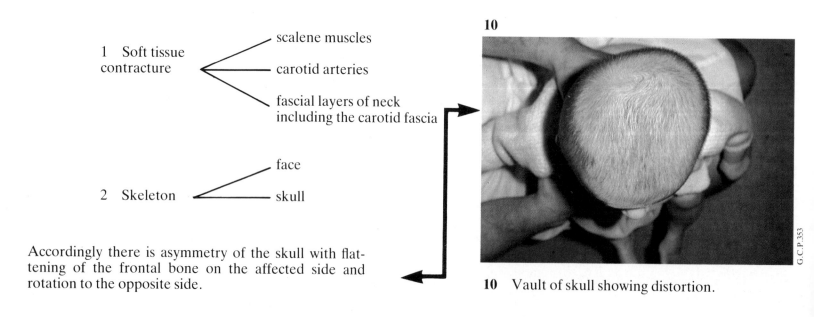

G.C.P.353

Accordingly there is asymmetry of the skull with flattening of the frontal bone on the affected side and rotation to the opposite side.

10   Vault of skull showing distortion.

Other conditions to be considered in differential diagnosis:

1 Congenital defects of the cervical spine such as hemivertebrae and abnormal fusion of vertebrae. These lesions are readily recognised radiologically.

2 Infections in the neck including spontaneous hyperaemic dislocation of the atlas.

3 Juvenile fibromatosis.

11

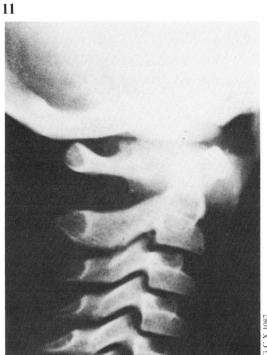

11 From a child of 4 years with a history of minor trauma resulting from a fall followed by a cervical inflammatory swelling during which period the development of torticollis was noted. Radiological examination confirmed the forward dislocation of the atlas with rotation and the absence of any bony disease.

Lymphangioma – cystic hygroma

12

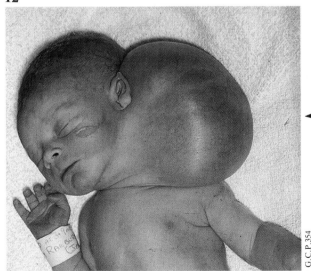

12 Tends to occur in the posterior triangle of the neck. Present at birth.

Possibly congenital obstruction of the lymphatics. Gives rise to multilocular infiltrating cysts in the neck extending into the tongue and larynx causing respiratory obstruction. Histologically these cysts are lined by flattened endothelium with focal nodules of lymphocytes. There may be evidence of thrombosis and calcification.

I.S. Kirkland

Syphilis

The Museum of the Royal College of Surgeons possesses many specimens illustrating the gross effects of syphilis. Many of these appear to be of historical interest only but they exhibit the appalling results of untreated disease.

Inherited syphilis

These lesions are now rare since syphilis is a manageable disease in the parents and there is widespread antenatal surveillance.

Craniotabes

In inherited syphilis the organisms attack and destroy the centres of ossification in the membranous bones of the skull which lead to imperfect ossification and resulting defects. These become manifest during the first two years of life.

Parrot's nodes have been attributed to syphilis but this is doubtful. These consist of bossing of the frontal or parietal bones and are due to subperiosteal spongy bone formation which is possibly syphilitic but may be due to subperiosteal haemorrhages caused by scurvy.

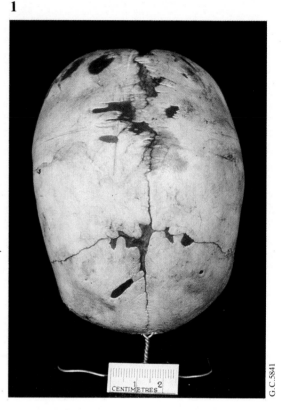

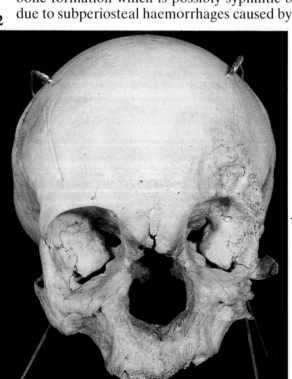

1 Skull demonstrating multiple areas of decalcification due to inherited syphilis.

Nasal bones

Saddle nose is a well recognised stigma of inherited syphilis. This is due either to failure of growth of the septum because of persistent syphilitic rhinitis in infancy, or to later gummatous destruction of the nasal bones. The palate may also be similarly affected.

2 Case of inherited syphilis demonstrating the wide nasal aperture and the absence of the nasal bone.

Hutchinson teeth

An abnormality in development of the medial upper incisor teeth resulting in a peg-shaped deformity often with notching of the narrowed cutting edge. These lesions may be accompanied by interstitial keratitis and corneal scarring and later by development of neurosyphilitic manifestation similar to those of the late adult disease.

The congenital lesions which develop in childhood are associated with malnutrition and the bony damages suggest that the lesion is often associated with recurrent rickets.

Acquired syphilis

Both the scalp and the underlying skull may be affected independently by the presence of gummatous lesions. These are late manifestations. In untreated cases as occurred in former times and which may still occur in some undeveloped areas of the world, gross lesions with hideous consequences may result. While such conditions are not seen today in the United Kingdom specimens in the museum show what can be the disaster of untreated syphilis.

A gumma of soft tissue is a yellow rubbery nodule resulting from coagulative necrosis of tissue probably as a result of a hypersensitivity reaction to the treponema. Few, if any micro-organisms can be found. The necrotic centre is surrounded by a zone of vascular granulation tissue, heavily infiltrated by inflammatory cells particularly plasma cells. A few multinucleated cells may also be present but are small and infrequent as compared with tuberculous giant cells. Endarteritis is a feature of syphilitic lesions. The syphilitic gumma ulcerates on the surface and secondary infection occurs. The underlying bone becomes involved with sequestrum formation.

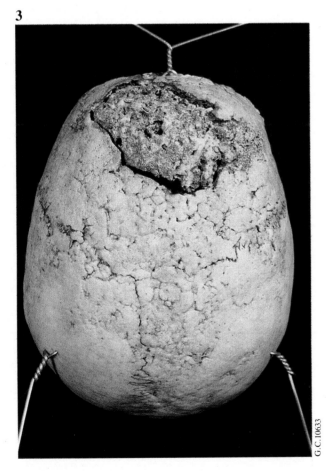

3

G.C. 10633

3 Calvarium of an adult showing osteitis and necrosis following acquired syphilis. The frontal bone is rough and irregular from extensive fissuring which divides the outer table into innumerable, small, irregular areas giving it a wormeaten appearance. The fissures have been formed by an ulcerative process destroying the outer table and affecting the diploe, and in the course of healing new bone has been deposited on the diploe in the depths of the fissures. There is a large frontal bone sequestrum perforated at numerous points. The sequestrum is adherent in part.

Tumours

Tumours of special surgical significance of the skin of the head, scalp and neck include squamous epithelioma, basal cell carcinoma and Kaposi sarcoma. These lesions are considered in detail in Part IV of this volume.

Primary tumours

Primary tumours of the skull are rare. Only two require mention here, the simple osteoma and osteo-clastoma. Simple osteomas usually occur on the inner surface as raised, sometimes elongated mounds of bone. This may cause pressure on a cranial nerve or on specific parts of the cerebrum. Osteomas also occur in the sinuses of the skull and maxilla. The osteoclastoma is much less common and on occasion has been attributed to preceding trauma.

Secondary tumours

Secondary tumours of the skull are much more common and are often multiple.

Those arising as distant metastases are most frequently derived from lesions of the breast, kidney or thyroid. Secondary tumours in childhood most usually are metastases from the suprarenal. Typically metastases from the breast appear as multiple small punched out areas in the skull with minimal surrounding bone reaction. Isolated tumours occur which may be quite large in size with pressure effects. Again the surrounding bone shows no reaction. Special note is made of thyroid metastases which are often highly vascular and pulsating and may simulate an aneurysm.

4

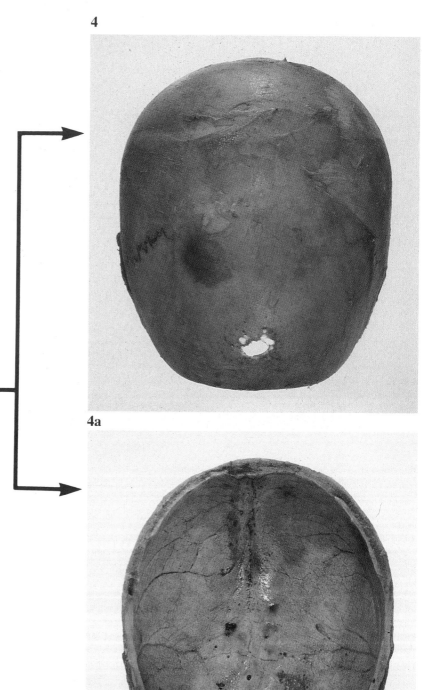

4a

4 and **4a**   Metastasis from breast car-cinoma. Exterior and interior views.

G.C. 8471

Tumours such as lymphoma, chloroma and eosinophilic granuloma may occur as part of a more generalised neoplasia which is frequently multifocal.

5 An example of chloroma in which the lesions occurred in the mandible and in the skull. This illustration, although imperfect, demonstrates the skull defects. (See p. 64)

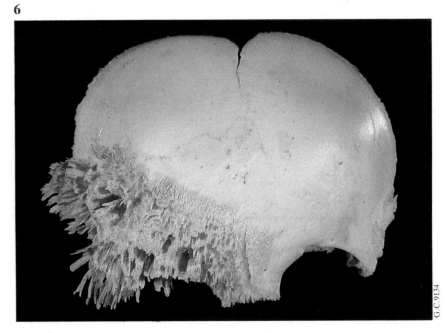

These lesions are usually first observed radiologically as a defect of the skull but the diagnosis requires fuller investigation including if necessary biopsy.

Defects of the skull which may also be recognised radiologically are found in the metabolic lesions of Hand-Schüller-Christian disease.

Two tumours which give rise to unique secondary lesions are the neuroblastoma and the meningioma. In both instances these result in the production of new bone.

Neuroblastoma

6 In the neuroblastoma spicules of bone projecting from the skull outwards are visible radiologically and are seen in the specimen. (See also p.296)

Tumours (*Continued*)

Meningioma

A meningioma causes a bone reaction in the adjacent skull with the production of projecting masses of bone which may present as spicules on both the inner and outer surfaces. Identification of these may not be easy. For example there are two museum specimens of the vault of the skull which have always presented difficulty in interpretation. They are dry specimens which antedate the days of histological examination and there are no clinical notes of the original cases. In both there are unusual outgrowths of bone from the surface of the vault of the skull. The interior of both skulls shows change. The naked eye appearances together with the radiological findings appear to establish the diagnosis of meningioma.

Case 1

7

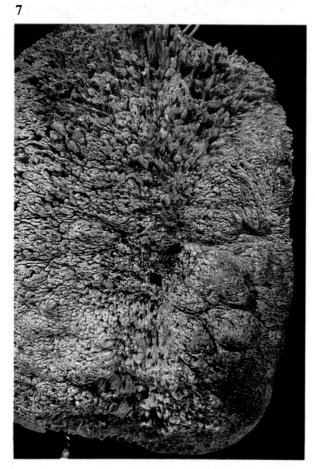

7 Exterior aspect

7a

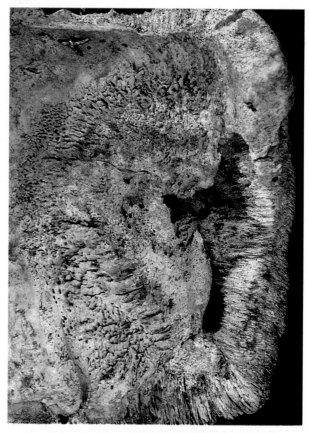

7a Interior aspect

7b

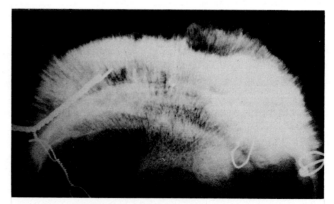

7b Radiological appearances

In this skull the inner table shows areas of erosion and formation of new bone projecting inwards simulating in structure, but in a more gross form, the spicules seen on the outer surface.

The specimen shows a layer of spicules of bone covering two thirds of the vault which involves the parietal bone on both sides.

G.C.2705

Case 2

8

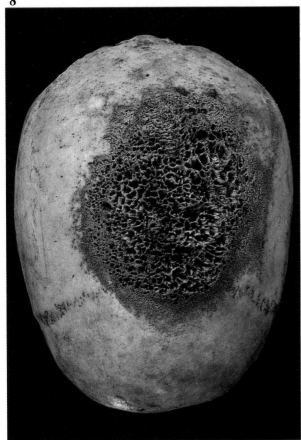

8   Exterior aspect

8a

8a   Interior aspect

In this case the external abnormality is an ovoid honeycombed area of protuberant bone measuring 10 × 8.5cm. There are diffuse areas of erosion of the inner table of the skull and a certain amount of new bone has been formed projecting inwards but to a much less degree than the reaction on the superficial surface. The area involved corresponds to the external lesion.

G.C.13262

8b

8c

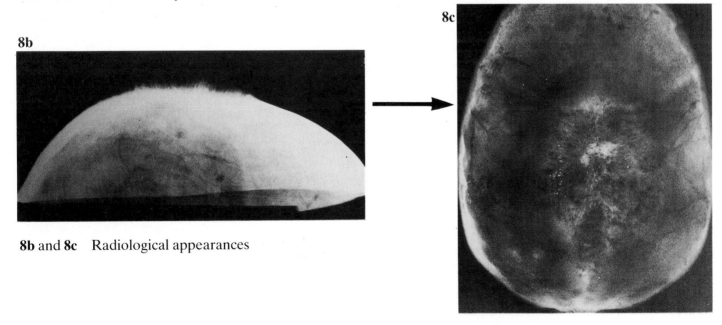

8b and **8c**   Radiological appearances

The pathology of these lesions occurring in association with an underlying meningioma is a hyperostosis of bone with infiltration of meningeal tumour cells into the inner table of the skull.

Cheek − infection

Hair follicle infection with staphylococcus aureus (boil or furuncle) is common on the cheek and lips but is more frequently seen on the back of the neck in adolescence.

The condition may be acute with rapid tissue necrosis and with general manifestations. There is a central core of necrotic tissue which is found within the abscess cavity and until this is discharged the inflammatory reaction continues. The surrounding tissue which forms the wall of the abscess becomes thickened and later fibrotic. Healing of a boil necessitates both the discharge of the necrotic core and the collapse inwards of the wall. Boils are frequently multiple, can occur in any part of the body and are typically seen in ill-nourished persons especially children.

Carbuncle

Staphylococcal infection may spread to involve the subcutaneous tissue especially in diabetics or in patients with other debilitating conditions to form a carbuncle. This consists of a honeycomb of abscesses separated by connective tissue and containing sloughs. These are most commonly seen on the back of the neck.

Septic cavernous sinus thrombosis

If septic infection occurs on the face it may spread along an emissary vein to the cavernous sinus and lead to septic cavernous sinus thrombosis. This is a rare, and potentially fatal complication.

Synergistic infections with mixed organisms, usually from the mouth, may occur on the cheek or in the submandibular region.

Cancrum oris (noma)

1 Cancrum oris is an acute ulcerative condition of the cheek caused by anaerobic micro-organisms including fusospirochaetes. It is usually encountered in the tropics in young children debilitated by malnutrition or acute infective disease such as measles. It is most commonly seen in girls between the age of 2 and 5 years. Noma begins as a blister on the inner surface of the cheek associated with marked oedema and swelling. As the blister bursts an ulcer forms and penetrates deeply. A black area of gangrene heralds the stage of total penetration. The disease spreads rapidly, may involve the floor of the mouth and mandible and is often fatal. Comparable lesions occur in the nose, vulva or scrotum (Fournier's gangrene).

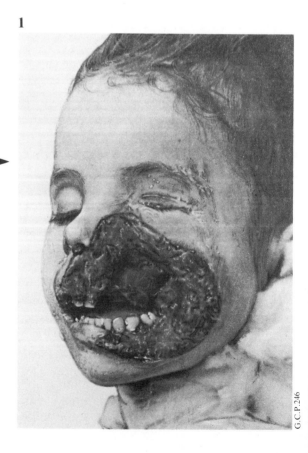

1

Lesions of the salivary glands including parotid, are dealt with in Volume I p. 10.

G.C.P.246

Epithelial tumours

Epithelial tumours both basal cell (rodent ulcer) and squamous epithelioma occur on the face and together form the most common neoplasms. These tumours occur in skin which is exposed to actinic radiation, especially in fair-skinned persons who live and work in the open air. It is particularly common in Australia. In the United Kingdom the incidence is highest in agricultural workers and fishermen. As the result of the actinic radiation the skin frequently shows a keratosis with a roughening and thickening. This forms a potential field of cancerous change and subsequent neoplasia may arise at many sites. Multiple tumours may be found in the same individual though usually not simultaneously.

The basal carcinoma or rodent ulcer is most commonly found below the lower eyelid and along a line extending from the inner canthus down the side of the nose. The tumour presents as an indolent button-like swelling with raised edges and often with a central depressed area. It expands slowly and as it does so the central area shows persistent ulceration. Occasionally these tumours undergo a sudden acceleration of growth. Initially the majority are superficial in location but an expanding invasive type occurs penetrating the deeper tissues and eventually the maxilla itself. The basal cell carcinoma may appear sometimes to undergo a transition and become a more squamoid type of lesion. The tumour is radiosensitive. The pathology of this condition is considered more fully on p. 388.

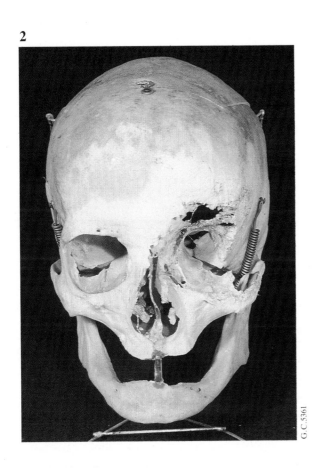

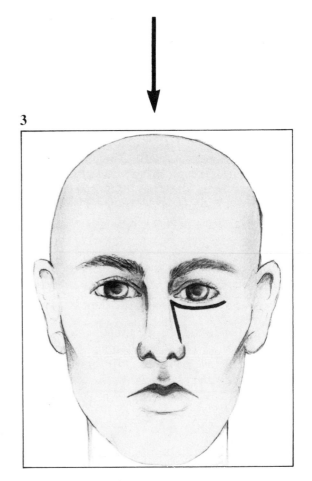

3 Maximal site incidence.

2 From a female aged 77 years. The illustration shows the destruction of the underlying bones of the face by the basal cell carcinoma which had originated in the neighbourhood of the frontal process of the zygomatic bone. Note that there has been destruction of most of the left zygomatic bone. There has also been partial destruction of the left frontal bone with penetration into the left frontal sinus and of the nasal bones and the left orbit.

The end result of the extensive tumour may be horrific and a specimen dating back to the period prior to radiotherapy and modern surgery is shown.

A.I.S. Macpherson

Maxilla

Fibro-osseous lesions of the maxilla occur in a variety of forms reflecting different proportions of osteoid and fibrous tissue. The clinical presentation is variable but classically may appear with unilateral facial swelling, deformity of the alveolar margin and loosening of the teeth. The aetiology of these lesions remains obscure.

Fibrous dysplasia

These lesions affect both or either the maxilla and the mandible with resulting deformity of the face. The disturbance commences during childhood and the process ceases to expand in later adolescence when general bone maturation occurs. The cause of the dysplasia is unknown.

The main feature is the development in the jaws of fibrous tissue and bony trabeculae showing irregularity of form. The consequent deformity of the bones may suggest tumour formation.

Radiological diagnosis is established by the deformity of the maxilla or mandible and by the bony texture which shows areas of irregularity. On occasion pseudo-cystic lesions to some of which the term 'ground glass' is applied are observed. Where the disease is of more limited character affecting only the maxilla or the mandible and is unilateral, the term monostatic (monosteotic) fibrous dysplasia is applied.

Dysplasia (cherubism)

This is an inherited disorder affecting both the mandible and the maxilla. The first evidence of the condition occurs during the 2nd and 3rd year of life. Progess thereafter may be comparatively rapid but becomes progressively less after the 7th or 8th year. The deformity resulting from the overgrowth of bone may show some diminution after puberty.

Radiological examination shows extensive areas of radiolucency involving the mandible and maxilla. There is disturbance of dentition.

Histologically there is proliferation of fibrous tissue which is seen as mature fibroblasts lying in an oedematous ground substance. Osteoclasts are present and may be in small clusters arranged around capillaries.

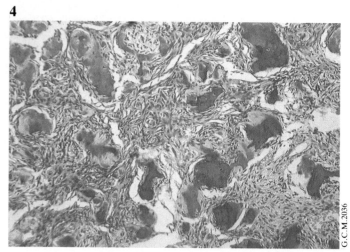

4

4 Fibrous dysplasia of the maxilla in a girl of 7 years who had a swelling of the right cheek for eighteen months. Numerous particles of cementum-like bone are set in a spindle-shaped fibrous stroma. This form of fibrous dysplasia has been referred to as 'osteocementoma'. (*H&E × 125*)

The essential feature of both fibrous dysplasia and cherubism is interference with the normal maturation of bone. The radiological picture varies according to the relative amounts of fibrous tissue proliferation and new bone formation and particularly in the early cases may resemble fibrosarcoma.

Osteitis fibrosa cystica

In hyperparathyroidism bony changes may occur both in the maxilla and mandible. There is disturbance of both the formation and resorption of bone. Cyst formation or the presence of a pseudoneoplasm resulting from marked proliferation of osteoclasts (giant cell tumour) may be a dominant feature.

The diagnosis will depend upon evidence of hyperparathyroidism.

Tumours

Tumours involving the maxilla are diverse. The clinical presentation is similar in many instances and the diagnosis may only be established after radiology and histological examination. The lesions may be classified as follows:

1. Tumours arising from fibrous or osseous tissue.
2. Tumours arising from lymphoid tissue − may be systemic.
3. Secondary tumours.
4. Tumours of dental origin.
5. Epithelial tumours arising from air sinuses.

The latter two may present as tumours of the maxilla. The lesions are considered separately.

Group 1

Primary tumours of the maxilla are rare but both fibromatous and chondromatous lesions are described and both simple and malignant types occur. The tumour may arise within the bone or from the bone surface. The tumour expands and the features depend upon its precise primary site. It may expand slowly upwards towards the orbit and erode the orbital plate, downwards to occupy the antrum and outwards giving bulging of the cheek. Inwards it involves the nasal cavity.

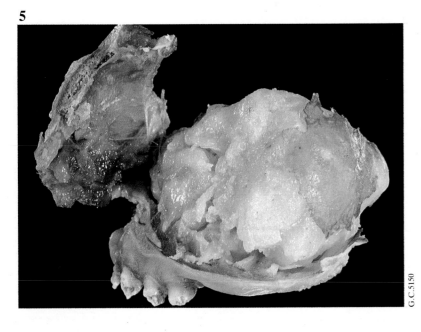

5

G.C.5150

5 An example of myxofibroma occurring in an adult. The tumour appeared to occupy the maxillary sinus and its precise point of origin was not determined.

The maxillary sinus is grossly dilated but the margins of the tumour are defined and osseous invasion is not evident.

Group 2

This group includes tumours of the lymphoma series. Of special significance is the tumour described by Burkitt which frequently demonstrates major lesions of the maxilla.

Maxilla (*Continued*)

Burkitt's lymphoma

Epidemiology

Burkitt's lymphoma is the most common childhood malignancy in tropical Africa and Papua New Guinea, and in both these areas its distribution appears to be dependent on climatic conditions – temperature and humidity. The tumour in Africa is found in those areas designated wet tropics and only rarely occurs where the mean temperature in the coolest month falls below 60°F or the rainfall is less than 40 inches per year. In these areas of every 2000 children born one will develop lymphoma before the age of 16 years. The tumour defined by histological and clinical features occurs sporadically elsewhere in the world but has a much lower incidence. Epidemiological studies in Africa have shown a time-space clustering. Variations of this clustering have been observed giving evidence of epidemic drift and also of seasonal fluctuations.

Age incidence

Burkitt's lymphoma is rare under the age of 3 years and has a peak incidence at approximately 7 years. Thereafter the incidence falls rapidly and the tumour is uncommon after the age of 15. Late teenage and adult cases of Burkitt's lymphoma are rare in tropical Africa and tend to occur in immigrants from highland areas where the tumour is uncommon. The age of onset of Burkitt's lymphoma appears to be inversely related to the frequency of the tumour in any one population group.

Sex incidence

The male to female sex incidence is approximately two to one, though under the age of 5 years the incidence in females is greater than in males.

Pathology

The anatomical distribution of Burkitt's lymphoma in most patients is strikingly different from that seen in other malignant lymphomas.

Face

Involvement of one or more quadrants of the jaw occurs in approximately 50% of the African cases. This is an age-related phenomenon being maximal at the age of 3 years and falling progressively thereafter. The earliest radiological lesion appears around the apices of erupted and developing teeth. Jaw involvement is considerably in excess of lesions in other bones.

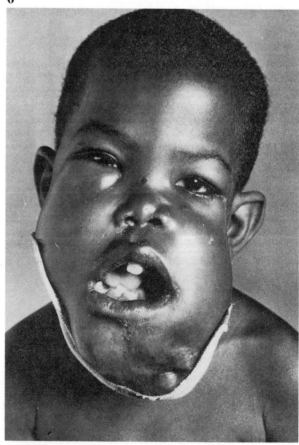

6

6 Burkitt's lymphoma involving all four quadrants of the jaw, with considerable displacement of the teeth.

The illustrations are from the collection of Professor D.H. Wright.

Lymphatic system

The tumour rarely involves the thymus or peripheral nodes and at autopsy only involved one third of the spleens of the Ugandan cases and often only to an extent that was trivial in comparison with other organs.

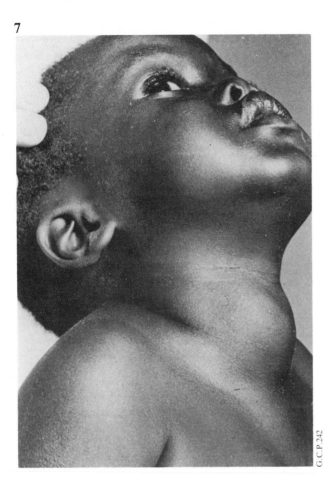

7 Infiltration of the thyroid gland causing a goitre in a child with Burkitt's lymphoma.

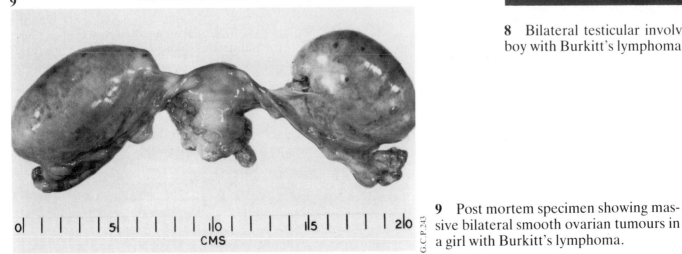

Gonads and breasts

Other characteristic sites of the disease are the gonads and the breasts.
Male – One or both of the testes are involved in 5–10% of patients.
Female – 80% of the Ugandan females suffering from Burkitt's lymphoma had ovarian infiltrations which were usually bilateral and frequently massive, whilst in young women during pregnancy and lactation, massive bilateral involvement of the breasts was often a dramatic manifestation of the disease.

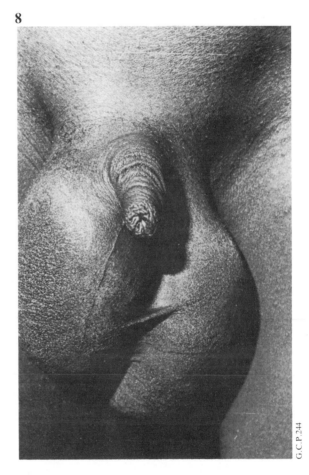

8 Bilateral testicular involvement in a boy with Burkitt's lymphoma.

9 Post mortem specimen showing massive bilateral smooth ovarian tumours in a girl with Burkitt's lymphoma.

Burkitt's lymphoma (*Continued*)

Kidney and liver

At autopsy almost all cases show renal tumours and the liver is involved in approximately 40% of cases. Retroperitoneal masses are common. Endocrine glands are often infiltrated and goitre may be a presenting feature of the disease.

Nervous system

The nervous system may be involved either directly by infiltration of the brain, meninges or nerves, or indirectly by retroperitoneal masses impairing the blood supply of the spinal cord and thus causing paraplegia.

Histopathology

In histological sections, the tumour shows monomorphic sheets of undifferentiated lymphoblasts with a well-defined intensely pyroninophilic cytoplasm. The tumour cells exhibit a high mitotic rate and also a high death rate with many pyknotic forms. Scattered between the lymphoid cells are non-neoplastic histiocytes with abundant clear or foamy cytoplasm that frequently contain ingested pyknotic cell remnants. These macrophages give the tumour the so-called 'starry-sky' appearance.

Electron microscopy

The tumour cells show rounded or indented nuclei with clumped heterochromatin and from 1 to 4 nucleoli visible in any one plane of section. Nuclear pockets are frequent. Cytoplasm contains occasional mitochondria and short runs of rough endoplasmic reticulum. Polyribosomes are abundant and occasional lipid vacuoles may be seen.

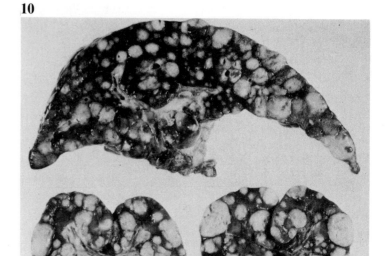

G.C.P.245

10   Post mortem specimens from a child with Burkitt's lymphoma showing massive nodular involvement of the liver and both kidneys.

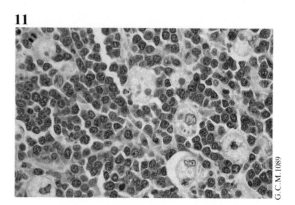

G.C.M.1089

11   Section of Burkitt's lymphoma showing uniform immature lymphoid cells interspersed with large foamy macrophages.

Electron microscopy is not particularly characteristic and is therefore rarely of great diagnostic value.

Cytology

Touch preparations of Burkitt's lymphoma stained by one of the standard Romanowsky methods provide a rapid and accurate means of diagnosing Burkitt's lymphoma. The tumour cells have the appearance of lymphoblasts with rounded or indented nuclei, 3 or 4 nucleoli, and moderately clumped nuclear chromatin. The cytoplasm is intensely basophilic and contains vacuoles corresponding to lipid droplets that have been dissolved out during fixation.

12

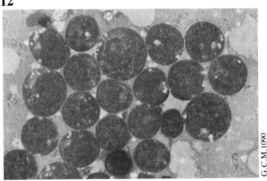

12 Imprint preparation of Burkitt's lymphoma showing immature lymphoid cells with deeply basophilic cytoplasm containing clear vacuoles.

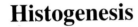

Histogenesis

The precise histogenesis of Burkitt's lymphoma is in dispute. It is clearly a B-cell lymphoma since the tumour cells have monotypic membrane immunoglobulin. In some classifications it is categorised as a lymphoblast and in others as a type of follicular centre cell.

Cytogenetics

Most African cases of Burkitt's lymphoma exhibit a characteristic 8–14q translocation. Non-African cases have been less well studied. Some show this characteristic feature but others have exhibited other translocations.

Aetiology

The Epstein-Barr virus was first discovered in cultured lymphoblasts from a Ugandan case of Burkitt's lymphoma. There is a strong association between this virus and African cases of Burkitt's lymphoma. Almost all African cases have high antibody titres to various EBV related antigens and the virus can be retrieved from tumour cells following appropriate culture techniques. DNA hybridisation studies have shown EBV genomes within the majority of African Burkitt lymphomas studied. The association between EBV and non-African cases of Burkitt's lymphoma is less close; only 20–25% show antibodies to the virus or have evidence of viral genomes within the tumour cells.

One of the main difficulties in accepting an aetiological role for EBV is the poor correlation between the sero-epidemiology of this virus and the distribution of the tumour. For this reason a number of workers have proposed that co-factors such as malaria may act together with EBV to produce the high incidence of Burkitt's lymphoma seen in the tropics.

Professor D.H. Wright

Mandible

Many lesions of the mandible are similar in aetiology and character to those already described as occurring in the maxilla. In this section the lesions which have a higher incidence in the mandible or which can be more readily illustrated from the material in the museum collection are considered.

Osteomyelitis

Osteomyelitis occurs both in the maxilla and mandible, more frequently in the latter. The infection may follow trauma but more often the initial lesion is in the gingival margin and results from dental sepsis. Note has already been made of the spread of dental infection to the maxillary sinus. This may occur as part of the picture. In the case of the mandible the blood supply to the bone is readily impaired with sequestration formation. It is to be noted that the lower margin of the mandible is composed of very dense bone and sequestration here is delayed. Sinus formation is common.

The mandible when destroyed shows repair with considerable new bone formation but the maxilla being a membranous bone shows only limited repair and subsequent deformity is common.

Sinus formation to the cheek and neck occurs. The condition then runs a chronic course of long duration.

13

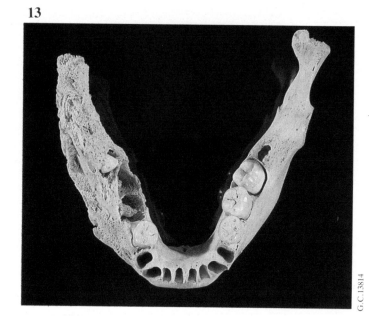

G.C.13814

13 An example of extensive osteomyelitis of the mandible in which there has been major destruction of bone in the right ramus with exposure of the third molar tooth socket. Elsewhere there is extensive periosteal reaction with new bone formation.

Radiation necrosis

Another cause of bone destruction of the mandible and always associated with some degree of infection is irradiation necrosis. This may follow radiation treatment of primary lesions of the mouth or lip in which bone has been insufficiently shielded.

Actinomycosis

The cause of actinomycosis is an anaerobic strepto-thrix, Actinomyces israelii, which is present as a commensal in the human mouth. Relatively rare in man, the disease is frequent in cattle, sheep and horses. Cervico-facial actinomycosis is the commonest form in man. Infection by the actinomyces is usually through an abrasion in the oral mucous membrane or through the socket of an extracted carious tooth. Sinuses form discharging pus characteristically containing small yellow masses of mycelium, the 'sulphur granules'. The sinuses sometimes heal spontaneously as others develop.

Histologically there is a chronic inflammatory reaction and fibrosis. Granulomas form around a central core of tangled mycelial filaments. The disease spreads directly through tissue planes and may involve the salivary glands, bone and other tissues of the neck.

Increasingly involvement of the paranasal sinuses has been found with widespread antibiotic use.

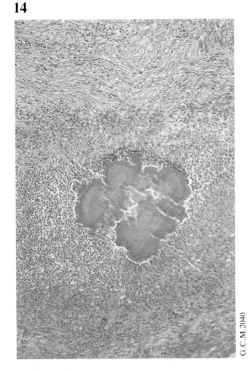

14

14 (*H&E × 100*)

Tumours

Neoplasms of the mandible are similar to those found in the maxilla and conform to the same classification:

1   Tumours arising from fibrous or osseous tissue.

2   Tumours arising from lymphoid tissue.

3   Secondary tumours.

4   Tumours of dental origin − odontomas.

Mandible (*Continued*)

Tumours — Group 1

Ossifying fibroma

This lesion is seen both in the maxilla and mandible but particularly in the latter. It would appear to be a variant of the fibro-osseous lesion already described in the maxilla but one in which the degree of ossification is carried to a greater extent. Trabeculae of bone rimmed by rows of active osteoblasts are seen and the structure may be very dense or one in which vascular connective tissue is more evident. Some of these lesions closely simulate osteosarcoma.

What appears to be a variant occurs when there is a degree of deposition of cementum. The bony trabeculae are extremely dense and are not surrounded as previously described by a margin of osteoblasts. These lesions closely simulate the odontomatous tumour known as a cementoma. The commonest site of these is the mandibular premolar or molar region.

Osteofibroma of right half of mandible. The tumour involves the whole of the body of the mandible, projecting both into the mouth and on the buccal surface. The 1st molar is carious, and the 3rd molar, unerupted, lies embedded in the bone. Microscopically there is intertrabecular fibrous tissue with trabeculae of bone. This is an innocent osteofibroma.

G.C.3419

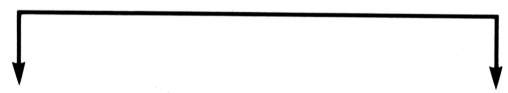

15   Superior and lateral aspects   15a   Medial (lingual) aspect

15

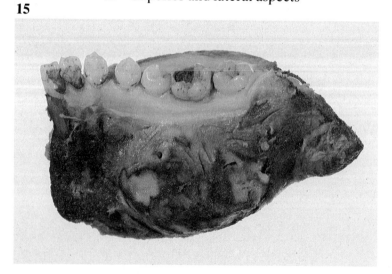

15a

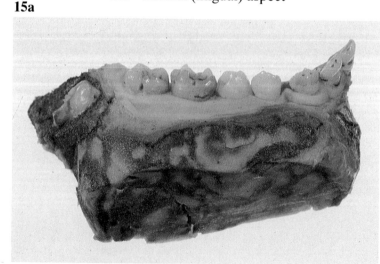

Osteoma

Simple osseous tumours are occasionally found.

16

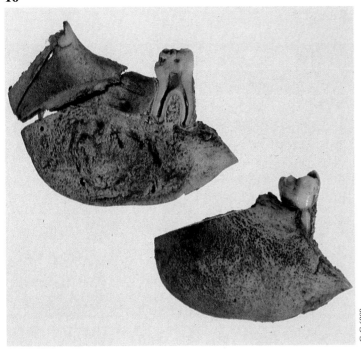

G.C.6989

16 From a child. The swelling had appeared at the angle of the jaw and consists of cancellous bone with an overlay of porous cortical bone. The 1st molar tooth is *in situ* and posterior to this is a small cavity which appears to be related to faulty eruption of the 2nd molar. The tumour has the appearance of a cancellous osteoma but probably pathologically is a reactive hyperostosis.

Osteosarcoma

The osteosarcoma of the mandible may arise as a complication of a fibrous dysplasia or without pre-existing disease. It causes destruction of bone and the diagnosis is based on both the clinical features and the radiological examination. It conforms to the general features of an osteosarcoma. Chondrosarcomas are also found.

17

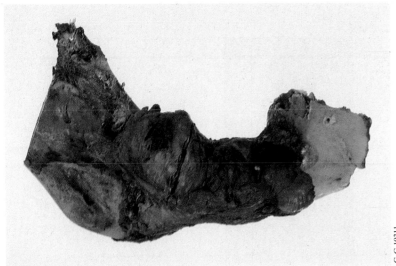

G.C.10311

17 Chondrosarcoma of the mandible. A man of 23 developed a tumour of the inside of the left mandible. It was excised through the mouth and was reported to be a sarcoma. Radiotherapy was advised but the patient defaulted. Two years later a resection of the mandible was carried out for recurrent tumour. Eight months after operation there was no sign of recurrence and part of the iliac crest was transplanted to bridge the gap in the mandible. The resection extended from the canine tooth to the tip of the coronoid process. A lobulated tumour measuring 5.5×3 cm covers most of the medial aspect of the horizontal ramus. Microscopically it has the appearances of a chrondrosarcoma.

Mandible (*Continued*)

Tumours — Group 1 (*Continued*)

Epulis

The word 'epulis' means a tumour of the gum. Under this heading are described lesions which may be either granulomatous or neoplastic. These lesions arise from the alveolus usually close to the gingival margin in relation to a tooth. The majority arise in the anterior part of the mandible (less commonly the maxilla) and the presence of an epulis is in only a minority of cases associated with any evidence of tooth decay.

Granulomatous

Structurally these are formed by fibroblasts and spindle cells occasionally showing myxomatous change. There is frequently marked giant cell (or osteoclast) infiltration and the condition has been mistaken for an osteoclastoma — a true tumour. The overlying epithelium may show hyperplasia. The vascularity of the lesion varies. These lesions are non-invasive and surgical removal is curative.

Occurring in childhood and commonly called a congenital epulis this lesion arises in relation to an unerupted tooth. Comparable to this is a tumour found in later life and generally known as a fibrous epulis. This presents as a smooth broadly pedunculated tumour which arises either from the periosteum or the peridental membrane. The adjacent teeth often show calcareous deposits.

It is most usually found in patients in the 4th decade and there is a female preponderance. It is also commonly found during pregnancy being active in the earlier months but becomes more fibrous after parturition. These lesions are generally covered by a small epithelial membrane but if traumatised by biting, ulceration occurs.

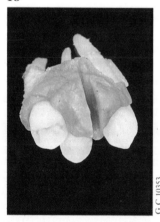

18 Female aged 16 years in whom a swelling developed over four months involving the lingual side of the left upper canine and two premolars. The tumour had grown between the teeth and a small portion is visible on the lateral surface. There is a shallow ulcer in relation to the 2nd molar. Elsewhere the mucosa is smooth and intact.

Microscopically the tumour consists of whorls of dense fibrous tissue extending up to the mucosa. There is plasma cell infiltration but no multinucleated cells are present.

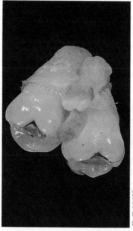

19 From a 25 year old female. The tumour developed during the early months of pregnancy. It lies between the 1st and 2nd molars. The epithelium shows hyperkeratosis and ulceration. Histology demonstrates angiomatous tissue with newly formed thin walled blood vessels and many plasma and lymphoid cells in the fibrous stroma.

Neoplastic

'True' epulis is a lesion which in all respects simulates an osteoclastoma, there being marked giant cell formation and the lesion is invasive to some degree.

Growth is slow initially but occasionally later more rapid with invasion — local malignancy.

Disputation as to the nature of this tumour is considerable and there are authorities who regard it as probably granulomatous.

20

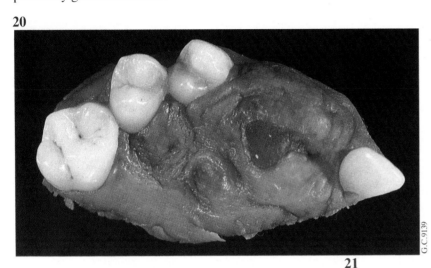

20 From a male aged 10 years. Swelling of the cheek had appeared seven months previously. Radiology showed a supernumerary tooth in the right maxillary air sinus. The tooth was excised from a pus-filled cavity. In spite of drainage the swelling did not diminish and excision was undertaken. The site of the right canine is occupied by a brown fleshy tumour which surrounds the two premolars and extends upwards into the maxillary sinus.

Microscopical examination shows this to be a giant cell tumour (osteoclastoma).

21

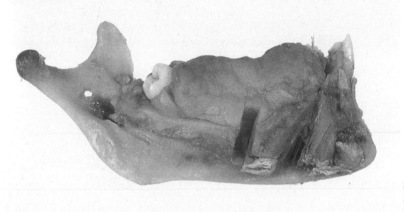

21 From a male aged 12 years. The tumour involves the alveolar border from the left canine tooth to the anterior border of the ramus. Anteriorly the 1st and 2nd premolar teeth are embedded into the tumour and displaced anteriorly. Posteriorly the tumour has displaced the 2nd molar tooth. The tumour is well defined and overlaps the superior half of the facial aspect of the body of the mandible. Microscopic examination shows a non-malignant giant cell tumour.

21a

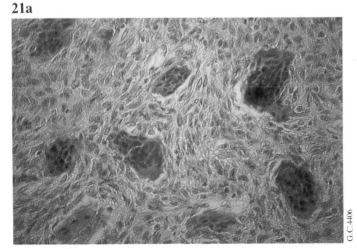

21a Jaw — giant cell tumour (benign reparative granuloma). Multinucleated giant cells of osteoclast type are set in a cellular fibroblastic stroma. (*H&E × 250*)

Mandible (*Continued*)

Tumours – Group 2

The mandible may be the site of lesions of lymphoid and myeloid tissues characterised clinically as an ovoid swelling with or without disruption of teeth and with radiological evidence of a defect of bone. Included in this group are lymphoma, plasmacytoma, chloroma and histiocytosis X.

When the initial lesion is in the mandible the radiological evidence will be a defect of bone often suggesting 'sarcoma' but not diagnostic. In such cases search should be made for other bony lesions especially in the skull. Haematological studies are also required.

Chloroma

22

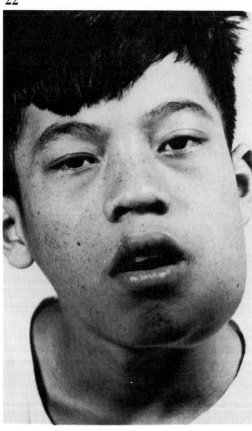

22a

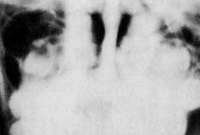

22 and **22a**   This 14 year old Chinese boy was admitted to hospital on account of the swelling on the left side of his mandible. The swelling was ovoid, firm and fixed.

Radiological examination gave the diagnosis of osteosarcoma. Half the jaw with the tumour was excised. When the tumour was sectioned the cut surface showed the vivid gross green colour establishing the diagnosis as that of chloroma. This was confirmed on histological examination. Subsequently an X-ray of the skull revealed two areas of neoplastic bone destruction.

G.C.10751

22b

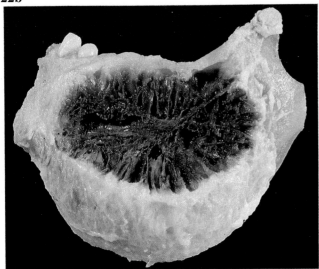

22b This specimen shows the tumour and demonstrates the green coloration. Unfortunately the specimen on removal from its primary fixation lost its colour and the appearance seen here has been approximately reproduced.

22c

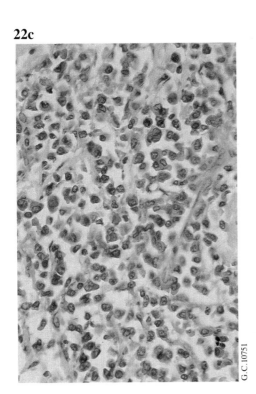

22c Jaw – chloroma. The tumour is composed of closely packed, poorly differentiated cells with little stroma. (*H&E × 400*)

23

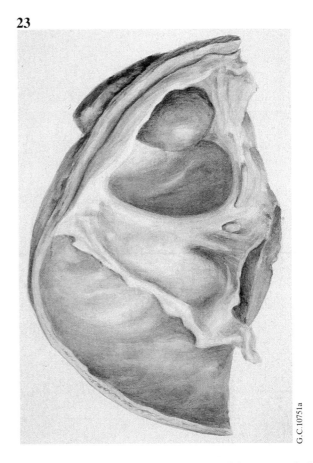

23 Water-colour drawing showing a chloroma of the skull. The tumour has invaded the base of the skull and has extended laterally around the auditory meatus and into the orbital fossa. There are no clinical notes of this case. The colour of the chloroma as shown in the drawing conforms closely to personal observation.

Mandible (*Continued*)

Tumours − Group 2 (*Continued*)

Histiocytosis X

A disease of unknown pathogenesis characterised by proliferation of histiocytes in various tissues.

Incidence

A rare disease mainly affecting children and young adults. M: F 2 : 1

Any tissue of the body may be affected. Bone and skin are involved most frequently, but lymph nodes, liver and spleen may also be infiltrated and enlarged. Infiltration of the pituitary may result in diabetes insipidus.

Three forms have been described differing in presentation and prognosis:

Type of histiocytosis X	Alternative name	Common initial presentation	Prognosis
Localised	Eosinophilic granuloma	Lytic lesion in bone − particularly skull	Limited lesions relatively benign
Chronic disseminated	Multiple eosinophilic granulomas or Hand-Schüller − Christian disease	Lesions in craniofacial and other bones Middle ear disease Loss of teeth Pituitary infiltration	Grave but may be brought under control
Acute disseminated	Letterer-Siwe disease	Skin involvement, with papules and later ulceration	Usually fatal

Histology

The affected tissue is infiltrated by histiocytes with nuclei which may be lobulated. Electron microscopy may reveal characteristic cytoplasmic structures − the Birbeck bodies (**25**). Lymphocytes, plasma cells and eosinophils are also present in varying numbers.

The histiocytes may contain lipid material derived from breakdown products of necrosis at the site of the lesion. By contrast the histiocytes in such storage diseases as Gaucher's disease results from a generalised metabolic disturbance.

24

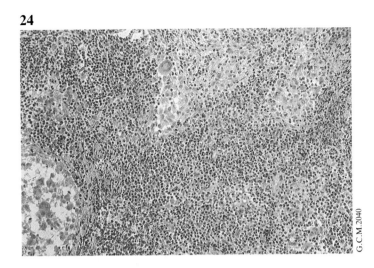

24 Bone – Eosinophilic granuloma. There is marked infiltration by eosinophilic leucocytes. The histiocytes, some multinucleated, here occur in groups. (*H&E × 125*)

24a

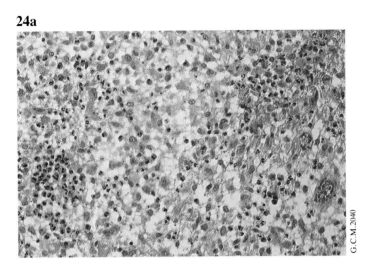

24a Same case. In this field eosinophils are less numerous. Histiocytes occupy the central area and many are vacuolated. (*H&E × 250*)

In their histology multiple eosinophilic granulomas resemble that of the solitary lesion. Involvement of the membranous bones of the skull may result in proptosis, diabetes insipidus or aural discharge (Hand-Schüller-Christian).

25

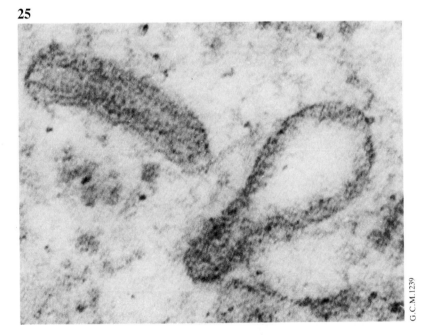

26

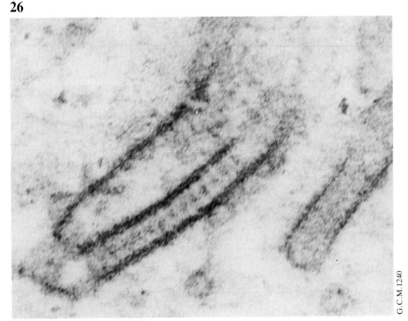

25 and **26** Electron micrographs of Birbeck bodies, rod-shaped and flask-shaped in the histiocytic cytoplasm.

By courtesy of Dr K.M. McLaren

Mandible (*Continued*)

Tumours — Group 3

Secondary tumours — local invasion

Epithelial tumours of the gum or floor of the mouth may invade underlying mandible. These are generally squamous epitheliomas. Occasionally the neoplasm infiltrates the bone deeply and may cause a disunion in the mandible.

27

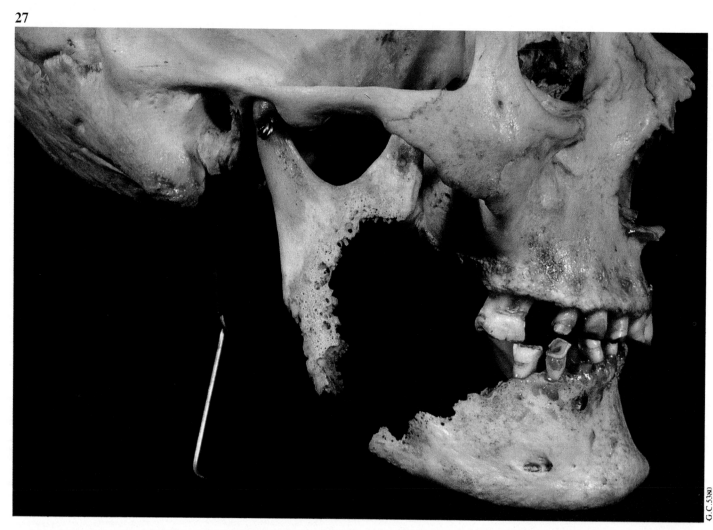

27 From a male aged 66 years who died of oral squamous-cell carcinoma fourteen months from the onset of pain. There had been progressive ulceration of the right glossopalatine arch extending on to the floor of the mouth and the lingual surface of the mandible accompanied by pain in the ear, impairment of hearing and progressive enlargement of the submandibular and cervical lymph nodes. The specimen shows destruction of the ramus, angle of the jaw and part of the body of the bone.

Secondary tumours – haematogenous

Metastases (haematogenous) of the mandible are rare. They usually appear as multiple areas of bone destruction.

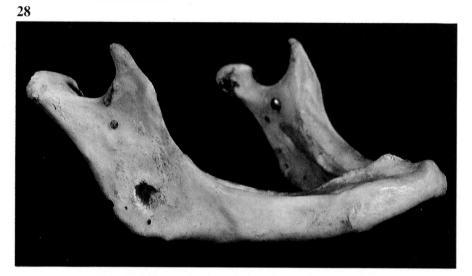

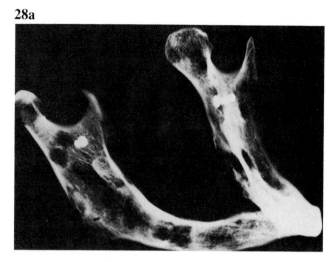

28 and **28a** From a female aged 68 years who died from widespread malignant disease arising from a carcinoma of the pylorus.

Note how in this specimen secondary deposits have occurred in each condyle and affecting also the ramus and angle of the jaw on both sides.

28b Enlarged radiograph to demonstrate in detail the manner in which the bone has been destroyed and replaced by malignant disease.

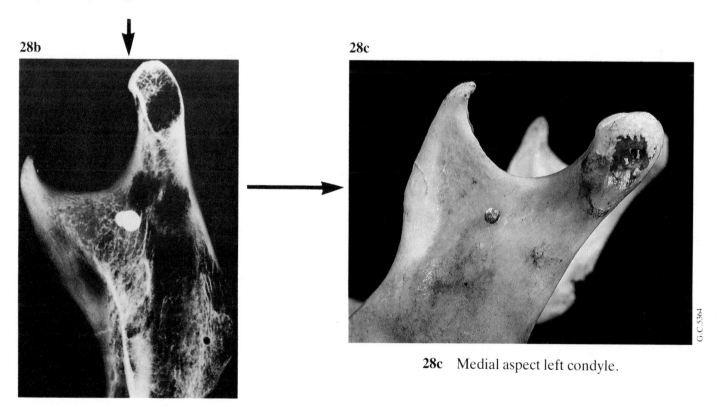

28c Medial aspect left condyle.

Development

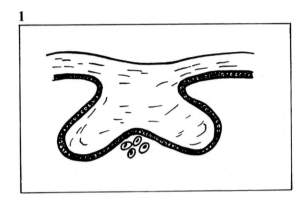

1   Deciduous tooth 12 week embryo

At approximately 6 weeks, epithelium thickens over the mesodermal tissue present and, growing inward, continues to develop as the primary tooth band. This extends deep into the mesenchyme and divides into two bands — the vestibular band which eventually degenerates separating the lip from the gum, and the dental lamina which gives rise to the tooth germ.

Each quadrant has a tooth band along which epithelial thickening or tooth buds appear at intervals starting from the point. These invest the mesenchymal condensations giving rise to the dental follicles which differentiate into the eventual dental tissues.

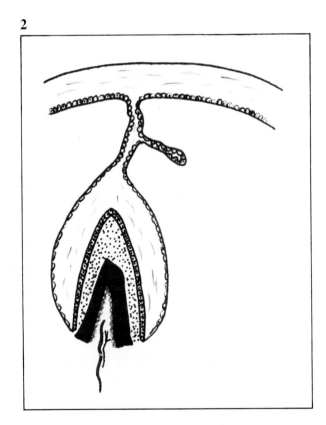

2   Deciduous tooth 17 week embryo

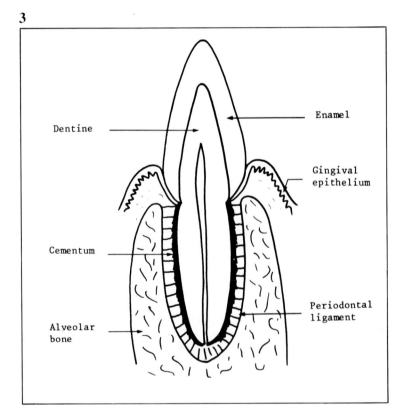

3   Tooth structure

Cysts

Cysts of the jaws are more common than in any other bone. They are classified into those cysts lined by epithelium derived from the tooth-forming organ (odontogenic cysts) and those cysts lined by epithelium derived from another source (non-odontogenic cysts). The various types of cyst may be listed as follows:

Odontogenic cysts

1 Developmental
    Dentigerous (follicular) cyst
    Lateral periodontal cyst
    Odontogenic keratocyst

2 Inflammatory
    Radicular cyst
    Residual cyst

Non-odontogenic cysts

Nasopalatine (incisive canal) cyst
Globulomaxillary cyst
Nasolabial cyst

Dentigerous cyst

This cyst encloses the crown of an unerupted permanent tooth and is attached to the tooth along the amelocemental junction. The teeth most commonly involved are mandibular third molars and then, in order of decreasing frequency, the maxillary canines, maxillary third molars and mandibular premolars. Although a tooth will be missing from the arch, a dentigerous cyst may be undetected until routine radiographic examination is carried out or until the cyst has enlarged sufficiently to produce a painless expansion of the jaw. Radiological examination shows a well-defined radiolucent area associated in some way with the crown of an unerupted tooth which may be displaced. A typical dentigerous cyst is lined by a thin, regular layer of non-keratinised stratified squamous epithelium supported by a fibrous connective tissue capsule devoid of inflammatory changes. Mucous cell metaplasia and epithelial discontinuities are not unusual. If secondary inflammatory changes occur, the epithelium may become hyperplastic and cholesterol clefts may be seen.

4

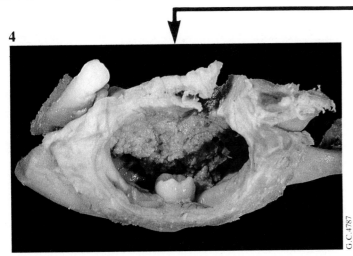

G.C.4787

5

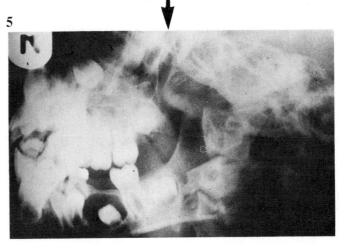

G.C.X.1088

71

Cysts (*Continued*)

Lateral periodontal cyst

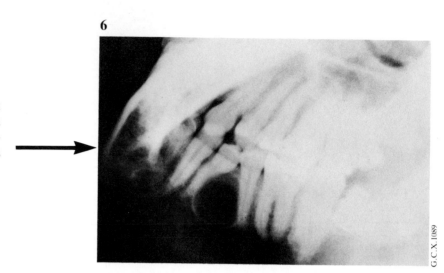

6 This unusual type of cyst is seen most frequently in the canine and premolar region of the mandible as a well-defined radiolucent area lying on the lateral surface of the root of a tooth and it only rarely causes expansion of the jaw. The pathogenesis is uncertain.

Odontogenic keratocyst

This type of cyst is thought to arise from remnants of the dental lamina. It occurs over a wide age range but there is a pronounced peak incidence in the second and third decades. About 80% of keratocysts occur in the mandible, most frequently in the third molar region and ascending ramus of the mandible. Keratocysts enlarge predominantly in an antero-posterior direction and so can reach a large size without causing bone expansion. Radiological examination shows a well-defined radiolucent area which may be unilocular or multilocular, sometimes in an apparent dentigerous relationship with an unerupted third molar although the crowns of such teeth are usually separated from the cyst cavity. A small number of patients develop two or more keratocysts which may be associated with multiple basal cell naevi – Gorlin-Goltz syndrome. Keratocysts are notorious for their high rate of recurrence after surgical treatment, recurrence of up to 50% having been described.

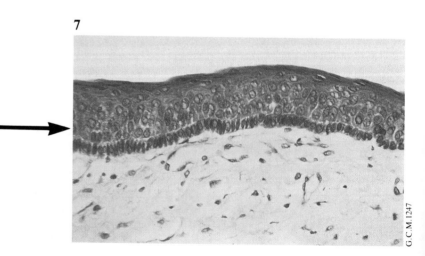

7 Diagnosis of an odontogenic keratocyst depends on histological examination. The wall is usually thin and covered by a regular layer of parakeratinised stratified squamous epithelium between five and ten cells in thickness. The basal cell layer is prominent and consists of palisaded columnar or cuboidal cells, above which the prickle cell layer abruptly changes into parakeratin. The cells desquamate into the cyst lumen which is packed with parakeratinised squames in varying states of autolysis with little free fluid and the contents have a low soluble protein level. Mitotic activity in the epithelium is higher than in other types of odontogenic cysts. The thin fibrous capsule is generally free from inflammatory cell infiltration and may contain small groups of epithelial cells resembling dental lamina residues.

Radicular cyst

This type of cyst is always associated with the root of a non-vital tooth and is by far the most common cystic lesion of the jaws. A radicular cyst develops from a periapical granuloma which follows inflammation or necrosis of the pulp. Epithelial cell rests of Malassez included within a granuloma may undergo inflammatory hyperplasia leading to cyst formation. When small, a radicular cyst may be symptomless, but as enlargement occurs, there may be associated bone expansion although gross expansion of the jaw is unusual. Pain is seldom a feature unless there is an acute exacerbation. Radiological examination shows a round or ovoid radiolucency in the bone at the apex of the involved tooth. The radiolucency is often well circumscribed but, unless large, cannot be distinguished from an apical granuloma.

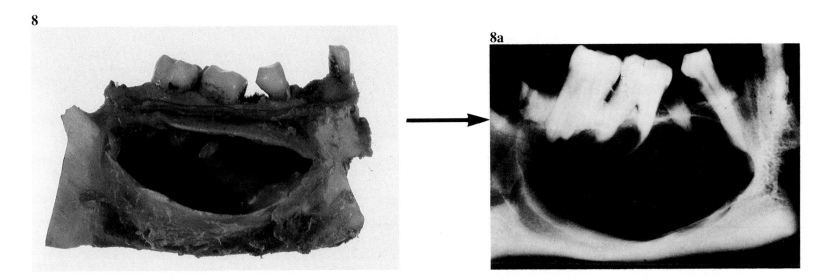

8 and **8a**   This specimen and its associated X-ray demonstrate a radicular cyst of an adult right mandible. The specimen has been opened by partial removal of the outer wall of the cyst and the photograph has been taken obliquely upwards and medially to demonstrate the roots of the teeth, which are projecting into the cavity. The gingival mucosa is intact. The last and 2nd molars are healthy, the 1st premolar is carious laterally at its neck and the central incisor is in a more advanced state of caries. The other teeth are represented by carious stumps and the roots of the three molars and of the 2nd premolar project into the cyst. The cyst extends from the alveolar to the inferior border of the mandible and horizontally from the ramus to the site of the canine tooth. Its lingual and facial walls are thin and translucent and its interior smooth.

G.C.6240

Cysts (*Continued*)

Radicular cyst (*Continued*)

The cyst is lined wholly or in part by non-keratinised stratified squamous epithelium supported by a chronically inflamed fibrous tissue capsule. The epithelium varies in thickness from being thin and even, to being irregularly hyperplastic with long anastomosing cords of epithelium forming complex arcades extending into the surrounding capsule. Mucous cells may be seen in the epithelial lining of up to 40% of cysts. Deposits of cholesterol crystals are common both in the wall and the cyst lumen, as are deposits of haemosiderin pigment and foam cells. The cyst contents are generally fluid with a soluble protein level much higher than that found in an odontogenic keratocyst.

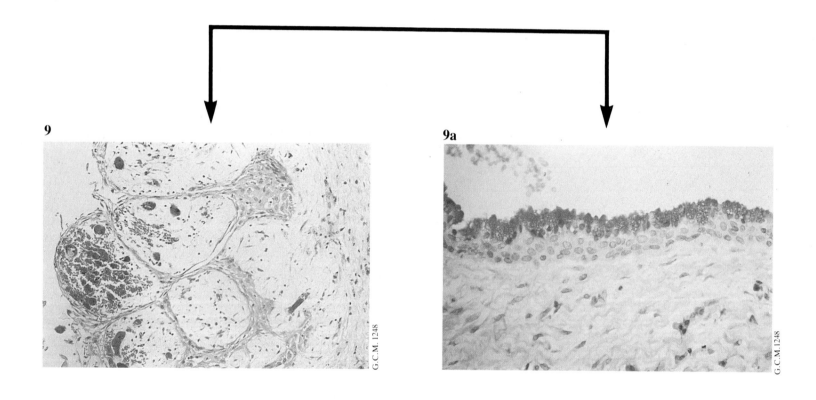

9

9a

Residual cyst

This is a radicular cyst that has remained in the jaw and failed to resolve following extraction of the involved tooth.

Nasopalatine duct cyst

This is the commonest type of non-odontogenic cyst that involves the jaws and is thought to be derived from epithelial remnants of the nasopalatine duct which connects the oral and nasal cavity in the midline of the embryo. Depending on whether the cyst arises within the bone in the nasopalatine canal or within the soft tissue of the incisive papilla, the cyst may be discovered as an incidental finding on radiological examination of the upper jaw or present as a slowly increasing swelling of the bone of the anterior maxilla or the soft tissues of the anterior midline of the palate. Many cysts become secondarily inflamed and may discharge into the mouth when the patient often complains of a salty taste. The epithelium lining a nasopalatine cyst may range from non-keratinised stratified squamous epithelium to respiratory epithelium with mucous and even ciliated cells. The supporting connective tissue may include prominent neurovascular bundles (long sphenopalatine) and collections of mucous cells.

Globulomaxillary cyst

This type of cyst occurs between the roots of the permanent maxillary lateral incisor and canine teeth. Previously thought to arise from epithelium entrapped in the fissure between the globular portion of the medial nasal process and the maxillary process, it is now not considered to be a separate entity. Cysts presenting in this way are thought to be radicular cysts, developmental lateral periodontal cysts or odontogenic keratocysts.

Nasolabial cyst

10

10 This rare type of cyst arises in the soft tissue of the upper lip just below the ala of the nose and is not strictly a cyst of the jaw. The wall is usually covered by pseudo-stratified columnar epithelium, but stratified squamous epithelium, mucous cells and ciliated cells may also be present.

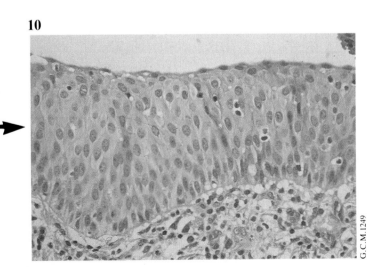

Odontomes

11 An odontome is a hamartoma containing calcified dental tissues. There is no consensus of opinion as to which dental anomalies and malformations fall into this classification except for the complex and compound odontomes presenting as lesions of the jaw. The complex odontome consists mainly of a mass of haphazardly arranged enamel, dentine and cementum, dentine usually forming the bulk of the lesion. The compound odontome consists of a collection of numerous tooth-like structures or denticles embedded in a small amount of fibrous tissue, each denticle consisting of enamel, dentine, cement and pulp arranged as in a normal tooth. Gradations between these extremes are often seen.

11

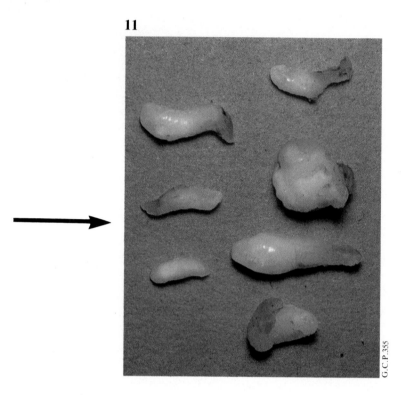

G.C.P.355

12 The odontomes are generally diagnosed in the second decade of life and are discovered as incidental findings when a patient with a tooth missing from the arch is investigated. Only occasionally is an odontome sufficiently large to cause expansion of the bone. Undetected odontomes may present in later life when they apparently erupt following resorption of the overlying alveolar bone. Radiographic examination shows a radiopaque mass, the compound odontome resembling a bag of small teeth and the complex odontome appears dense or with a radiating structure.

12

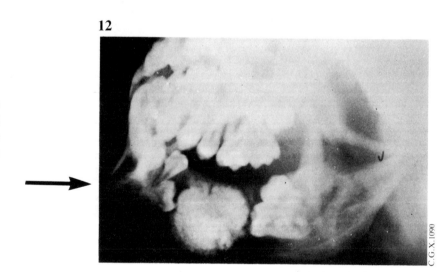

C.G.X.1090

The majority of odontomes arise in association with the permanent dentition and no further growth takes place after the time of formation of the dentition.

Odontogenic tumours

Tumours arising from the odontogenic tissues are uncommon lesions and cannot always be distinguished from lesions which are probably hamartomatous or dysplastic in origin. The term 'tumour' in this context indicates a localised, non-inflammatory swelling without any implication regarding neoplasia. The classification of odontogenic tumours is controversial, and the one used here is based on the behaviour and suspected origin of the tumours. The classification characterises different tumours quite narrowly and precisely, but it is accepted that one type of tumour may merge with another type to form a continuous series and that this classification will have to be changed in the light of future knowledge.

Classification of odontogenic tumours

Benign

1 Epithelial lesions

   Ameloblastoma
   Adenomatoid odontogenic tumour
   Calcifying epithelial odontogenic tumour
   Calcifying odontogenic cyst
   Squamous odontogenic tumour

2 Mesenchymal lesions

   Odontogenic myxoma
   Odontogenic fibroma
   Cementoma group
      (a) Cementifying fibroma
      (b) Periapical cemental dysplasia
      (c) Benign cementoblastoma
      (d) Gigantiform cementoma
   Dentinoma

3 Epithelial − Mesenchymal lesions

   Ameloblastic fibroma
   Ameloblastic fibro-odontoma

Malignant

1 Epithelial lesions
   Odontogenic carcinoma

2 Mesenchymal lesions
   Odontogenic sarcomas

Ameloblastoma

This tumour accounts for 1% of all oral tumours and is by far the commonest type of odontogenic tumour. An ameloblastoma may occur at any age, from childhood to old age, but is usually diagnosed in the fourth and fifth decades of life. The vast majority arise in the mandible, the molar region and ascending ramus being the commonest sites involved. It is a slow growing, painless tumour which usually presents as a gradually increasing facial deformity with expansion of the jaw bone. In the early stages it may be asymptomatic and discovered as an accidental radiological finding. The enlargement is usually bony hard and ovoid or fusiform in outline, but in advanced cases the overlying bone may be so thin that egg-shell crackling can be elicited. Teeth in the area of the tumour may become loosened.

13

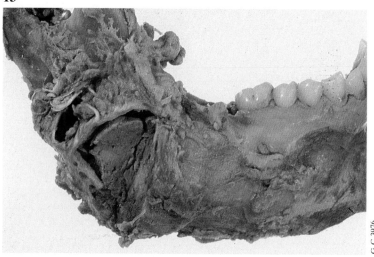

G.C.3976

13 The posterior part of the body and half the ramus (Rt) are expanded. The tumour has been incised on the facial aspect to demonstrate its cystic character with fibrous septa and irregular masses of epithelium.

Note with one exception the teeth are all present and in perfect condition.

14

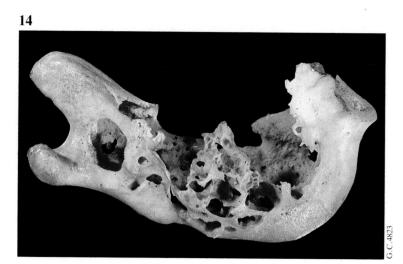

G.C.4823

14 A macerated specimen demonstrating the effects of an ameloblastoma on the bony structure of the mandible.

15

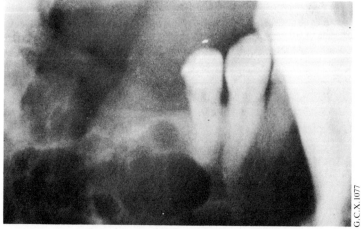

G.C.X.1077

15 The radiographic appearance of an ameloblastoma is either a unilocular or multilocular radiolucency which may be associated with an unerupted tooth and so mimic a dentigerous cyst.

There is considerable variation in the histopathology of ameloblastoma but two main patterns are usually described, the more common being the follicular type and the less common being the plexiform type.

16 The epithelium in the follicular type is arranged in discrete rounded islands or follicles, each consisting of a central mass of loosely connected, angular cells surrounded by a layer of columnar or cuboidal cells with the nuclei situated away from the basal ends of the cells. The central cells are thought to resemble the stellate reticulum of the normal enamel organ, and the peripheral cells resemble ameloblasts. The follicles are separated by various amounts of fibrous connective tissue stroma. Microcyst formation in the centres of the follicles is common and large cystic areas may develop by coalescence of smaller cysts. Squamous metaplasia in the centres of some follicles is not unusual. Gross cystic change may occur and the tumour may then consist of a fluid filled cavity lined by flattened and compressed epithelium with the typical histological appearances confined to one part of the cyst wall.

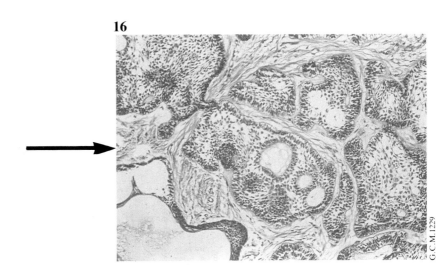

16

17 The epithelium in the plexiform type is arranged as a network of anastomosing strands and irregular masses, the strands having an outer layer of cuboidal cells surrounding cells resembling stellate reticulum. Microcyst formation is common but is due to stromal degeneration and large cystic spaces are not usually seen.

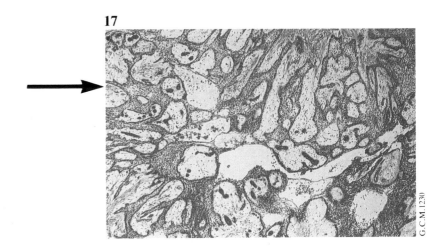

17

There is no difference in clinical behaviour between the various histological types. All are benign but locally invasive tumours. Extension of the tumour into adjacent soft tissues is a late feature, and an extra-osseous origin of a tumour has been rarely reported.

Adenomatoid odontogenic tumour

18 This tumour usually presents during the second and third decades of life, the majority of tumours arising in the anterior maxilla and presenting as a slowly enlarging swelling. Radiological examination shows a well-defined radiolucency, often with faint radiopacities within the tumour due to calcification. The tumour is often associated with an unerupted tooth and may simulate a dentigerous cyst.

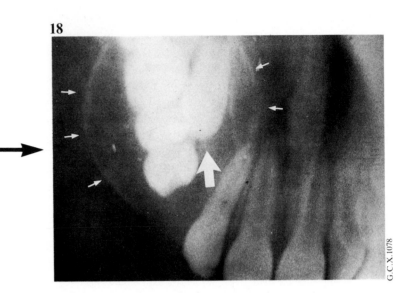

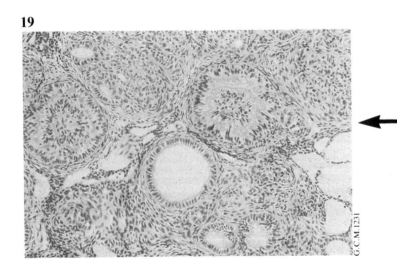

19 Histological examination shows a solid or cystic lesion consisting of sheets, strands and whorled masses of epithelium with little supporting stroma. In places the epithelial cells differentiate into columnar cells resembling ameloblasts which form ducts or tubule-like structures. Small foci of calcification are scattered throughout the tumour.

It is thought to be a hamartomatous and not a truly neoplastic lesion. Recurrence following local curettage is very unusual and the lesion does not require radical excision.

Calcifying epithelial odontogenic tumour

20 This rare tumour occurs over a wide age range and arises in the mandible much more frequently than in the maxilla, the molar-premolar area being the usual site. Radiographs show an irregular radiolucent area containing varying amounts of radiopaque bodies. Histological examination shows that the tumour consists of sheets and strands of epithelial cells lying in a fibrous stroma, the epithelial cells often showing prominent intercellular bridges and marked nuclear pleomorphism. A characteristic feature is the presence within the epithelial cells of homogeneous, amyloid-like material which may become calcified. The tumour has a similar behaviour to an ameloblastoma, being benign but locally invasive.

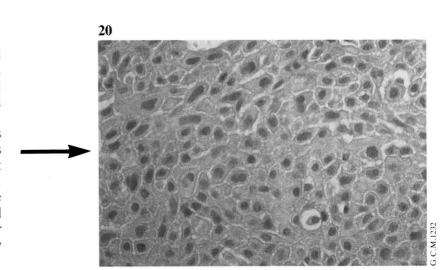

Calcifying odontogenic cyst

21 The nature of this lesion is not clear, but it is probably not neoplastic and recurrence is rare after enucleation. It occurs over a wide age range and either jaw may be involved, the lesion generally arising anterior to the molars. Radiographic examination shows a well-defined radiolucent area containing varying amounts of radiopaque, calcified material.

Histological examination usually shows a cystic cavity lined by epithelium with a well-defined basal layer of columnar cells resembling ameloblasts supporting loosely arranged cells. A characteristic feature is the presence within the epithelium of keratinising cells with the original cell outlines retained. These are described as 'ghost cells' and calcification of these cells is common. Occasionally no cyst cavity is present.

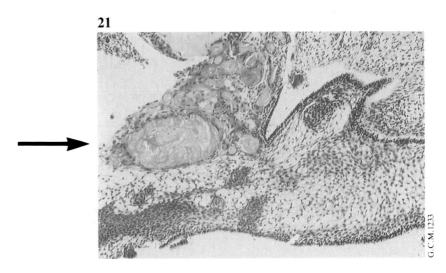

Squamous odontogenic tumour

This unusual lesion has only recently been described. It appears to be a benign tumour and is thought to be derived from the cell rests of Malassez. Histologically the tumour consists of follicles of squamous epithelium lying in a fibrous stroma, the follicles often showing keratinisation but with no evidence of stellate reticulum-type tissue.

Odontogenic myxoma

22 A myxoma of the jaws is a benign but locally invasive neoplasm which arises from mesenchymal dental tissues, most probably the dental follicle. Radiographically, it typically appears as a multilocular radiolucency, usually with a well-defined border, and the roots of teeth involved by the tumour may show resorption. Histologically the tumour consists of stellate fibroblast-like cells separated by abundant connective tissue ground substances rich in glycosaminoglycans. Variable amounts of collagen may be present as well as a few strands of odontogenic epithelium. Although radiographically it may appear well-defined, the tumour is locally invasive which makes local removal difficult and predisposes to local recurrence.

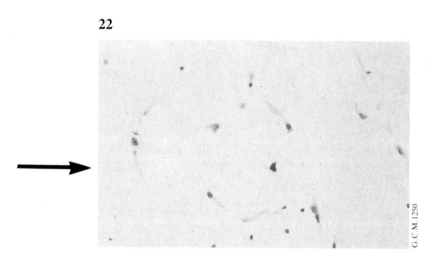

22

Odontogenic fibroma

23 This odontogenic mesenchymal tumour is much less common than the odontogenic myxoma and is a benign fibroblastic neoplasm containing varying amounts of odontogenic epithelium. It is not locally invasive and is readily enucleated.

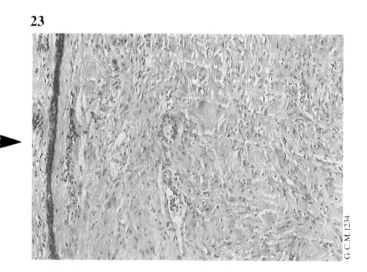

23

The cementoma group

The World Health Organisation (1971) has defined four types of lesion within this group but in practice it may be difficult to ascribe a particular case to any one of these types. It may be difficult to distinguish cementomas from hypercementosis, and the histological distinction between cementum and bone may be difficult or even impossible, so that distinction from some primary lesions of bone may not be clear. The following lesions may be identified.

Cementifying fibroma

This lesion may be related to ossifying fibroma of bone and presents most frequently in the molar and premolar areas of the mandible. In the early stages of its development, it presents as a well-demarcated radiolucent area composed of fibroblastic tissue but increasing amounts of calcified, acellular cementum-like tissue arranged in round or ovoid islands are deposited in the fibrous tissue as it matures so that finally a dense, sclerotic and radiopaque mass is formed.

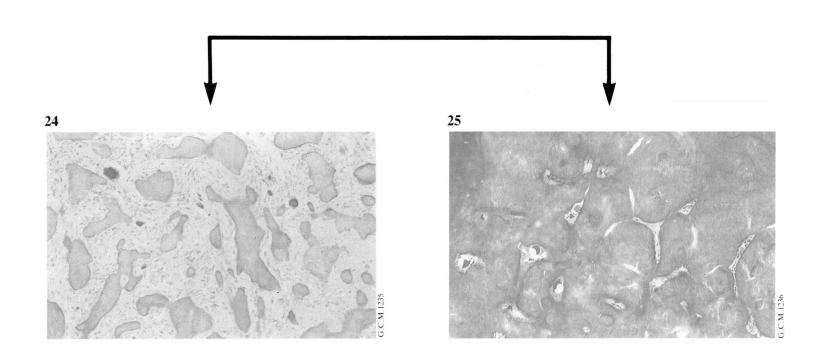

24

25

Periapical cemental dysplasia

This condition is usually symptomless and discovered as an incidental finding on routine radiographs, almost invariably associated with the apices of the mandibular incisor teeth. It evolves in a similar manner to that described for cementifying fibroma, ill-defined radiolucent areas consisting of cellular fibrous tissue being seen in the initial stages. Increasing radiopacity is then seen due to the deposition of cementum-like tissue as the lesion evolves. The condition may be a variant of cementifying fibroma.

Benign cementoblastoma

26

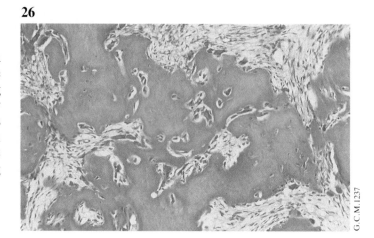

26 This benign neoplasm is attached to the root of a tooth, usually in the premolar or molar area of the mandible, and presents as a slowly enlarging swelling which sometimes gives rise to pain. Radiographs show a well demarcated, mottled or dense radiopaque mass with a radiolucent margin. Histologically the neoplasm consists of a mass of calcified, cementum-like tissue containing scattered cells lying in lacunae and showing numerous, irregular cementing lines.

Gigantiform cementoma

This is a rare type of tumour, usually seen in middle aged Negro females and there may be a family history. The lesions are often multiple and symmetrically distributed in the jaws. They present as slow-growing painless swellings which consist of dense, highly calcified and almost acellular cementum. The lesions are probably dysplastic or hamartomatous rather than being truly neoplastic.

Dentinoma

This very rare tumour is composed of dentine-like tissue lying in connective tissue which in some cases resembles the dental pulp. Strands or islands of odontogenic epithelium may also be present.

Ameloblastic fibroma

27 This is a mixed tumour in which both the odontogenic epithelial and odontogenic mesenchymal tissues are neoplastic. It presents at a younger age than the ameloblastoma as a slowly increasing, painless swelling usually involving the premolar or molar area of the mandible. Radiologically it appears as a well-defined radiolucency, usually unilocular.

Histologically the tumour consists of cellular fibroblastic tissue resembling the dental papilla of the developing tooth, with scattered clumps and strands of odontogenic epithelium. The tumour does not show the locally invasive growth pattern of the ameloblastoma, and curettage rather than radical excision is the preferred treatment.

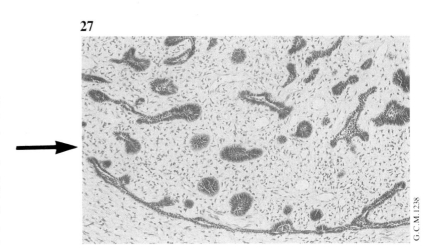

Ameloblastic fibro-odontoma

In some tumours with the features of ameloblastic fibroma, dentine and enamel matrix also may be present and such lesions may be designated ameloblastic fibro-odontoma.

Odontogenic carcinoma

A malignant ameloblastoma is a very rare neoplasm in which both the primary growth in the jaws and a metastatic growth show the features of an ameloblastoma.

Odontogenic sarcoma

This is a neoplasm with a structure similar to an ameloblastic fibroma, but in which the mesodermal component shows the features of a sarcoma.

Professor J.C. Southam

Many lesions of the cervical lymph nodes arise from infections of the mouth, nasopharynx, pharynx, face and scalp resulting in types of lymphadenitis which vary in their histology according to the nature of the infecting micro-organisms. Pyogenic bacteria generally give rise to a non-specific histological picture. Others such as Microbacterium tuberculosis excite a characteristic reaction.

Cervical lymphadenopathy may also result from metastasis of carcinoma of the head and neck, or less commonly from the various forms of malignant lymphoma. The incidence of the causes of cervical lymphadenopathy will obviously vary in different age groups.

For the diagnosis and treatment of these lesions it is necessary to understand the pathways of spread of infections and tumours and to be familiar with the anatomy of the lymphatics of the neck.

Anatomy

Lymphoid tissue in the head and neck is arranged in two rings and a vertical chain of nodes. At the entrance to the pharynx lymphoid tissue is present in the roof of the pharynx (adenoid), the lateral walls (faucial tonsils) and at the base of the tongue (lingual tonsil). Collectively these are known as Waldeyer's ring and they play an important part in preventing the entrance of infection into the body. Drainage from Waldeyer's ring is into the vertical chain of lymph nodes.

The second ring of lymph nodes is situated superficially around the base of the skull and in the submandibular region.

Cervical lymph nodes — second ring

Lymph nodes	*Drainage area*
Occipital and posterior auricular	Occipital and temporal regions of the scalp
Pre-auricular anterior to the tragus	Lateral surface of pinna and anterior temporal region of the scalp
Parotid	Nasopharynx
Submandibular under deep fascia lying on or even within the submandibular salivary gland	Cheek, upper and lower lips, the gums and side of tongue
Submental	Tip of tongue and adjacent part of floor of mouth; central part of lower lip
Two groups of superficial nodes (not illustrated).	
a On the sternomastoid along the external jugular vein	Parotid region and external ear
b In connective tissue antero-lateral to the larynx and trachea	Thyroid gland, larynx and trachea

Vertical chain

The vertical chain lies deeply along the carotid sheath in close contact with the internal jugular vein. It consists of a large number of nodes of which two require special mention because of their importance in the lymphatic drainage of the fauces and tongue:

1 The tonsillar or jugulo-digastric node in the angle between the internal jugular and facial veins.
2 The lingual node situated below the tonsillar gland at the level of the intermediate tendon of omohyoid.

The deep cervical chain receives afferents from the whole head and neck either directly or via intermediate nodes in the lymphatic rings. The efferents from the deep cervical chain form one or two large trunks which drain on the left side into the thoracic duct and on the right into the junction of the internal jugular and subclavian veins.

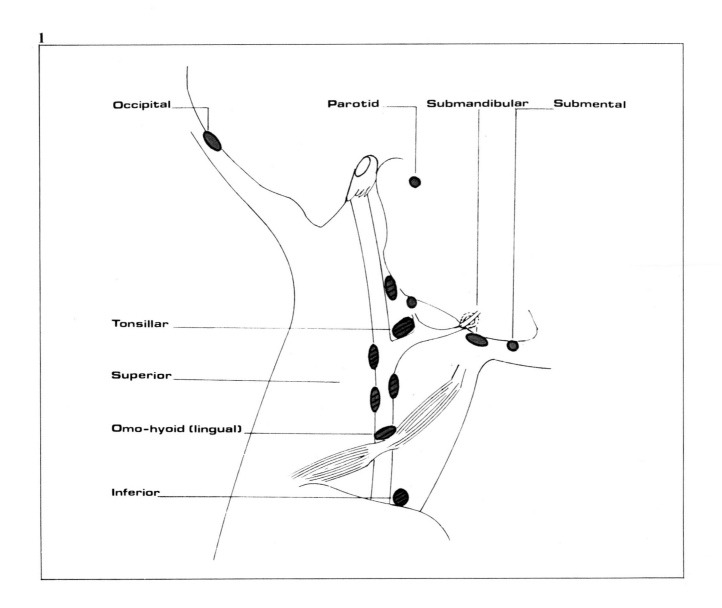

Infections

Anthrax

Anthrax derives its name from the black (coal-like) gangrenous centre of the malignant pustule. It is caused by B. anthracis, a large, gram-positive, encapsulated sporing bacillus. The disease is acquired from handling infected animals or their products e.g. hides, bone meal, which may harbour viable animal spores for a long time. The disease still occurs in the tropics but in Europe industrial legislation and hygiene have made it rare. Anthrax occurs in two forms, pulmonary and cutaneous, and both may be associated with septicaemia.

The common cutaneous form of the disease occurs most often on the head and neck which are infected either by direct contact with an infected hide or by rubbing the perspiring face or forehead with hands contaminated by B. anthracis. After a few days an itchy papule develops, blisters and becomes gangrenous centrally to form a black or grey slough surrounded by extensive oedema.

Lymphadenopathy is common but septicaemia is much less frequent than in the pulmonary form. Here the inhaled bacilli lead to pneumonia and septicaemia which are often fatal.

2

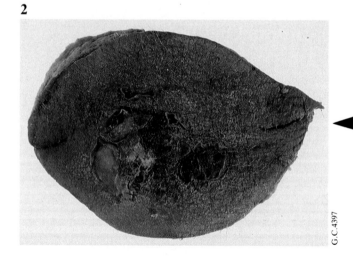

G.C.4397

2 The patient was a vanman (and therefore in contact with horses). He developed a small papule on the left side of his neck. Following abrasion there was increase of swelling and fever. A black patch then appeared which became necrotic and there was surrounding vesication.

Lymphadenitis

Acute lymphadenitis affecting nodes of the cervical chain may be secondary to a superficial or deep infective focus in the drainage area of the affected nodes. The enlargement is painful and tender and is localised. There is a marked inflammatory reaction the node becoming congested and oedematous. The inflammatory process may resolve or progress to suppuration, depending on the type and severity of the infection.

Tuberculosis

Tuberculous lesions of the cervical lymph nodes were common in the United Kingdom until the control of bovine infection was effected in the first half of the 20th century. The lesion is still common in some parts of the world. The disease occurs in two forms, lymphogenous and haematogenous.

Lymphogenous

In this form the tubercle bacillus has probably gained access through Waldeyer's ring, usually the tonsil. The organisms are carried by lymphatics from the point of entry to the tonsillar node and are arrested in the subcapsular space. Tubercles develop at this site and go on to caseation. The caseous areas enlarge and coalesce until the whole node is replaced by yellow cheesy material. Inflammation around the node fixes it to the surrounding tissue and to adjacent nodes which become secondarily involved. In general the progress of the disease is slow. It may be arrested at any stage and the affected part of the nodes replaced by fibrous or calcified tissue; or it may form a cold abscess which tends to track forwards and downwards to pierce the deep fascia and reach the skin on the line of the anterior border of the sternomastoid. The skin over a cold abscess is thin, has a bluish glazed appearance and is very likely to break down and a tuberculous sinus is formed. Where the disease is more extensive involving many nodes, an adherent, ill-defined matted mass forms and becomes attached to adjacent tissues making operative excision difficult and hazardous.

Haematogenous

This is much less common and is part of a generalised infection with involvement of the lymph nodes. Because it results from haematogenous spread the first lesion in the node lies in the centre of the lymphoid follicles. The disease may be widely distributed and is frequently bilateral.

Syphilis

Generalised lymphadenopathy may occur in tertiary syphilis and involve the cervical nodes.

Sarcoidosis

Sarcoidosis is a generalised condition which frequently affects the lymph nodes. The nodes enlarge and are painless and mobile. Histologically they show a granulomatous picture very similar to tuberculosis except that caseation seldom if ever occurs. The tuberculin test is negative and the Kveim test positive.

Infections (*Continued*)

Glandular fever

A condition usually characterised by malaise, sore throat, pyrexia, lymphadenopathy – particularly cervical, and by mononucleosis. Formerly thought to be identical with infectious mononucleosis caused by the Epstein-Barr virus it is no longer regarded as a single entity. Many of the symptoms are common to infectious mononucleosis, cytomegalovirus infections and acquired toxoplasmosis.

Infectious mononucleosis

Acute cervical lymph node enlargement may occur often associated with a persistent tonsillitis and sore throat, widespread lymphadenopathy and splenomegaly. The liver is also frequently involved and isolated cranial nerve palsies may occur. The diagnosis is confirmed by demonstrating atypical lymphocytes in the peripheral blood and by positive Paul-Bunnell and Monospot tests. Histological examination shows a proliferation of plasma cells and immunoblasts in the lymph node.

Epstein-Barr virus

The Epstein-Barr virus (EBV) is a herpes-like virus first isolated by Epstein and Barr from cultures of cells in cases of Burkitt's lymphoma (see p. 57).

It has also proved to have a relationship with nasopharyngeal carcinoma (see p. 137) and with infectious mononucleosis.

The relationship of EBV to these diseases is complex. Infection with EBV is common, worldwide and apparently does little harm in most cases. A high proportion of adults, therefore, are immune to the EBV. It would appear that these three diseases generally occur in non-immune subjects and that antibodies to the virus develop during the course of the disease.

Tumours

Branchial carcinoma

The development of carcinoma in a pre-existing branchial cyst or arising from isolated remnants of the branchial cleft is recognised. It occurs usually in males over the age of 40 and is situated high in the neck, lying deep to the anterior border of the upper part of the sternomastoid and extending towards the angle of the jaw. The tumour may be either solid or cystic and is by nature a squamous epithelioma. It may spread deeply and become fixed. Its presentation is almost identical to that of secondary malignant disease of the upper cervical lymph nodes especially when the primary lesion is in the pharynx where its identification is difficult.

The only other primary tumour in the neck which presents as a solid palpable mass is that which arises in the carotid body (see p. 304).

The vast majority of neoplasms of the neck occur in the lymphatic nodes and may be in the nature of a lymphoma, but more commonly are secondary to carcinomas arising in the mouth, nasopharynx, larynx, etc.

Lymphoma

Enlarged lymph nodes which are painless, rubbery in consistence, discrete and mobile are a common feature of both Hodgkin's and non-Hodgkin's lymphoma. Hodgkin's lymphoma is a progressive disease but it may remain localised to a group of nodes for a considerable time.

The staging of Hodgkin's lymphoma and the histological appearance in it and in non-Hodgkin's lymphoma are described under the section on lymphatics.

Lymph borne malignant cells tend to be arrested in the subcapsular sinus of the lymph node and are frequently destroyed there. Should they survive and multiply they gradually replace the normal architecture of the node, causing a firm or even hard rounded enlargement which eventually becomes fixed to adjacent structures.

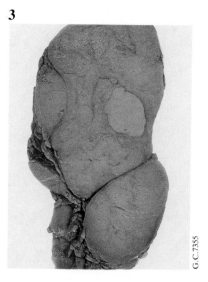

3 This is an example of a typical Hodgkin's disease. Note the uniform, relatively avascular cut surface, greyish pink in appearance with one small area of necrosis but no abscess formation. Typically the capsule shows no evidence of adhesion formation. These nodes feel firm and rubbery but are not hard.

Lymphangioma

Lymphangioma is a developmental anomaly of lymph vessels. As with haemangioma, it may occur in capillary or cavernous forms. In the neck a type with very large lymphatic spaces is found and is called cystic hygroma. Cystic hygroma is usually present at birth. It may be circumscribed or may ramify deeply between the muscles and extend into the mediastinum. It may disappear spontaneously but is more likely to require surgical care because of infection or pressure effects.

Secondary carcinoma

Secondary malignant disease of the cervical lymph nodes is common. It occurs as the result of lymphatic spread from a primary carcinoma in the soft tissue of the head and neck, including thyroid, nasopharynx and larynx. The mass formed is a hard fixed lesion, usually lobulated. As the malignant cells spread through the capsule of the nodes, the overlying skin is invaded and ultimately ulceration occurs. Malignancy arising at special sites is followed by early involvement of the jugulo-digastric (tonsillar) and the lingual nodes (omohyoid). The third node of significance lies immediately above the clavicle at the lower end of the vertical chain. This node on the left side is occasionally the site of malignant disease secondary to carcinoma of the stomach. It is close to the entrance of the thoracic duct into the subclavian vein.

A.I.S. Macpherson

Buccal mucosa

Structure

The mucosa of the mouth, nasopharynx and pharynx is structurally a squamous epithelium which is characterised by the orderly arrangement of cells in layers. These layers demonstrate a transition from the basement membrane to the surface.

The mucous membrane and mucous glands of the lips, cheeks, gums, anterior two thirds of the tongue, part of the floor of the mouth, the palate and of the nasal cavities and paranasal sinuses, are derived from the ectoderm of the stomatodaeum. The mucosa of the nasopharynx and pharynx including the posterior third of the tongue is derived from the endoderm of the foregut. At first the stomatodaeum is separated from the cranial end of the foregut by a diaphragm – the buccopharyngeal membrane. The diaphragm ruptures in the 3rd week of embryonic life thus establishing continuity between the two components. The line of the primitive buccopharyngeal membrane is not readily defined after the 3rd week, but can be described as an imaginary plane descending from a point anterior to the body of the sphenoid downwards to the floor of the mouth at the junction of the anterior two thirds and posterior third of the tongue.

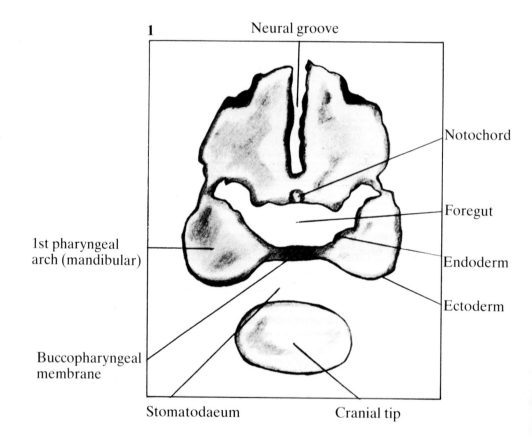

The cells of the basal layer in general are cubical. These cells form the active proliferating layer and on mitosis divide in a plane parallel to the basement membrane. The daughter cells adjacent to the basement membrane remain *in situ* reforming the proliferating layer but the more superficial cells slowly pass towards the surface and while so doing undergo transition.

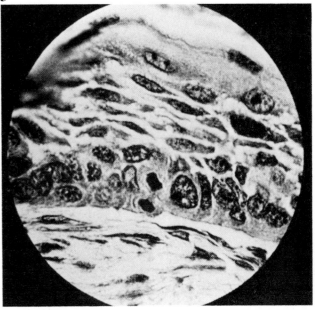

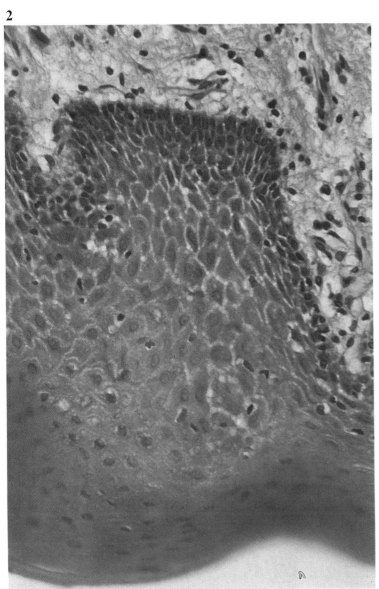

Further superficial migration of the cells follows and as this occurs the cells and their nuclei both increase in size. Ultimately the cell becomes considerably enlarged and polyhedral in shape. Simultaneously separation from adjacent cells occurs with the formation of an intercellular space crossed by protoplasmic filaments, the so-called prickles. Within this space serum circulates.

At the next stage of superficial migration the cytoplasm shrinks so that the cells again assume a fusiform shape. The nuclear membrane ruptures and nuclear debris is extruded while at the poles eosinophilic staining properties become evident. This is the first evidence of the process of keratinisation.

The next stage of migration is associated with keratinisation of the cytoplasm which fuses with that of adjacent cells to form continuous laminae.

Buccal mucosa (*Continued*)

The thickness or depth of the mucosa shows considerable variation according to site. This is attributable either to an increase in the layer of prickle cells or to the thickness of the keratin laminae. In some areas the superficial keratin layer may be defective or absent.

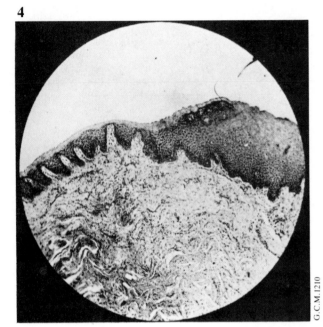

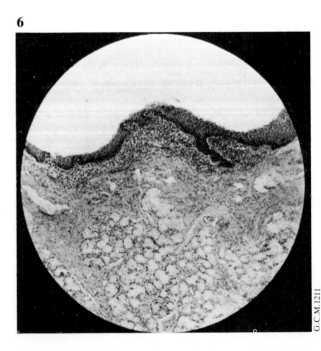

5 The epithelium in the section illustrated is from the dorsum of the anterior two thirds of the tongue and shows well marked keratinisation.

4 The illustration shows the variation which occurs at the lateral margin of the tongue. The thicker epithelium is that seen on the dorsum. The thinner part is that of the gingivo-lingual sulcus.

Pharyngeal mucosa

The mucosa which is derived from the endoderm of the foregut shows little or no keratinisation and beneath the epithelial layer aggregations of lymphoid cells are frequently present. To such epithelium the term lymphoepithelium has been applied in the past.

See also nasopharyngeal carcinoma p. 135.

Squamous carcinoma

The majority of tumours arising from the surface epithelium of the mouth, nasopharynx and pharynx are squamous carcinomas and their features are essentially similar irrespective of the precise site at which they arise. It is therefore convenient to consider the factors which are common to all in the first instance.

Carcinoma of the mouth and of the pharynx is a disease the incidence of which in the United Kingdom is diminishing.

Age incidence

All forms of carcinoma of the mouth and pharynx are rare below the age of 40 in the United Kingdom but their incidence increases with advancing years.

Sex incidence

Carcinoma of the mouth is more common in males than females. In the past this may be explained by the greater degree of injury which the male inflicts upon the buccal mucous membrane by such irritants as spirits, tobacco and dental caries. Women were probably more careful about their teeth and oral hygiene.

7

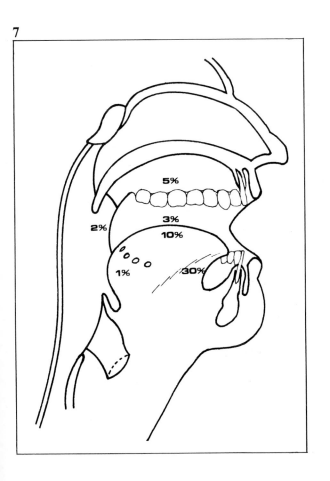

7   There is variation of the incidence of carcinoma according to precise site. The percentages shown were part of a series which included the pharynx.

8

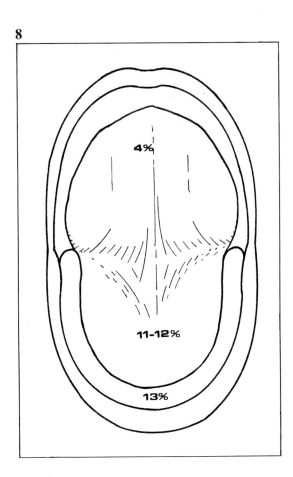

8   Floor of mouth and under surface of tongue.

Squamous carcinoma (*Continued*)

Predisposing factors

Local irritation or injury

Damage to the mucosa by physical or chemical agents is important in relation to the development of carcinoma of the mouth and pharynx. These factors, which will be discussed later when consideration is given to carcinomas arising in certain sites, may be responsible for the variation of site incidence of the disease.

Leucoplakia

The term leucoplakia refers to the development of white thickened patches on the mucosa. In the mouth it is seen principally on the dorsum of the tongue, the lip and occasionally the inner surface of the cheek. The patches represent areas of increase of the intermediate layers of the epithelium and keratinised laminae. The lesions may be small with round edges or more widespread with serpiginous margins especially on the dorsum of the tongue. Fissures develop with some frequency.

Syphilis

In older studies it was evident that syphilis was an important aetiological factor. In one such series 14% of mouth tumours had evidence of an antecedent syphilitic infection. In carcinoma of the tongue there was an even closer relationship (40%), and where the tumour occurred on the dorsum of the tongue the relationship was as high as 80%.

9

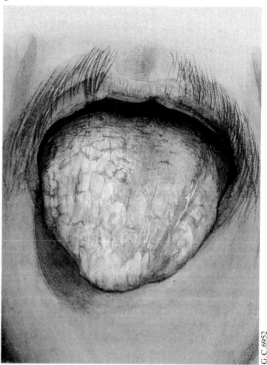

The introduction of antibiotic treatment of syphilis resulted in a fall in the incidence of tertiary syphilis and this was associated with a corresponding reduction in the incidence of carcinoma of the tongue. More recently the control of syphilis has been less effective and presently there is an increasing incidence of the disease.

It may be noted that leucoplakia of squamous and transitional epithelium has been described in sites other than the oral cavity, notably oesophagus, the urinary tract and female genital tract.

Causation

Many instances of leucoplakia have been attributed to local irritation by the mechanical friction of irregular teeth or faulty dentures. Other examples have been attributed to the presence of dental fillings in which dissimilar metals have been used. One example has been described as occurring in an electrician who had acquired the custom of testing battery leads on his tongue. Other instances are attributed to chemical irritation or to burns, chemical or thermal. In this respect pipe smoking has been blamed. Betel nut chewing is also a cause of leucoplakia (vide infra) but in this instance an associated vitamin A deficiency is implicated.

In the earlier stages of leucoplakia the thickening of the intermediate layers of the epithelium results in the formation of downward projections of masses of intermediate cells which pass into the corium. The superficial layer of keratin may or may not increase. The basal layer retains its normal formation and shows no evidence of increased mitosis. In the subepithelial corium infiltration by inflammatory cells is common.

Later, signs of dysplasia may become evident. Variation in nuclear and cell size together with increased mitotic activity appears. In the advanced stage there is loss of surface epithelium with the formation of fissures. The epithelium becomes greatly thinned, only the basal layer remaining and showing irregularity. Prolonged dysplasia may be followed by invasive carcinoma.

10

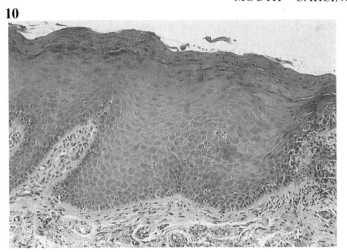

10   Leucoplakia of lip. The rete is thickened and there is mild hyperkeratosis. Inflammatory infiltrate is slight. (*H&E × 100*)

10a

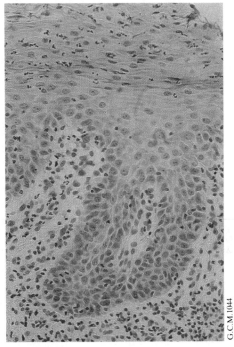

10a   Same case. Here the rete pegs are elongated.

There are more immature cells and mitotic activity is increased. The inflammatory infiltrate is more marked. (*H&E × 200*)

Widespread leucoplakia also occurs as a complication of tertiary syphilis but spirochaetes cannot be demonstrated in the affected mucosa. In cases of advanced leucoplakia the deep white plaques may diminish and be replaced by raw wide fissures (the raw beef tongue).

Squamous carcinoma (*Continued*)

Macroscopic features

Carcinomas of the mouth vary in their gross morphology according to their degree of differentiation. The best differentiated tumour, the verrucous carcinoma, occurs almost exclusively in men with leucoplakia induced by chewing tobacco. At first resembling a squamous papilloma it later invades and becomes locally destructive but seldom metastasises.

More often the squamous carcinoma is less well differentiated, flatter, ulcerated and invasive. Lymph node metastases are common.

In the early stages the ulcer may be superficial but the majority of these tumours present as a frank malignant ulcer with rolled edges. As the ulcer expands adjacent tissues are involved and the tumour becomes fixed. Haemorrhage, occasionally considerable, is common. The mucosa around the tumour may show leucoplakia or carcinoma *in situ*. Sometimes the carcinoma occurs as a deeply penetrating fissure. Such tumours tend to be poorly differentiated and they may escape detection. This is especially true where the lesion is located in sites such as the pyriform recess. The first manifestation of such a tumour may be enlargement of the related lymph nodes.

Histology

11

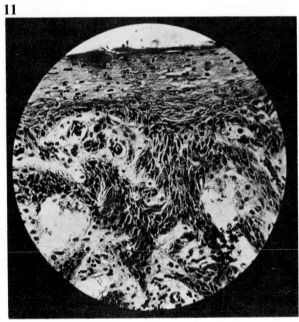

Surface layer

11 Basal layer showing evidence of irregularity and hyperchromatism indicating malignancy.

Downgrowth of tumour cells

The squamous carcinoma cells arising from the basal layer show variation in shape, size and staining properties and mitotic figures become more evident. The method of downgrowth into the subjacent tissue varies with the degree of malignancy. In the less malignant group clumps of cells or thicker downward growing columns are seen. These demonstrate changes comparable in character to those already described as occurring in normal epithelium. The cells which lie at the margin of the clumps or columns in contact with the surrounding stroma have the essential features of basal layer cells.

Tracing the cells to the centre of the clump or column the changes ending in keratin formation are observed. Clumps of cells which have undergone this change are described as 'cell nests' (**12**). In more malignant forms the process of differentiation is less complete or may be absent. The degree of differentiation has been used as the basis for grading the malignancy of tumours.

Differentiation

The degree of differentation which occurs in squamous epithelial tumours varies from that in which cell nest formation is marked to that in which no keratinisation occurs.

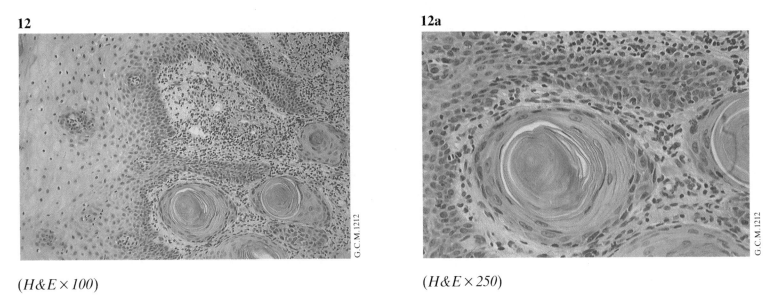

12

(*H&E × 100*)

12a

(*H&E × 250*)

12 and **12a**   Highly differentiated carcinoma. Marked cell nest formation.

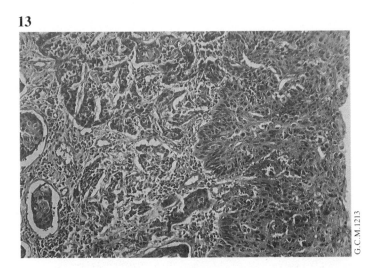

13

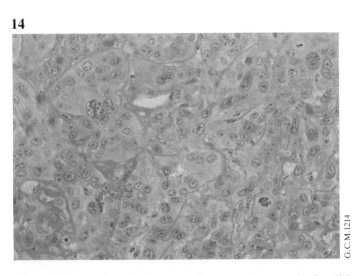

14

13   Intermediate stage of differentiation. The tumour is still recognisably squamoid but no cell nests can be seen. (*H&E × 100*)

14   Poorly differentiated carcinoma composed of solid masses of cells showing nuclear pleomorphism and mitotic activity. (*H&E × 250*)

Squamous carcinoma (*Continued*)

Carcinomas of the mouth and pharynx all show an invasive propensity, locally by direct invasion and more widely by lymphatics or haematogenous dissemination. The spread may be late or early according to the degree of malignancy of the initial lesion. In some instances lymphatic dissemination in particular may be clinically evident before the primary lesion is detected.

Fascial spread

Local invasion tends to follow connective tissue planes but where connective tissue condenses to a definite fascial plane the malignant cells may spread along one surface and only transgress the fascial plane where it is penetrated by anatomical structures.

15

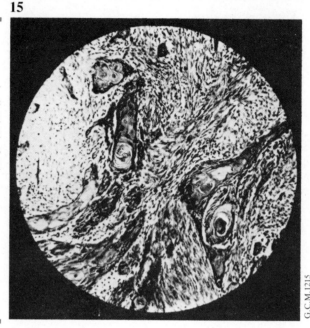

15 Invasion of fascia by malignant cells. Note that where the cells have 'clumped' keratinisation or cell nest formation has occurred. The clumps, however, are connected by narrow strands of malignant cells.

Lymphatic spread

Lymphatic spread is the commonest form of dissemination and may be found even when the primary lesion is small. The earliest lymph nodes to be involved depend upon which area of the mucosa is primarily affected but eventually the final pathway for lymphatic drainage, the deep cervical chain of nodes, is invaded by secondary tumour and may become a large and fixed mass.

16

17

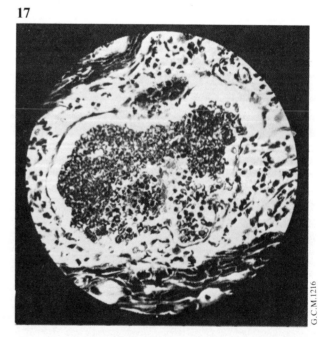

16 A clump of malignant epithelial cells lying within a thin-walled lymphatic channel deep to a primary malignant lesion.

17 A small lymphatic lying adjacent to the wall of a venule and containing neoplastic cells.

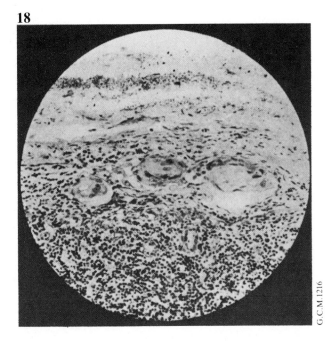

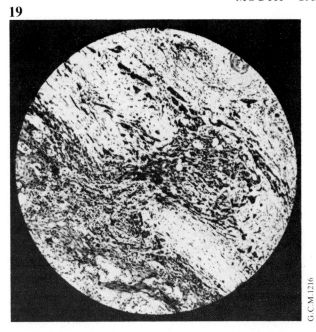

18 A section of a lymph node showing the presence of three small groups of malignant cells lying in the subcapsular sinus (gland corridor) situated between the capsule and the lymphatic follicle.

19 The section shows rupture of the capsule of a lymph node with invasion of the surrounding tissues. This leads to fixation.

Periductal spread

Involvement of salivary glands, especially the submandibular, is relatively common in squamous carcinoma involving the tongue or the floor of the mouth. There is periductal spread from the primary lesion to reach lymph nodes which lie within the capsule of the salivary gland. Comparable periductal spread occurs with involvement of minor submucous glands.

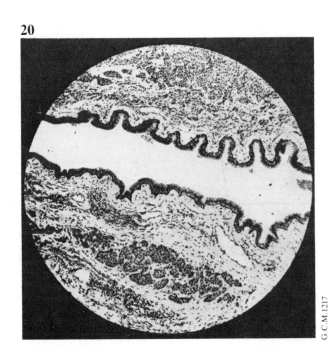

20 Subepithelial mucous gland. Periductal lymphatics contain malignant cells.

Squamous carcinoma (*Continued*)

Involvement of nerves

A special feature of carcinoma of the tongue or pharynx is severe radiating pain often referred to the ear or radiating along the line of the jaw and resulting from direct invasion of sensory nerves.

21

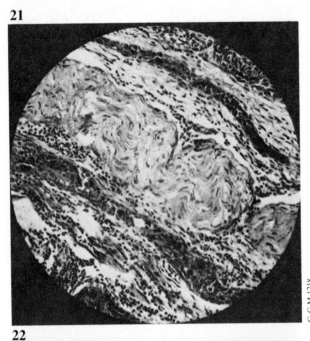

G.C.M.1218

21　A nerve fibre with perineural invasion by malignancy. The malignant cells lie in relation to the nerve sheath forming a distinct layer of malignant tissue.

22

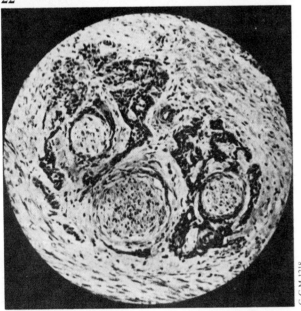

G.C.M.1218

23

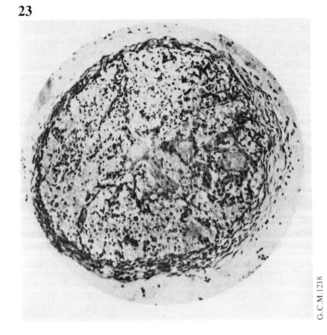

G.C.M.1218

22　A comparable section showing an even greater degree of infiltration by malignant cells separating the nerve fibres within the nerve sheath.

23　Transverse section of a nerve demonstrating nerve bundles surrounded by malignant cells.

Haematogenous spread

Haematogenous spread is relatively uncommon. Malignant cells appear to enter venous channels from perivascular lymphatics. Distant metastases are few in number, appear late and are seldom diffusely scattered.

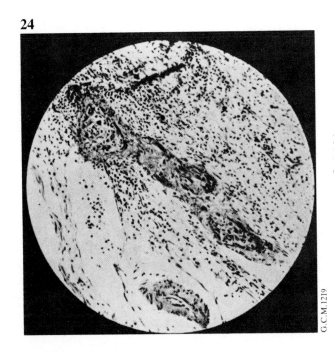

24 This section shows a venule, the lumen of which has been completely occupied by malignant epithelial cells.

25 Transverse section of a vein, the lumen of which contains a mass of malignant cells.

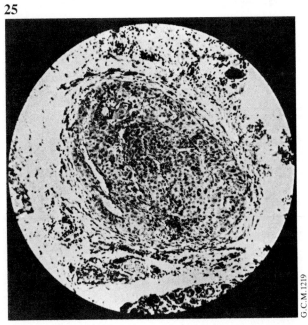

Squamous carcinoma (*Continued*)

Variations according to site

The incidence of squamous carcinoma in the mouth shows considerable site variation. This is attributable to differences in the exposure of the mucosa to a variety of irritants which are of aetiological significance. There is also variation in the character of the mucosa.

Note must also be made of the differing routes of lymphatic drainage according to the location of the primary site.

Lip

The mucosa of the normal lip shows little or no keratinisation. On the outer surface of the lip the mucosa is closely applied to the underlying muscle. On the inner surface the mucosa is more loosely attached to the underlying tissue and there are numerous mucous glands.

A large majority of these carcinomas arise in the lower lip but it is uncommon to find them originating at the midline or angle of the mouth. There is a high male preponderance (90%). Tumours of the upper lip are rare and occur relatively more frequently in females.

The disease is frequently preceded by a chronic roughening and cracking. This may be due to exposure to sunlight (actinic cheilitis) and is therefore particularly common in men who are engaged in outdoor activities (farmers, fishermen). It possibly also explains the high incidence of the disease in Australia. Clay pipe smoking was previously a recognised causal factor and cases have been reported where the condition has been found in tar workers.

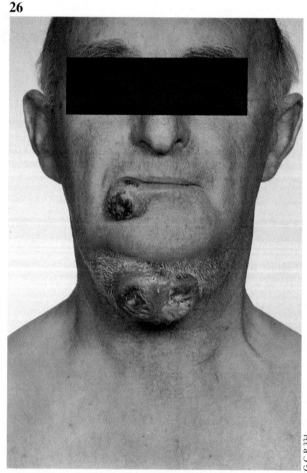

26

26 From a male aged 76 years who presented in 1978 with a swelling of the lower lip which rapidly proceeded to ulcerate. A few months later there was an evident tumour arising in relation to the submental and submandibular glands. This too rapidly became ulcerated. Histological examination showed an infiltrating squamous cell carcinoma (grade II). The tumour responded to radiotherapy.

By courtesy of Professor W. Duncan.

G.C.P.334

Carcinoma of the lip is slow growing and frequently of protruding papilliferous type with scab formation and later ulceration. As the ulcer expands tissue destruction gives rise to a foul smelling discharge.

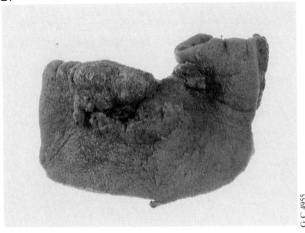

27 Typical ulceration on the lateral part of the lower lip with some infiltration and swelling.

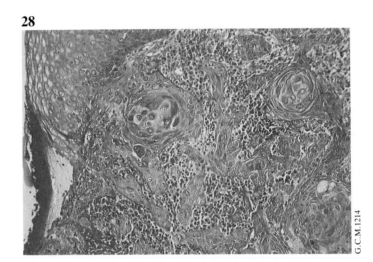

28 Squamous carcinoma of lip. A moderately differentiated tumour showing some keratinisation and attempt at cell nest formation. (*H&E × 110*)

Spread

Lymphatic spread is not so rapid as in neoplasms of other parts of the oral cavity. It is generally unilateral to the submental and submandibular nodes. In tumours which involve the midline the spread is bilateral to the submental nodes.

Prognosis

Since these tumours are well differentiated and diagnosis is made early the prognosis is good.

Squamous carcinoma (*Continued*)

Cheek

Squamous carcinoma of the inner aspect of the cheek is rare and has been held to be the result of chewing tobacco.

29

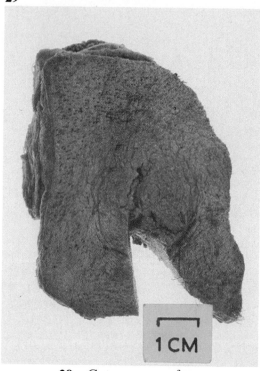

29   Cutaneous surface

The patient was admitted to hospital complaining of a tumour on the buccal aspect of the cheek. No aetiological factor was noted. The mucosa of the cheek is partly replaced by a papillomatous, ulcerating carcinoma and the tumour has extended deeply through soft tissues to reach the skin of the cheek. This has produced on the cutaneous surface a circular thickening which slightly projects beyond the adjacent skin level.

G.C.3815

29a

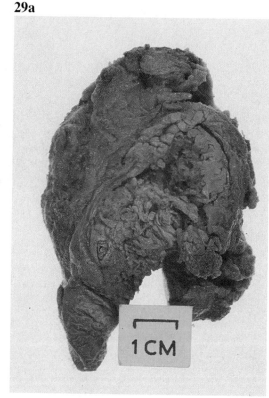

29a   Buccal surface

Betel nut carcinoma

Much more significant is a carcinoma resulting from betel nut chewing in the Far East.

It is a common social custom in adult males in the orient to chew constantly a 'quid' lodged in the inside of the cheek or under the tongue. The practice is particularly common in southern India, Sri Lanka and the Philippines and to a lesser degree in other countries in South-east Asia. The quid consists of a mixture of betel or areca nuts, tobacco, spices and lime wrapped in buyo leaf. The mouth is constantly stained a bright red from the juices of the betel nut. The association of betel nut chewing with a high incidence of carcinoma in the inner surface of the cheek, alveolus and tongue has long been recognised.

A betel nut tumour is typically a radiosensitive keratinising squamous carcinoma usually with gross sepsis and a foul smelling discharge. Lymph nodes draining the area are enlarged but this is often attributable to the sepsis rather than to secondary malignant invasion.

The 'quid' or 'pan' causes constant localised irritation of the mucosa especially of the cheek, alveolus and the side of the tongue. In addition, the teeth become worn and jagged and thereby cause mechanical injury. Oral hygiene is often poor. The consequential initial reaction in the mucosa is a localised meta-plasia with the formation of white patches (leucoplakia). Areas of ulceration, cracking and fissure forma-tion occur later and evident malignant change supervenes.

30

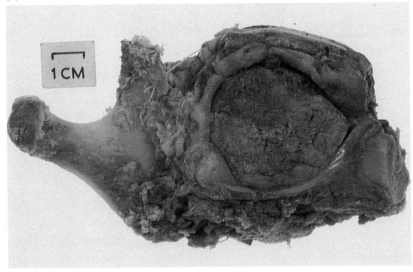

30a

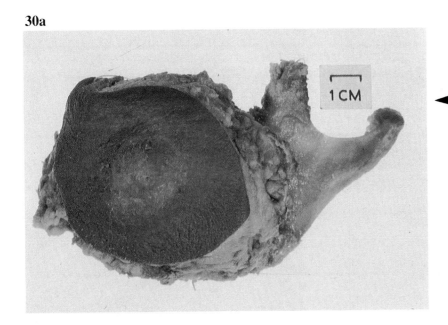

30 and **30a**   This is a typical case of betel nut carcinoma from a male aged 76 years, a native of Travancore (S. India). The specimen, the left half of the jaw and cheek, shows a malignant ulcer in the gingivobuccal sulcus and extending over the alveolus.

The tumour has invaded the soft tissues of the cheek and is commencing to involve the skin where a small nodule is present. The skin around the nodule **is** indurated but not ulcerated. Later ulcera-tion develops with eventual fistula for-mation.

G.C.6229

Much research has been carried out in an endeavour to identify the carcinogenic agent. Attention has been paid to the geographical and social incidence and to variations in the content of the quid. Three factors have been the subject of special study:

1   The use of certain coarse types of tobacco.
2   The caustic effect of lime and the apparent greater carcinogenicity of lime derived from sea-shells.
3   The greater susceptibility of the oral mucosa to damage in groups of people subject to impaired nutrition. Vitamin A deficiency in particular has been implicated.

Squamous carcinoma (*Continued*)

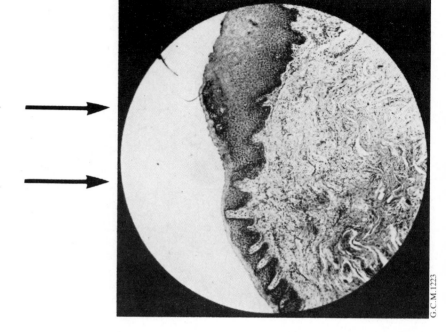

Tongue – mucosa

31 The mucosa of the dorsum of the anterior two thirds of the tongue is thick due to the increase of the intermediate layers of the epithelium. In addition the mucosa has a fur-like coat due to the presence of numerous filiform papillae and is adherent to the underlying muscle.

At the margins of the anterior two thirds the mucosa becomes much thinner, without filiform formation and extends down to and is continuous with the mucosa of the floor of the mouth (gingivo-lingual sulcus) where it finally sweeps upwards to form the mucosa covering the alveolar margins.

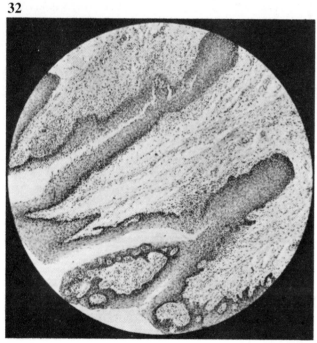

32 Of special significance is the folia lingula which is an atavistic remnant of a prominent taste bud observed especially in ruminants. The folia lingula is situated at the posterior end of the lateral margin of the tongue and is represented by vestigial clefts. This site is also the point where the anterior pillar of the fauces merges with the margin of the tongue. The folia lingula may present as an elevated area of mucosa.

33 The posterior third or pharyngeal part of the tongue which lies behind the level of the foramen caecum is covered by mucosa which is not adherent to the underlying muscle. It is relatively thin with minimal or no keratin formation. It contains numerous mucous and serous glands. In addition, closely related to the overlying epithelium are numerous aggregations of lymphoid tissue, the so-called lingual tonsil.

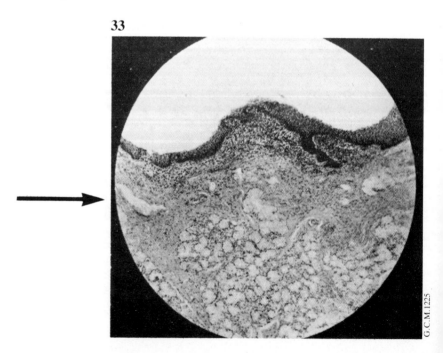

The most common site of oral carcinoma is the tongue.

The incidence of these tumours is decreasing. This may be attributed to changing social habits, reduction of smoking and improved dental care. It has been noted that carcinoma seldom occurs in the edentulous. The disease has been described as occurring at all ages but is rare below the age of 50 years, after which there is a progressive increase. There is a marked male preponderance (90%). Tumours arise most frequently on the lateral margin of the anterior two thirds especially in relation to the folia lingula.

The mucosa of the anterior two thirds of the tongue originates from the epiblast of the oral pit, whilst the posterior third is derived from the cephalic end of the foregut. In this section only lesions of the anterior two thirds of the tongue are considered since they differ from the posterior third. However, for convenience and comparison, note is made of the distinctive features of the mucosa in both areas.

Lateral margin − clinical presentation

34

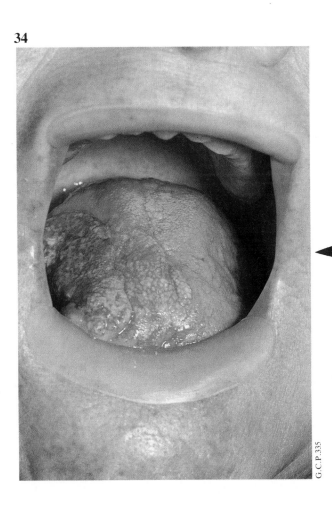

34 From a female aged 47 years. The initial lesion was a small patch of leuco-plakia on the right side of the tongue which was excised. Six years later she returned to hospital with an infiltrating carcinoma of the tongue. No nodes were palpable in the neck. Histology of the lesion showed an invasive keratinising squamous cell carcinoma. The tumour completely resolved following radio-therapy. She died of a cardiovascular accident four months after completion of radiotherapy.

By courtesy of Professor W. Duncan.

Squamous carcinoma (*Continued*)

Tongue – lateral margin

Tumours on the lateral margin of the tongue are probably the most malignant of oral carcinomas and it is commonly held that the early ulcerative lesion is caused by adjacent septic or irregular teeth.

The classical lesion is seen as an ulcerating tumour with fixed and hard everted edges. A majority arise in relation to the folia lingula. The tumour extends into the substance of the tongue and into the floor of the mouth and may become fixed to the mandible. Invasion of the sensory nerves may result in severe pain frequently radiating upwards into the ear. It is associated with a foul discharge.

The tumour may be well differentiated but a considerable percentage of lesions are undifferentiated to a varying degree. Those arising in relation to the folia lingula are often less differentiated.

It is important to differentiate between malignancy and simple swellings of the folia lingula due to chronic irritation which may require biopsy.

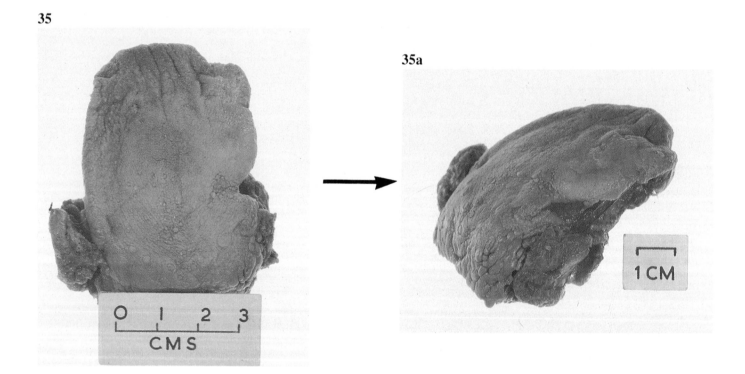

35 and **35a** Two views of a carcinoma of the tongue from a female aged 36 years in whom the submandibular lymph nodes were considerably enlarged.

The right margin of the anterior two thirds of the tongue is almost wholly replaced by a deep ulcer with irregular, undermined edges and a granular-looking, necrotic floor. Though ceasing some little distance from the tip, the ulceration was found to extend posteriorly into the posterior third of the tongue. The central portion of the dorsal surface appears unusually smooth.

G.C.3936

Tongue – dorsum

Tumours arising on the dorsum of the tongue are much less common and the majority are clearly associated with leucoplakia especially of syphilitic origin. Since the tumour involves both halves of the tongue the lymphatic spread is bilateral.

36

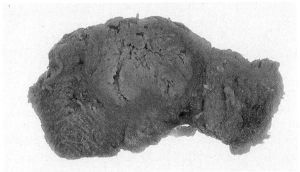

36 Section through tumour (33mm × 25mm) from the medial side.

36a

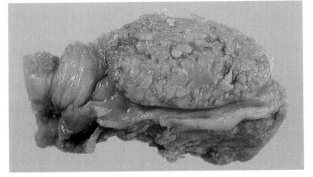

36a Lateral surface.

From a woman of 86 who had suffered from a papillary lesion of the tongue for many months before carcinoma was diagnosed and a hemiglossectomy was performed.

The specimen consists of most of the excised portion of tongue and shows a surface papillary growth protruding from the mucous membrane. The cut surface also reveals that the tumour is invading muscle and is therefore malignant. Microscopically the tumour proved to be a well-differentiated squamous carcinoma with considerable keratinisation. Most tumours of the tongue ulcerate and it is unusual for a tumour to attain the size in the present specimen without ulceration.

G.C.14436

Spread

Lymphatic spread occurs early. The affected lymph nodes include the submandibular nodes. Other tumours show early spread to the lymph node which lies on the anterior border of the jugular vein where it is crossed by the omohyoid muscle. This is sometimes referred to as the lingual or jugulo-omohyoid node. On occasion there appears to be direct lymph spread to this node from the primary tumour without involvement of intervening lymph nodes. The spread is unilateral unless the primary tumour has crossed the midline raphe or involves the tip of the tongue. In the latter case involvement of the submental nodes may occur.

Squamous carcinoma (*Continued*)

Floor of mouth

Carcinoma arising in the gingivo-lingual sulcus is relatively uncommon. It has been held that an ill fitting lower dental plate may be of aetiological significance. The usual lesion is one which has initially been located at the margin of the tongue and spread laterally. In this situation carcinomas usually ulcerate deeply, spread early to gum and involve the mandible. Early spread to the submandibular lymphatic nodes occurs.

37

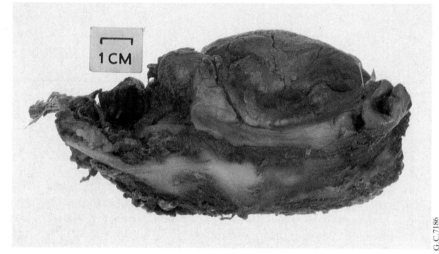

G.C.7186

37 From a male gardener aged 67 years, a heavy smoker. Three weeks after complaining of pain in the gums, teeth and tongue, especially on the right side, he had several teeth removed. Death occurred on the tenth day after operation.

A carcinomatous ulcer replaces the mucosa from the right canine tooth to the right glossopalatine arch and extends on to the gum where it incorporates the periosteum. It involves the right edge and inferior surface of the tongue.

38

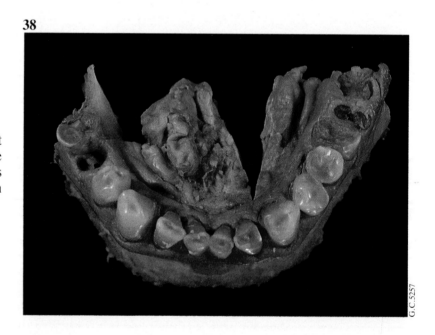

G.C.5257

38 Portion anterior to the molar teeth of an adult mandible showing a squamous-cell carcinoma of the floor of the mouth. The tumour forms an irregular mass ulcerated on its surface and adherent to the periosteum of the lingual surface of the body of the mandible.

Carcinoma of the palate is rare. Cases have been described attributable to wearing artificial dentures. There are no pathological features of special significance except that there is destruction of the underlying palatal bone.

Tumours – miscellaneous

Melanoma

Melanomas occurring in the palate or in relation to the gingival sulcus of the mandible are rare and constitute not more than 1% of all melanomas. These tumours are characterised by pigmentation and are associated with a high mortality. Pre-malignant melanosis of the lip and gingival margins has been described.

39

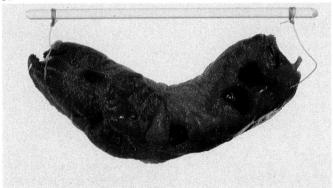

G.C.7663

39 Specimen removed by operation from a female aged 30 years whose maxillary incisor teeth had been extracted seventeen years previously as they were 'unsightly and arranged in two irregular rows'. At 27 years of age a maxillary sinusitis was operated on and shortly after that a nasal polypus was removed. A year later she noticed black spots on the gum and these had gradually increased in size. A biopsy showed the structure of a melanoma. Later the discoloration extended becoming prominent and nodular.

The black patches are irregular and their outline somewhat ill defined with here and there outlying black spots. The pigmentation varies in density.

40

40 From a female aged 80. The specimen demonstrates a melanoma of the alveolar margin of the maxilla. Note the patchy pigmentation extending along the gingival mucosa and on to the palate.

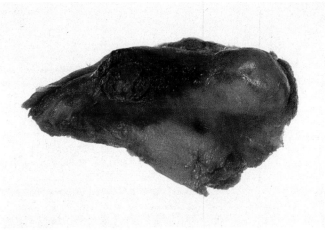

G.C.6390

Salivary gland
Tumours exhibiting the features of neoplasms arising from salivary gland tissue are occasionally found. (See p. 14 Volume I.)

Haemangioma and lymphangioma
Both haemangiomas and lymphangiomas occur and the latter type is one of the causes of macroglossia. The lesion may be either unilateral or bilateral. These tumours represent either innocent neoplasms or hamartomas.

Tumours – miscellaneous

Abrikossof

The histogenesis of this tumour is debatable. Origin from myocytes or fibroblasts has been suggested but it is now becoming accepted that these tumours arise from Schwann cells. The tumour, usually solitary and localised, has rarely been known to metastasise. It is composed of packed masses of large pale granular cells. The nuclei are relatively small and show little or no mitotic activity. The cytoplasm is abundant and contains small, slightly eosinophilic granules.

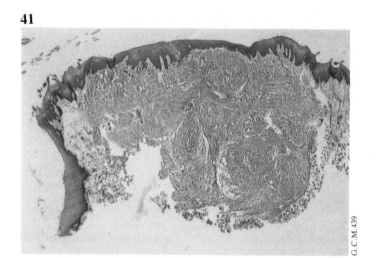

41 Tongue – Abrikossof tumour. The subepithelial tumour is composed of whorls or strands of eosinophilic cells. (*H&E × 15*)

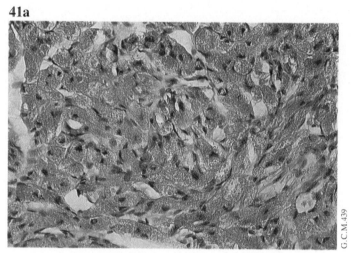

41a Same case. The cytoplasm is packed with eosinophilic granules. The nuclei are small and darkly staining. There is no mitotic activity. (*H&E × 250*)

Cysts – miscellaneous

Retention cyst

The mucosa of the lips, tongue and mouth contains numerous small mucous glands which may become the site of retention cysts. Initially these are small swellings located in the mucosa but by trauma, e.g. from the teeth, they may become infected and ultimately show ulceration.

Ranula

This is a cystic swelling arising in the floor of the mouth which may be located on either side of the fraenum. Occasionally it may arise in the midline and be hour-glass in shape, presenting as masses on both sides of the fraenum. The cystic swelling arises from smaller salivary glands in the mucosa of the mouth and under surface of the tongue and has a thin lining (sometimes defective of mucosa) which may be cuboidal or ciliated. In the defective areas the lining appears to be solely fibrous tissue. The content of the cyst is jelly-like and has been compared to the contents of a ganglion. In tumours of greater size the swelling may pass downwards through the myelohyoid muscle and appear in the submental triangle. On occasion the lesion arises in early childhood and may cause deformity of the mandible.

Infections – miscellaneous

Infections of the mouth and nasal cavities initially may be viral but secondary infection by pyogenic organisms occurs. These infections may be localised or extend. In the mouth, nasal cavities and pharynx, either by the increase of mucus secretion, sometimes purulent, or by mucosal swelling due to engorgement and oedema interference with breathing and swallowing occurs. The mucosal swelling may also lead to the occlusion of the natural channels of drainage from the sinuses. These lesions may be associated with generalised systemic disturbances.

Non-specific, including pyogenic, infections may spread:
(a)   along fascial planes leading to a cellulitis
(b)   involvement of the neighbouring and cervical lymph nodes. This may occur as a chronic ailment and is important in differential diagnosis.

Chronic infections of the mouth may result from ill fitting dentures or dental sepsis. Chronic infection, which is usually ulcerative, may result from continuing irritation of dental origin. It may be granulomatous and may simulate tumours, e.g. lingual tonsil.

Occasionally chronic lesions originally inflammatory are associated with giant cell proliferation (so-called Giant Cell Granuloma).

Infections – miscellaneous (*Continued*)

Ludwig's angina

Ludwig's angina is a cellulitis of the submandibular space usually from an infected tooth. The space is limited superficially by the attachment of the superficial and tougher investing layer of the deep cervical fascia to the mandible and deeply by the small muscles of the tongue covered by the deeper layer of fascia. Because of this the inflammatory oedema is confined and tension in the space rises. The tongue is pushed upwards and backwards into the mouth and fatal oedema of the glottis may ensue before pus has begun to form. The infection is commonly mixed with streptococcus predominant.

Tuberculosis

Tongue

Involvement of the tongue is a rare complication usually associated with tuberculous laryngitis and an open pulmonary lesion. The organisms reach the tongue from infected sputum. The typical lesion is a well defined but not deeply penetrating ulcer on the dorsum close to the tip.

42

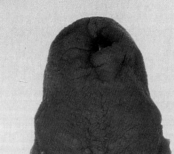

G.C.10005

42 Tongue – tuberculous ulcer. From a male aged 27 years the subject of bilateral pulmonary tuberculosis.

The ulcer is situated on the dorsum of the tongue close to the right side of the mesial plane, about 1cm from the tip. The crater is about 1cm in diameter and 1cm deep, with overhanging edges and a necrotic base. The epiglottis and larynx are healthy.

The tuberculous nature of the lesion was demonstrated histologically.

Syphilis

Primary

The primary lesion (chancre) may rarely develop on the lips, tongue or face. It starts as a papule which breaks down to form a painless ulcer with induration of its base and a well defined margin. As in other primary syphilitic granulomas large numbers of treponema pallidum are present.

Secondary

The mouth is commonly affected. White mucous patches, snail track ulcers and superficial glossitis may all be found. Numerous treponema are present and the lesions are highly infective. Lymphadenopathy is common and may affect the cervical lymph nodes.

Tertiary

Tongue – the condition may present as a diffuse syphilitic glossitis resulting in superficial ulceration or as leucoplakia. Treponemas can seldom be demonstrated. If long continued, cracks and fissures form. In the pharynx, syphilitic ulceration may simulate carcinoma.

Gumma of the palate may result in perforation. Gummas arising in the maxilla may simulate tumours of the antrum.

43

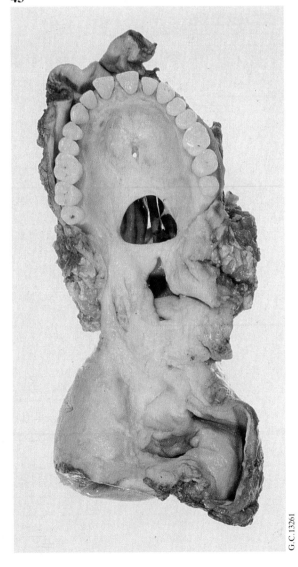

43 This subject was a known syphilitic. The palate shows a small circular perforation a little to one side of the midline of the hard palate anteriorly, and a large rounded opening posteriorly. There is complete destruction of the epiglottis and greater part of the soft palate. The anterior lesion in the palate shows an ulceration in association with an underlying gumma. The posterior lesion has smooth margins suggesting that this was an earlier manifestation of the disease which has become quiescent and the margins have become epithelialised.

G.C.1326I

117

Hypopharynx

Tumours of the hypopharynx (post-cricoid) and the upper oesophagus are of similar nature. Lesions frequently transgress the theoretical anatomical line of division and accordingly while post-cricoid tumours are frequently classified as tumours of the hypopharynx they commonly involve the upper end of the oesophagus. The hypopharynx extends from the hyoid bone above to the cricoarytenoid joints below where it becomes continuous with the oesophagus. Important lateral relations of the hypopharynx are the lobes of the thyroid gland and the carotid sheath. Anteriorly lie the epiglottis, the glottic aperture, and this is bounded on both sides by the aryepiglottic folds. At the same level, lateral to the aryepiglottic folds, lies the piriform recess which is bounded laterally by the thyroid cartilages and thyrohyoid membrane. Upward boundary of the piriform recess is the pharyngo-epiglottic fold.

Incidence

The majority of carcinomas arise in relation to the piriform recess (60%), or are located in the post-cricoid region (40%).

The special feature of post-cricoid tumours is that they occur chiefly in women and at an earlier age period than other tumours of the hypopharynx and oesophagus. The sex ratio gives an 80% female incidence and the common age is between 35 and 55 years. Tumours of the anterior and lateral hypopharynx show a male preponderance and occur in the sixth and seventh decades.

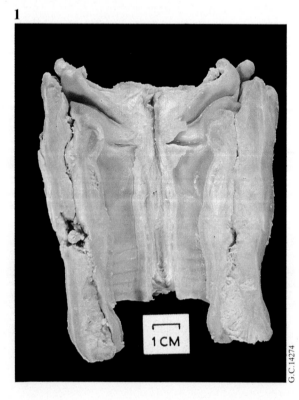

1

1 CM

G.C.14274

1 Female aged 51 years. Dysphagia for two months followed by midline fistula due to post-cricoid squamous carcinoma. Symptoms relieved by radiotherapy but recurred more severely three months later. Barium meal – full length of oesophagus involved by tumour. Radical removal was carried out.

The operation specimen has been split posteriorly in the midline showing the total involvement of oeso-phagus and post-cricoid region by tumour. The tumour infiltrates deeply and at the lower end grows into the lumen in a polypoid fashion. On microscopic examination the tumour proved to be a keratinising squamous carcinoma throughout its length. At the lower end it was papillary and highly vascular. The prevertebral fascia was involved but no tumour was found in the paratracheal lymph nodes.

Pathology

The majority of tumours of the hypopharynx are epidermoid carcinomas and may be either typical squamoid lesions showing cell nest formation or especially in those which arise in the piriform recess the lympho-epitheliomatous variant is frequently found. Since commonly these tumours are extensive when first seen it may be difficult to define the precise point of origin. These tumours are ulcerative in character and invade and destroy surrounding structures.

Tumours arising anteriorly involve the glottis. Those which extend medially involve the aryepiglottic space and lead to fixation of the glottis. Lateral extension of these tumours leads to destruction of the thyroid cartilage and may be palpated in the neck simulating secondary carcinoma. Upward extension leads to invasion of the base of the tongue. Lymphatic spread to the upper cervical nodes occurs and may be bilateral.

2

G.C.X.104

2 Female aged 50 years who suffered from dysphagia. The radiograph illustrates an extensive post-cricoid carcinoma with an associated large soft tissue swelling.

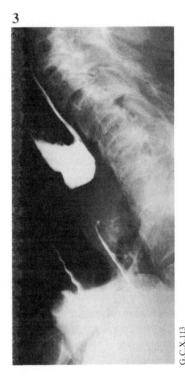

3

G.C.X.113

3 Male aged 78 years who suffered from dysphagia. The radiograph demonstrates pharyngeal stenosis with retention of barium indicative of a carcinoma.

In many of these patients a syndrome associated with the name Plummer-Vinson has been present for a considerable period of time. The syndrome is characterised by long standing and progressive although sometimes intermittent dysphagia, which is attributable to a generalised mucosal atrophy with loss of sensibility. There is consequent disturbance of the deglutition reflex with spasm of the cricopharyngeus. An iron deficiency anaemia (hypochromatic) is present. There is usually achlorhydria. In long standing cases the atrophic mucosa develops patches of leucoplakia and a later carcinoma may develop.

In approximately 50% of female patients suffering from post-cricoid carcinoma there is a preceding history of the Plummer-Vinson syndrome. The condition has been studied extensively in Sweden but occurs rarely in the United Kingdom.

Nasal sinuses

Anatomy

Paranasal sinuses

The paranasal sinuses are cavities within the cancellous bone of the facial skeleton. The maxillary antrum, frontal sinus and anterior ethmoidal cells communicate with the middle meatus of the nose and the posterior groups, the sphenoid and posterior ethmoidal cells, drain into the spheno-ethmoidal recess and the superior meatus respectively.

Maxillary sinus

The floor of the maxillary antrum is in close proximity to the roots of the secondary dentition; the posterior wall is adjacent to the infratemporal and pterygo-palatine fossae; the medial wall is the lateral wall of the nasal cavity; the roof is the floor of the orbit and the anterolateral walls are superficial. The orifice for drainage is situated high in the sinus and opens into the middle meatus of the nose.

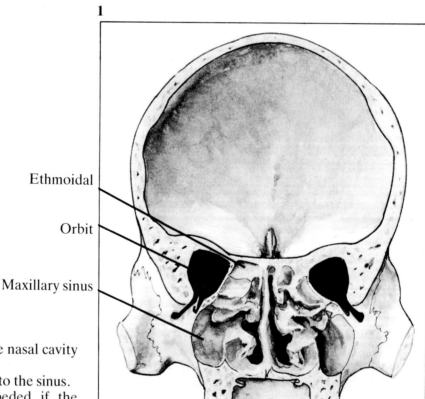

1

Ethmoidal

Orbit

Maxillary sinus

The nasal sinuses all communicate with the nasal cavity by relatively small channels. Accordingly:
(a) Infection from the nose can extend into the sinus.
(b) The drainage may be readily impeded if the mucosa of the communicating channel becomes congested or swollen.

Ethmoidal – frontal

The ethmoid sinuses constitute a cell labyrinth between the upper half of the nasal cavity medially and laterally are separated by the lamina papyracea from the orbit.

The frontal sinus should be regarded as part of the anterior ethmoidal system. The anterior wall is formed by the outer table of the frontal bone, the posterior inner table forms part of the floor of the anterior cranial fossa and the orbital roof forms the floor of the sinus. Medially lies a bony septum which separates the two frontal sinuses. The opening is anteroinferiorly and leads to the middle meatus through the fronto-nasal duct.

Sphenoidal

The sphenoidal sinus occupies the body of the sphenoid bone. The lateral wall is closely applied to the internal carotid artery and the cavernous sinus, the roof to the frontal lobe, the pituitary gland and the floor of the pterygoid canal. A medial septum separates it into two and the drainage ostium is situated high in the sinus.

2

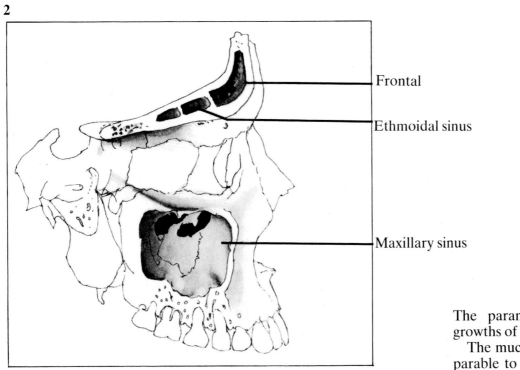

Frontal

Ethmoidal sinus

Maxillary sinus

The paranasal sinuses arise as outgrowths of the buccal mucosa (oral pit).

The mucosa lining the sinuses is comparable to the epithelium of the buccal cavity with some modification. There are many mucus-secreting cells.

Nasal sinuses (*Continued*)

Tumours

Osteoma

The osteoma commonly occurs in the frontal sinus and is often discovered on routine radiography. Such tumours are of a dense ivory nature or of less compact cancellous bone. They are slow growing and symptoms only supervene when some structure is involved, e.g. the fronto-nasal duct with superimposed infection.

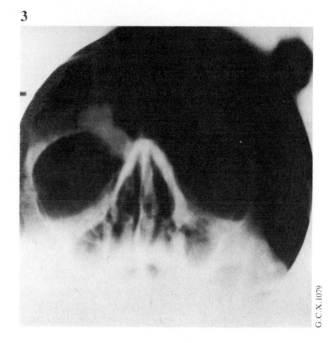

3

3   Osteoma – frontal sinus

Carcinoma

Carcinoma of the maxillary sinus is a well recognised lesion. The tumour is bulky and occupies the sinus cavity eventually occluding the nasal drainage and superadded infection is therefore common. As the tumour expands it leads to medial bulge into the nasal cavity, downward displacement of the palate and disruption of the dentition, lateral bulging of the cheek, and by upward displacement distortion of the eye and compression of the infraorbital nerve which lies in the floor of the orbit.

The condition may simulate either a chronic sinusitis or rarely, a gumma.

Histologically these tumours present considerable variation. They may present an essentially epidermal structure or as an adenocarcinoma arising from mucous cells; and occasionally a mixed pattern which some have regarded as suggestive of salivary gland tumours. Similar lesions occur in the ethmoid sinus and in the frontal sinus.

Aetiology

A strong correlation exists between adenocarcinoma of the sinuses and woodworkers. The carcinogen appears to be a particular type of wood dust. The high incidence of antro-ethmoidal cancer in South African Bantu peoples may be attributed to home-made carcinogenic snuff. A correlation has also been shown between workers in the chrome and nickel industries.

The presenting features include pain, nasal obstruction, purulent or bloody nasal secretion, dental or oral cavity symptoms, swelling of the cheek or ocular symptoms. Radiology and intranasal biopsy confirm the diagnosis. Sixty per cent of sinus cancers show evidence of bony destruction and the tumour limits should be defined with polytomography.

4

4a

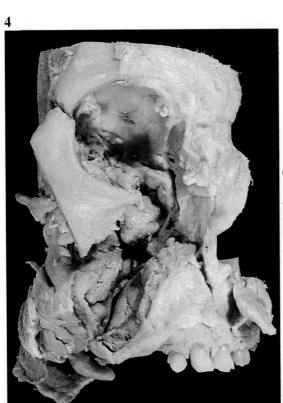

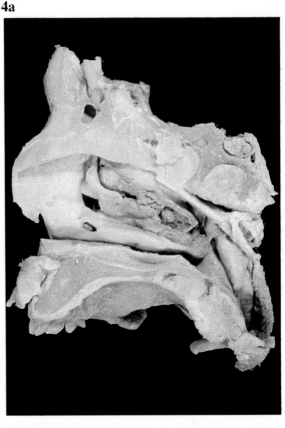

Carcinoma of the maxillary sinus.

The specimen is from an elderly man who died three months after experiencing the first symptoms of illness. The destruction caused by his aggressive tumour was latterly complicated by infection.

G.C.969

4 The brown vascular tumour had eroded into the orbital cavity, destroyed the facial plate of the maxillary sinus, and penetrated through the maxilla to enter the mouth in the molar region.

4a On the medial aspect of the maxillary sinus the tumour has invaded the nasal cavity. The frontal and sphenoidal air sinuses are distended with mucus.

5

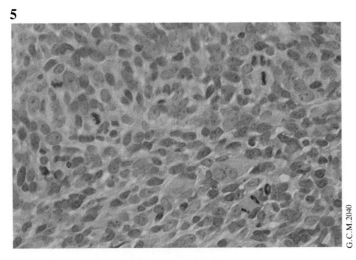

5 Paranasal sinus carcinoma. A poorly differentiated tumour composed of fusiform cells showing much mitotic activity. (*H&E × 400*)

G.C.M.2040

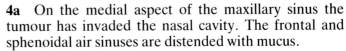

Spread

Nodal spread is to the retropharyngeal, upper deep cervical and mandibular nodes.

Most carcinomas of the paranasal sinuses are squamous carcinomas. Transitional cell and anaplastic carcinomas also occur and occasionally adenocarcinomas.

Nasal sinuses (*Continued*)

Acute sinusitis

Acute sinusitis may follow viral respiratory infections. The commonest affected sinus is the maxillary antrum. The ostium of this sinus is disadvantageously placed for gravity drainage as it enters the middle meatus. Infection of the antrum may involve the frontal and anterior ethmoidal sinuses owing to the confluence of their drainage ducts in the middle meatus (pan-sinusitis). Obstruction to the natural drainage of the sinus by local oedema or congestion is the commonest cause of sinusitis. Other predisposing conditions include pharyngeal infection, dental infections, sinus trauma, baro-trauma, swimming in infected water and anatomical abnormalities, e.g. a deviated nasal septum.

The initial infection is usually viral and the commonest viruses responsible are rhinovirus, para-influenza, echo, coxsackie and respiratory syncytial virus; secondary bacterial invaders include pneumococci, streptococci, staphylococci and haemophilus influenzae. Less common pathogens include anaerobes and fungi. Fungal infections, e.g. aspergillosis, usually occur after multiple antibiotic therapy or in immunosuppressed patients.

6

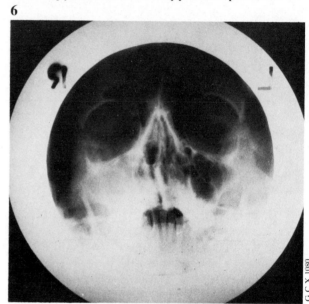

6 X-ray of acute right maxillary sinusitis.

Chronic sinusitis

Chronic sinusitis may follow an incompletely resolved acute sinusitis, or may appear insidiously following a 'cold' or dental infection. The responsible organisms are similar to those in acute sinusitis. The histological changes seen in the mucosa are classified into two types:
(a) Hypertrophic or polypoid sinusitis in which the inflammatory changes mainly affect the veins. The lymphatics and soft tissues are secondarily affected.
(b) Atrophic sinusitis where the increase in tissue is much less and is due to submucosal fibrosis instead of stromal oedema.

7

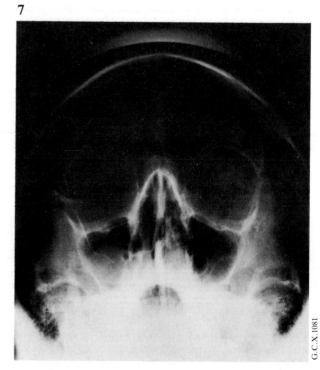

7 Chronic sinusitis. Polyp in right maxillary antrum.

Complications

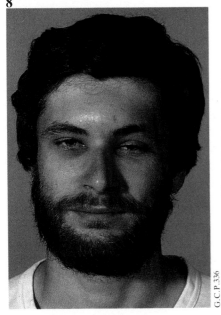

Complications of sinusitis have diminished since the advent of antibiotics. Orbital cellulitis and subperiosteal abscess which may result from ethmoidal or frontal infection produce eyelid oedema, conjunctival chemosis and displacement of the eyeball with impairment of its mobility. Posterior ethmoidal infection may produce retrobulbar neuritis, optic atrophy and ocular muscle paralysis.

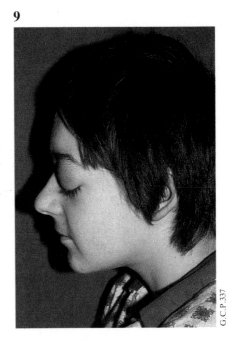

8   Left acute ethmoiditis

9   Left orbital cellulitis

Osteomyelitis from infected sinuses is more common in young people. The ethmoid sinuses in infancy are relatively larger than the ethmoid sinuses in later life and are more prone to be a source of infection. Pus under pressure may produce a septic bone, or an osteitis of the non-diploetic bones. A swinging temperature and undue tenderness of the affected area are enough to make the diagnosis, as radiological changes may not mirror the true course of the disease.

Intracranial complications include meningitis and brain abscess as a direct extension of the disease. Haematogenous spread may lead to thrombophlebitis and cavernous sinus thrombosis which is characterised by gross facial swelling, ocular palsies and high fever.

10

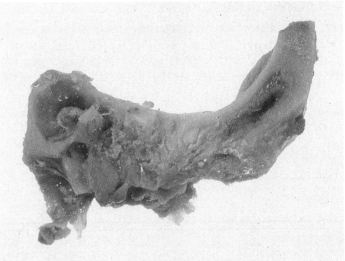

10   From an adult who died of septic leptomeningitis. The specimen is that of the anterior fossa of the skull showing septic inflammation of the right frontal air-sinus.
    Pus is present in the right frontal and anterior ethmoidal sinuses. There is thickening of the mucosa of the sphenoidal sinus.

Acute sinusitis frequently presents with characteristically located pain attributable to the rise of tension within the sinus. The pain is relieved by drainage.
    Chronic sinusitis is less frequently associated with characteristic localised manifestations and the diagnosis may depend on radiological examination and biopsy of the mucosa.

Nasal sinuses (*Continued*)

Mucocoele

This is commonly a cystic swelling of the frontal sinus. It occupies the whole of one sinus and by progressive enlargement erodes into the ethmoidal sinuses and into the orbit; or it may expose dura in the anterior cranial fossa. It is lined by cubical epithelium and contains thick tenacious white mucus. Occasionally the contents are straw coloured and serous, but are always sterile. The pathogenesis is thought to be a mucous retention cyst or blockage of the fronto-nasal duct from infection, allergy or trauma which leads to accumulation of secretions. Headache may or may not be a prominent feature, but more often a painless swelling appears above the medial canthus and slowly enlarges. Eventually the orbital contents may be displaced to produce diplopia. Radiology shows thinning of the bony walls of the frontal sinus, loss of scalloping of the walls and a depressed superomedial wall of the orbit. If untreated the condition progresses to optic atrophy or intracranial extension. Mucocoele of the maxillary sinus is rare.

Nasal polyps

Nasal polyps are pedunculated pieces of oedematous upper respiratory tract mucosa. They arise from any part of the nasal or sinus mucosa and are often bilateral. Most arise from the ethmoidal labyrinths and are multiple, but the antrochoanal polyp of adolescence originates from the maxillary sinus and is single.

The differential diagnosis of a simple nasal polyp is legion and includes neoplasms and meningocoeles. The clinical features are obstruction and hyposmia, and sinusitis may be superimposed. With continued growth of the polyps eventually the nose may broaden and in the young the nasal bone sutures separate.

Polyps are the result of vascular derangements of the mucosa induced by vasomotor instability. Evidence of the allergic component in the pathogenesis is provided by the eosinophilic infiltrate and the high levels of immunoglobulins in polyps. The allergic reaction is a type I immediate hypersensitivity reaction involving immunoglobulin E. The common allergens include pollens, animal dander, house dust, mites and moulds. An area of simple oedema becomes filled with blood and the oedematous mucosa becomes polypoid and hangs into the nose. Initially the surface of a simple polyp is covered with ciliated columnar epithelium, but exposure to air currents may produce transitional or later squamous metaplasia. The association between nasal polyposis and cystic fibrosis is well established.

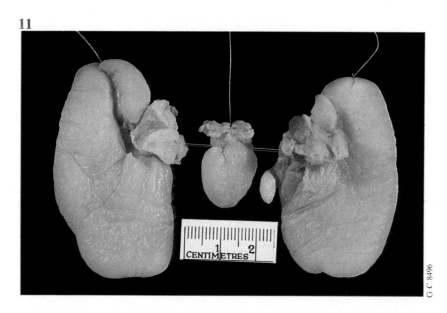

11 Polypi from the nose. From a male aged 50 years who complained of nasal obstruction. The affection was bilateral. The polypi probably involved the maxillary air sinuses as well as being naso-choanal. The polypi are three in number and are flattened and ovoid. The largest measures 60mm in length, 30mm in breadth and 10mm in maximum thickness. Each arises by a comparatively narrow and fleshy-looking pedicle and expands into a gelatinous looking semi-translucent mass.

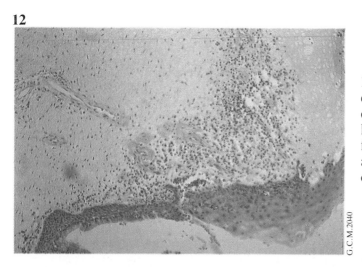

12 Nasal polyp. The portion of the polyp illustrated is covered by squamous epithelium (right) and partly by columnar cell respiratory epithelium (left). The underlying tissue is oedematous particularly to the left of the field, and there is a heavy infiltration by lymphocytes and plasma cells. The small vessels show hyalinisation of their walls.

Nasal cavity

Tumours

Benign tumours of the nasal cavity are many and diverse. They may be mesoblastic or epithelial in origin and they exhibit features common to comparable tumours seen elsewhere.

Malignant tumours are likewise numerous. Note is made of the most common variety of neoplasms encountered.

Benign	Malignant
Nasal polyp	Squamous carcinoma
Squamous papilloma	Adenocarcinoma
Haemangioma	Adenoid cystic
Angiofibroma	Melanoma
Olfactory neuroblastoma	Lymphoma

Papilloma

13

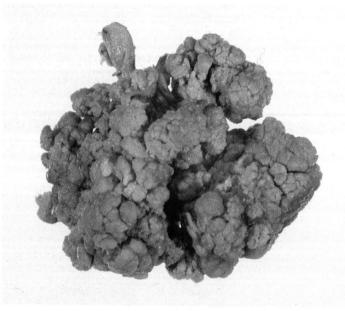

G.C.8888

13 From a male aged 52 years. History of nasal obstruction and epistaxis over 3 years. The naked eye appearance of the specimen which appears to grow from the thickened mucosa, is evident. The tumour forms a many-branched warty excrescence from thick hypertrophied mucosa. Microscopic examination showed it to be a simple papilloma with delicate connective tissue cores containing many thin-walled blood vessels and covered with epithelium which is stratified and squamous where it has been exposed to pressure. In other areas which have been free from pressure the epithelium has retained its columnar type and has remained ciliated.

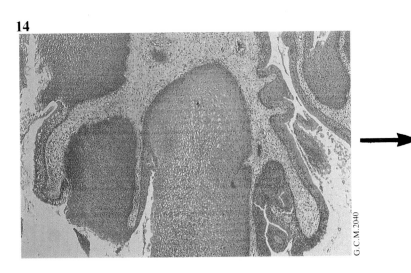

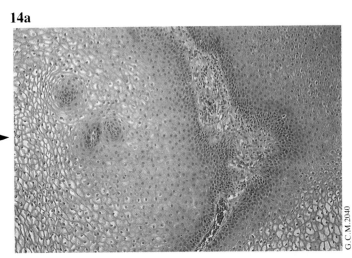

14 Nose – squamous papilloma. From the columnar cell respiratory epithelium, keratinised squamous epithelium dips down into the underlying stroma – inverted papilloma to form eventually a complex papillomatous tumour. (*H&E × 40*)

14a Same case. A higher power view of the complex mass produced by the ingrowing papilloma. (*H&E × 100*)

Juvenile angiofibroma

Juvenile angiofibroma is a rare condition mainly of adolescent males which is a mixture of vascular and fibrotic elements. It may present with epistaxis or obstructive symptoms and if untreated may erode the skull bone. The neoplastic nature of this lesion has been questioned.

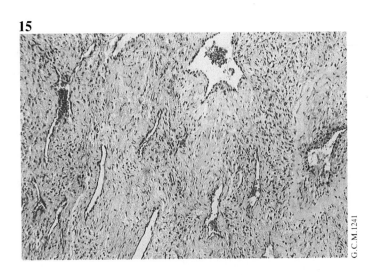

15 Nasopharynx – angiofibroma. Blood vessels usually lined by a single layer of hyperplastic endothelial cells are widely separated by the fibromatous component of the tumour. (*H&E × 100*)

Nasal cavity (*Continued*)

Of special significance in diagnosis are 'tumours' arising high in the nasal cavity and in the roof of the upper nasopharynx. As the result of failure of closure of the sutures at the base of the skull an area of weakness in the midline can exist. In consequence certain lesions of congenital origin arise or as the result of the line of weakness, CNS elements can protrude. From before backwards these are:

Dermoid cyst; Meningocoele; Glioma.

and more posteriorly in the roof of the nasopharynx tumours arising from remnants of Rathke's pouch — adamantinoma (see p. 78), and at a still lower level — chordoma.

16

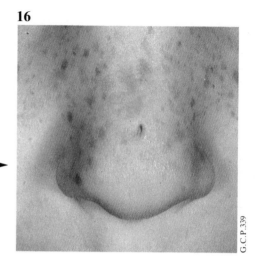

Dermoid cyst

16 Dermoid cyst is a superficial external midline cyst on the dorsum of the nose which contains hair and amorphous material. The hair distinguishes it from an external glioma but extension of the cyst under the nasal bones to the base of the skull may make removal difficult.

Meningocoele

17

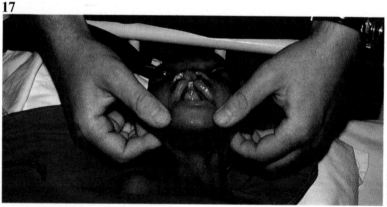

17 Infant with cleft palate and palpable meningocoele in roof of mouth.

19

18

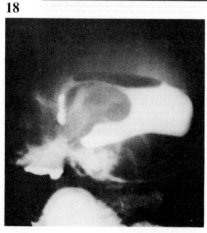

18 and **19** Radiological confirmation of the meningocoele by contrast.

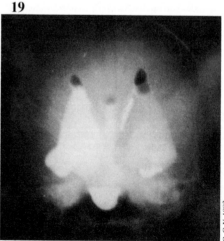

Encephalocoele

Encephalocoele is a herniation of dura mater which enters the nose through the foramen caecum or through a dehiscence in the cribriform plate. It contains CSF (meningocoele) and occasionally brain tissue (encephalocoele). The swelling may project downwards or forwards producing a deformity comparable to the elephant man described by Treves.

20

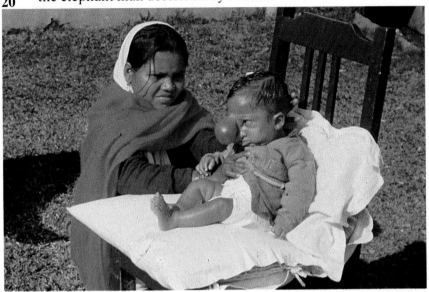

20 This child was born in Assam and it was over two years before he was first examined. The swelling obviously contained both brain tissue and CSF. There was an evident cranial defect.

This child had been exhibited publicly as representing the Hindu elephant god Ganish. Fits of unconsciousness suggesting divine trances could be induced by compressing the swelling.

By courtesy of Dr G.B. Young.

Glioma

A glioma is a solid tumour which may present externally either at the root of the nose, which becomes broadened, or intranasally from the roof or the lateral wall. It arises from a failure of the dura to become sealed off in the foramen caecum during foetal development. The glioma is composed of neuroglial tissue and astrocytes and is a true tumour.

Both the meningocoele and the 'glioma' must be treated by an approach from above to avoid the risk of infection.

Adamantinoma

More posteriorly behind the level of the buccopharyngeal membrane remnants of Rathke's pouch may persist and from these simple cysts or a tumour exhibiting the features commonly regarded as similar to those of an adamantinoma may arise.

Adamantinomas (ameloblastomas) are considered on p. 78.

Chordoma

Still more posteriorly and lying in front of the body of the sphenoid a chordoma may arise.

This is a slow growing tumour which arises from the remnants of the notochord. Peak incidence is between 20–40 years of age. They present with nasal obstruction and are locally aggressive with destruction of the basisphenoid.

Nasal cavity (*Continued*)

Infections

Lupus vulgaris

21 Lupus vulgaris probably results in most cases from haematogenous infection of the skin by tubercle bacilli. It may develop on any part of the body but the face alone is affected in the majority of cases.

Occurring mainly in children and young adults it is seen both in the skin and related mucosae. It is particularly prone to develop in the nares. The characteristic lesion is a small scaly nodule. When it is compressed under glass it has a yellow-brown translucent appearance (apple-jelly nodule). As the nodules increase in number they tend to coalesce, spreading peripherally and scarring centrally. Untreated lesions may become infected with other micro-organisms, break down, and ulcerate. Eventually extensive ulceration involving cartilage and bone may result in destruction of the nose, eyelid, external ear, or other part of the face.

Microscopically the typical early lesion consists of an aggregate of non-caseating tubercles in the corium. Later the histological picture is complicated by ulceration, secondary infection, and scarring.

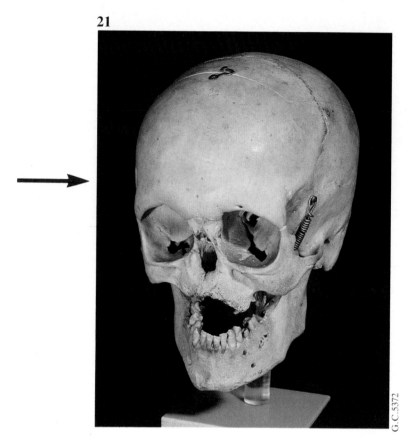

Lupus carcinoma

This is a late but well recognised complication of lupus vulgaris arising frequently many years after the lupus has been recognised. Either in the area of ulcerative disease or in the scar tissue a hyperplastic lesion develops, often multicentric, which may be difficult to diagnose as malignant change and histological study may be required. The tumour is a squamous carcinoma of irregular appearance with relatively rapid growth causing increasing local destruction of tissue. Lymph node metastases occur. In such cases the prognosis is always grave.

Granulomas

Nasal granulomas are uncommon in the Western World but must always be remembered in a differential diagnosis of unusual nasal masses.

Wegener's granulomatosis is an unusual potentially fatal disease. It is characterised by a focal necrotising vasculitis which may represent an unusual auto-immune response. Commonly the disease is of slow onset but on occasion may be fulminant and overwhelming due to bronchitis, pneumonia and glomerulonephritis. Clinically the condition may present as a painful nasal ulcer with a high ESR. Biopsy is necessary for the diagnosis.

The midline (lethal) granuloma disease is rare and characterised by ulceration and induration of the nose or nasopharynx. Biopsy shows dense polymorphic infiltration of the tissues by atypical lymphoid and reticulum cells with granulation tissue and neutrophils in the areas of active ulceration. In contrast to Wegener's there is no giant cell reaction, vasculitis or renal manifestations.

Atrophic rhinitis was the scourge of nasal surgery in the early twentieth century but has now diminished in civilised societies. The characteristic features include chronic inflammation, atrophy and fibrosis. The result is wide nasal passages with a crusting atrophic respiratory membrane. There is total anosmia but a foetid odour and foul mucus emanate from the nose. The aetiology of this condition was thought to be too radical intranasal surgery, but recently immunosuppression is considered the more likely cause.

Tropical lesions

Leprosy presents in the nose as red granular ulcerations of the mucous membrane of the cartilaginous septum. These ulcers enlarge, perforate the septum and totally destroy it. The end result is atrophic rhinitis.

Rhinoscleroma is endemic to Asia, Africa, Central and South America and Eastern Europe. The bacterial agent is Klebsiella rhinoscleromatis; poverty and poor hygiene may be additional factors.
  Several stages of the disease are recognised. Initially the mucous membrane undergoes atrophy, but there is no loss of smell. Following this the granulomatous reaction occurs and progresses to tuberculoid plaques and the formation of large masses within the nose. The end stage is submucosal fibrosis, consequent cicatrisation and stenosis and anosmia.

Fungal infections

Mucormycosis is a fulminant opportunistic infection caused by Rhizopus oryzae. It usually occurs in debilitated patients and if unchecked is rapidly fatal. Presenting symptoms include headache, nasal blockage and serous sanguineous discharge. Radiology confirms bony destruction and death occurs with intracranial involvement.

Aspergillosis has a characteristic greenish-brown discharge. This infection is encouraged by debilitation and death follows intracranial spread.

Rhinosporidiosis occurs mainly in India, Sri Lanka and parts of Africa. It is usually found in the young adult male and clinically presents with nasal obstruction or epistaxis due to an irregular pinkish nasal polyp which bleeds on touch.

J.A.M. Murray

The nasopharynx develops from the cephalic end of the primitive alimentary canal and accordingly the mucosa develops from endoderm and not from the epiblast (ectoderm). The line of demarcation in the embryo has already been noted (the buccopharyngeal membrane). This disappears after the third week of foetal life. In the adult the line of the buccopharyngeal membrane can be represented by an imaginary plane which passes from the basisphenoid immediately posterior to Rathke's pouch along the anterior pillar of the fauces to the V-shaped sulcus terminalis on the dorsum of the tongue which separates the anterior two thirds and posterior third of the tongue i.e. posterior to the foramen caecum.

The areas of mucosa derived from these two separate sources are illustrated in the accompanying diagrams.

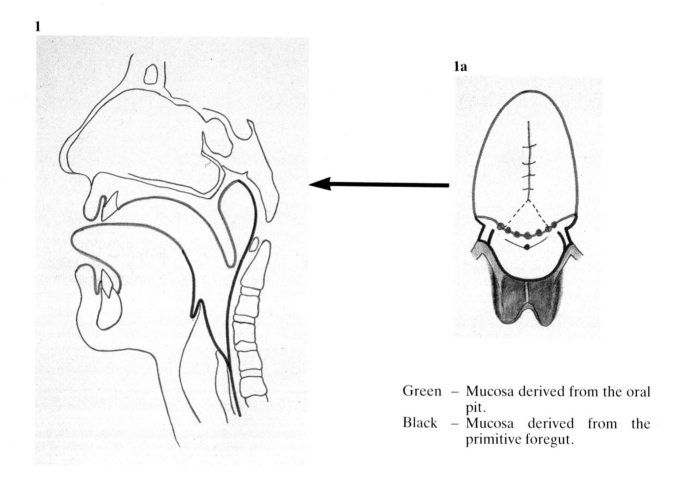

Green – Mucosa derived from the oral pit.

Black – Mucosa derived from the primitive foregut.

The mucosa arising from the ectoderm is *squamous* with intercellular channels and ultimately producing a superficial layer of keratin. The mucosa arising from the endoderm of the primitive canal has a *squamoid* formation but separation of the cells by channels is less marked. Keratinisation may occur but is not a uniform feature and there is frequently a close relationship of the basal cells of the epithelium with lymphoid tissue. These features have already been described (see p. 92).

Nasopharyngeal carcinoma

Geographical incidence

Nasopharyngeal carcinoma, a rare neoplasm in most countries, is one of the common cancers in China and in South-East Asia and has attracted intensive and important research studies.

The highest incidence rates (20–30 per 100 000 per year in males) occur in the southern provinces of China, Hong Kong and in emigrant Chinese communities in South-East Asia, USA and elsewhere.

Elevated rates (approximately 5–15) are found in Eskimos and in several racial groups in South-East Asia – Indonesians, Malays, Dyaks, Kadazans, Filipinos and Vietnamese. The incidence levels in Malta and in parts of northern Africa (Tunisia, Algeria and Sudan), although lower than in the countries mentioned previously, are appreciably higher than in Europe and America. The rates are low (less than 1) in virtually all other parts of the world.

2

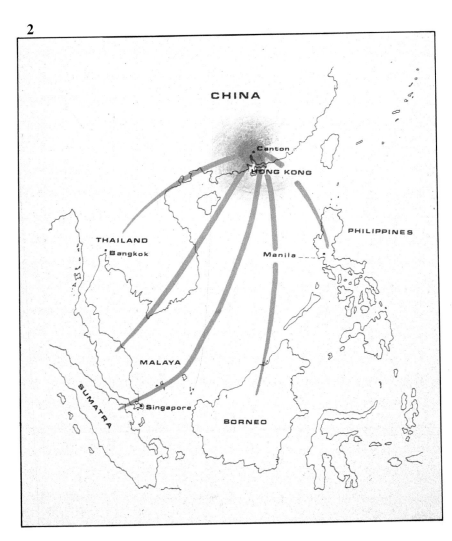

Migrant status

In the United States nasopharyngeal carcinoma risks among US-born Chinese, while considerably higher (approximately 20 times) than in Caucasians, are significantly lower (approximately half) than among foreign-born Chinese.

In Singapore there are no significant differences in risk between China-born and Singapore-born Chinese.

2   Map illustrating the southern migration from mainland China.

Nasopharyngeal carcinoma (*Continued*)

Incidence

Even when this tumour is studied in relatively localised regions the peculiar variation of incidence is observed. Thus amongst the Chinese community in Hong Kong the highest incidence is found among the Tanka or boat people. In Singapore the incidence among Cantonese from Guangdong province (30.4 in males and 10.9 in females) is approximately double that among Hokkiens from Fukien province, Teochews from the Swatow district of Guangdong province, Hiananese and Hakkas; similar differences have been observed among Chinese in West Malaysia.

Age and sex incidence

The sex ratios of nasopharyngeal carcinoma in most countries are closely similar, the risk in males being some 2−3 times higher than in females.

The age incidence of nasopharyngeal carcinoma in high risk Chinese populations is different. The incidence begins to rise at an earlier age, reaches a plateau around the 4th to 6th decades and does not exhibit any continued rise in the older age groups.

In Chinese, nasopharyngeal carcinoma is rare below the age of 15 years and only a small proportion of cases occurs in the 15−19 age group. On the other hand, the proportion of cases in the first two decades is appreciably higher in Tunisia (15% under the age of 16 years), Uganda, Sudan, India and among the Kadazans in East Malaysia and in US Blacks; the occurrence of a bimodal distribution, with an additional peak in the second decade, in some of these populations with intermediate or low risks for nasopharyngeal carcinoma suggests the influence of different aetiological factors.

Racial incidence

Racial differences in incidence are found even in the same geographical area. Thus the relative incidence in Singapore is:

	Males	Females
Chinese	19.2	7.3
Malays	5.1	1.1
Indians	0.9	0.0

In Hawaii the rates are high in Chinese, intermediate in Filipinos and Hawaiians and low in Caucasians.

Time trends

There has been no demonstrable change in incidence among Chinese in China or South-East Asia since their high risks for the disease were recorded some 50 years ago. It may therefore be inferred that the environmental risk factors are probably of a traditional type. The reported decline of nasopharyngeal carcinoma mortality among Chinese in the United States during 1950−1969 would allow the same inference. The risks for nasopharyngeal carcinoma in most countries have been fairly stable over a long period.

Occupation and socio-economic status

No specific occupation has been shown to be associated with high risks for nasopharyngeal carcinoma. Associations with lower socio-economic groups may be attributable to more traditional life styles.

The Epstein-Barr virus

There is growing evidence that the Epstein-Barr virus (EBV) is aetiologically implicated in nasopharyngeal carcinoma. Patients with nasopharyngeal carcinoma have consistently shown high antibody titres to various EBV-related antigens and EBV-DNA has been identified in the tumour cells. This virus has the capacity to induce lymphoproliferation and transformation *in-vitro* and to induce lymphoid malignancies in experimental animals.

It is reasonable to expect that carcinomas of the nasopharynx, like those of the rest of the respiratory tract, may be induced by inhaled carcinogens. Carcinogens may also reach the nasopharynx by routes other than inhalation; upper respiratory tract cancers have been produced experimentally by the administration of nitrosamine compounds by the oral, subcutaneous and intravenous routes. It has been proposed that salted fish, a traditional food item in several high risk areas, may be an important risk factor; nitrosamines and mutagens have been identified in preparation of salted fish. Several botanical products, some of which are components of traditional medicines, have been shown to have EBV activating properties. The possibility that such agents may act as co-factors in nasopharyngeal carcinoma is under investigation. Case-control studies on several other inhaled and ingested substances have so far yielded negative results.

Genetic factors

A genetic predisposition has been suspected on the basis of racial patterns of incidence and reports of familial clustering. Significant differences have been observed between the HLA antigen profiles of nasopharyngeal cancer patients and controls in some populations. Increased frequencies of the HLA-B locus alleles BW46 and BW17 and the HLA haplotypes A_2-BW46 and AW19-BW17 have been found in Chinese patients with nasopharyngeal carcinoma. These findings raise the possibility that the development of the neoplasm may be related to genetically determined differences in immunological responses to EBV or some other environmental agent.

Nasopharyngeal carcinoma (*Continued*)

Pathology

Since the initial lesion is small, failure to seek treatment results in the patient first presenting at hospital with a large, bulky, infiltrating tumour either in the nasopharynx or often because of enlarged metastatic deposits in the cervical lymph nodes.

3

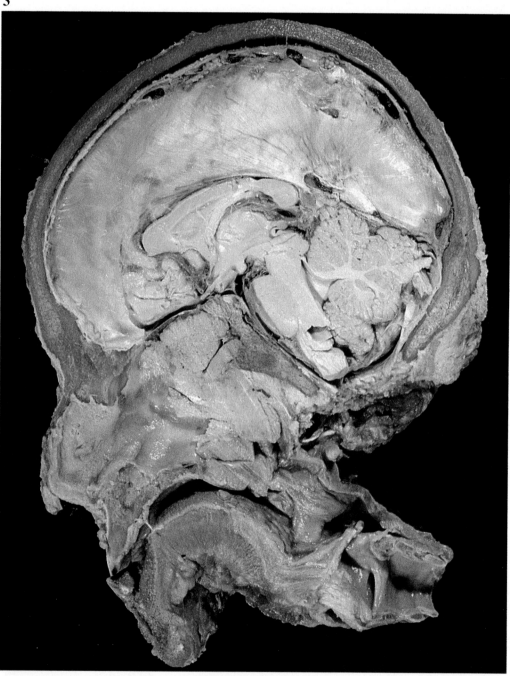

G.C. 10262

3 From an adult Chinese male who was admitted to hospital with intense headache, nasal obstruction and internal strabismus. The patient died shortly after admission to hospital.

On section the nasopharynx is seen to be occupied by a large irregular tumour which extends forward into the nasal cavity and presses below on the soft palate. Superiorly the tumour has destroyed the walls of the sphenoidal air sinus, and extended through the base of the skull into the sella turcica. The pituitary has been displaced backwards and compressed, but microsections reveal no definite evidence of invasion of the pituitary. The histological examination demonstrated the nature of the tumour as shown on the opposite page.

The tumour may be polypoid, ulcerative or present as a fissure. Infiltration may be the main feature. The majority of tumours arise in the lateral walls of the nasopharynx especially from the pharyngeal recesses (fossae of Rosenmuller) and Eustachian cushions. The tumour may also arise in the supero-posterior walls but only rarely in the anterior and inferior walls. It is markedly invasive and spreads directly and by lymphatic and vascular channels.

Local tumour infiltration may involve the Eustachian tubes, lateral parapharyngeal spaces, oropharynx, nasal fossae, paranasal sinuses, orbital cavities, parotid gland and base of skull. The neoplasm may extend into the cranial cavity or intracranial venous sinuses by invading bone, or more frequently, by traversing the cranial foramina; these intracranial extensions are usually extradural. The neoplasm may involve the cranio-occipital articulation reaching the extrathecal space through the occipito-atlantoid ligament. The atlas may be destroyed. Rarely metastatic involvement of the lower lumbar spine has been noted in patients with intracranial metastasis. This may represent transthecal dissemination. The cranial nerves may be involved at the base of the skull and the lateral parapharyngeal spaces. Lymphatic spread is exceedingly common; lymph nodes most frequently involved are the retropharyngeal and the upper and posteriorly placed deep cervical nodes. Blood-borne metastases may occur in any organ but are most frequently found in the bones, liver and lungs.

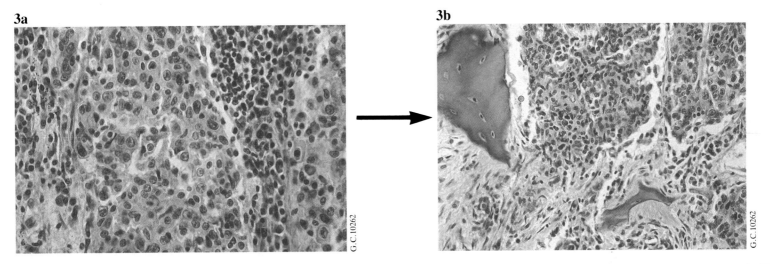

3a Nasopharynx − carcinoma. Trabeculae of poorly differentiated carcinoma cells occupy the right and mid portion of this field. The septa between the tumour trabeculae are heavily infiltrated by lymphocytic cells (*H&E × 400*)

3b Same case. Poorly differentiated carcinoma infiltrating the basisphenoid bone. (*H&E × 250*)

Nasopharyngeal carcinoma (*Continued*)

Symptomatology

The main symptoms in order of frequency are:

(a)   Cervical lymphadenopathy. This is the presenting symptom in more than 50% of cases and is particularly true in cases of the small infiltrating fissure type of tumour in the pharyngeal recess; it is present in almost all cases in the late stages of the disease. The lymph nodes most frequently affected are those lying behind the angle of the jaw.

(b)   Nasorespiratory symptoms such as bleeding and nasal obstruction.

(c)   Neurological symptoms such as headache which may be intense and aggravated by movement. Cranial nerve palsies are found in approximately 30–40% of all cases; the nerves most commonly involved are VI and V; next in frequency are III, IV, IX, X, XI, XII and the cervical sympathetic nerve.

(d)   Auditory symptoms such as earache, tinnitus, conduction deafness and otitis media; these are due to involvement of the Eustachian tubes.

(e)   Symptoms referable to other forms of local invasion. These include exophthalmos and enlargements of the parotid gland and soft tissues of the head and neck.

(f)   Symptoms referable to distant metastases such as bone pains, hepatomegaly, cough and haemoptysis.

These tumours are radiosensitive and the 5-year survival rate is approximately 25–30% for all cases of nasopharyngeal carcinoma and 60–70% in cases where the tumour is confined to the nasopharynx.

4

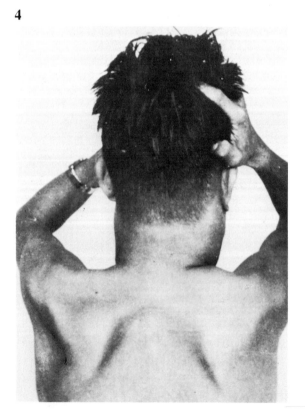

4a

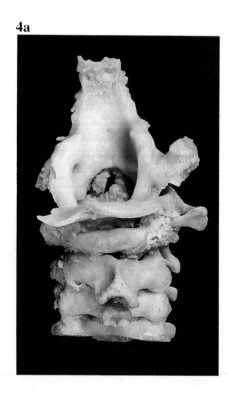

4 and **4a**   From a Chinese male aged 23 years. This patient illustrates invasion of the atlas resulting in instability of the head which was firmly held to prevent movement and to ease intense head-ache. The patient also had an internal strabismus.   G.C.10473

Histology

The following histological types of nasopharyngeal carcinoma may be recognised:

(a) Squamous cell carcinoma. This type exhibits evidence of squamous differentiation (intercellular bridges and/or keratinisation) over most of its extent. It may be subdivided into well differentiated, moderately differentiated and poorly differentiated types.

b) Non-keratinising carcinoma. The tumour cells have well defined cell margins and show an arrangement that is stratified or pavemented and not syncytial. There may be a plexiform pattern.

(c) Undifferentiated carcinoma. The tumour cells are undifferentiated and generally have vesicular nuclei and prominent nucleoli. The cell margins are indistinct and the tumour has a syncytial appearance.

The term 'lymphoepithelial carcinoma' (lymphoepithelioma) is used to describe non-keratinising and undifferentiated nasopharyngeal carcinomas in which numerous non-neoplastic lymphocytes are found among the tumour cells. All the histological types of nasopharyngeal carcinoma described previously have consistently shown ultrastructural evidence of squamous differentiation.

In comparison with squamous cell carcinomas, undifferentiated carcinomas have been reported to have better 5-year survival rates, comprise a larger proportion of cases in young persons and in high risk groups, and are associated with higher serologic reactivities to the Epstein-Barr virus.

5

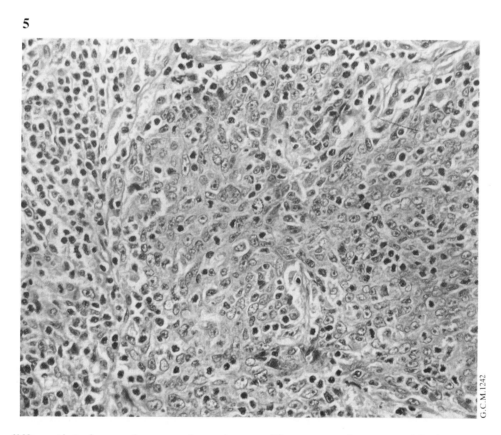

5 A poorly differentiated nasopharyngeal carcinoma. The tumour is composed of large cells often with poorly defined margins. The nuclei are vesicular and have prominent nucleoli. A focus of lymphocytes can also be seen (left). (*H&E*)

Professor K. Shanmugaratnum

The pharyngeal tonsil lies lateral to the posterior third of the tongue in the fossa between the pillars of the fauces. This fossa expands upwards to the palate and downwards into the pharynx. In structure the tonsil has a covering layer of squamous epithelium thrown into fissures and crypts. These extend into a subjacent closely related layer of lymphoid tissue and often harbour bacteria.

The tonsils and adenoids are masses of lymphoid tissue in a part of the lymphoid ring of Waldeyer. Until the age of 1 year they appear to have an immunological role. The adenoidal size is dependent on age as well as the presence of infection. There is spontaneous regression with the onset of puberty. Tonsil size also varies with age. Occasionally in very young children extremely large tonsils may embarrass respiration and make swallowing difficult.

Tumours

Neoplasms of the tonsil are frequently ulcerative and bulky. A variety of types occur including squamous epithelioma, lymphoepithelioma and malignant lymphoma. The differential diagnosis depends upon histological studies.

The most common malignant tumour of the tonsil is a squamous cell carcinoma. The presenting features are usually pain or dysphagia, but spread to nearby lymph nodes is extremely common. The tumour is fast growing. The condition is more common in North America than in the United Kingdom.

In the Far East the tumour is more closely allied to nasopharyngeal carcinoma already described.

Lymphoma of the non-Hodgkin's type is the other common malignancy of the tonsils. In both the diagnosis is made by inspection, but palpation of the tonsil is often necessary. The firmness of the tonsil may indicate malignancy despite a relatively normal appearance of the organ.

Infections

Tonsillitis

Acute
Acute infections of the tonsils initially are caused by viruses but secondary bacterial infections rapidly intervene. The common viruses are the EB virus, adenoviruses and rhinoviruses. The commonly encountered bacteria are the streptococci.

Chronic
Chronic tonsillitis, which gives a low grade contact sore throat and recurrent acute tonsillitis, is also commonly the result of streptococcal infection but recently with the increasing use of antibiotics, fungal infections of the tonsil are becoming more common.

Quinsy

This is a collection of pus in the peritonsillar space and like any other collection of pus in the body it requires to be drained.

Retropharyngeal infection

Lying anterior to the bodies of the vertebrae is a layer of fascia – the prevertebral fascia – which extends from the base of the skull downwards into the mediastinum. Enclosing the lateral and posterior aspects of the pharynx is another layer of fascia, the buccopharyngeal fascia, which is fused in the midline to the prevertebral fascia and divides the retropharyngeal space into two compartments. The lateral extensions of the retropharyngeal spaces are the site of special surgical lesions and have been designated by some as the parapharyngeal spaces. Within these latter spaces lie the deep lobe of the parotid, internal carotid artery, internal jugular vein, cranial nerves IX, X, XI and XII and lymph nodes. These nodes participate in the lymphatic drainage of the tonsil and the alveolar margins. About the carotid vessels and jugular vein fascial elements arising from both the buccopharyngeal and the prevertebral fasciae are condensed to form the carotid sheath. Retropharyngeal abscesses arise most commonly from lymph nodes (the node of Rouvière) and lie between the buccopharyngeal fascia and the prevertebral fascia (A). Because of the fusion of these two layers in the midline, such an abscess presents as a unilateral swelling postero-lateral to the pharynx. Abscesses arising from lesions of the vertebrae lie behind the prevertebral fascia and therefore can spread across the midline (B).

Chronic retropharyngeal abscesses are usually tuberculous and present as a bilateral swelling.

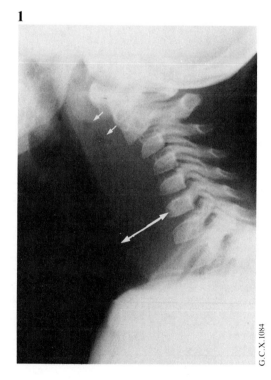

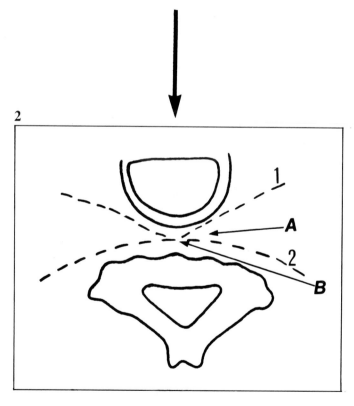

2 1 Retropharyngeal fascia
2 Prevertebral fascia.

1 The X-ray shows the prevertebral space to be widened and occupied by an abscess containing both pus and gas.

J.A.M. Murray

Phylogenetically the larynx is first and foremost a sphincter protecting the lower respiratory tract from inhalation of foreign material. Phonation is a secondary acquisition, but a change in this function may be the first sign of serious pathology. Hoarseness lasting more than 2 weeks demands further investigation. Other serious symptoms include prolonged sore throat, dysphagia and referred pain, e.g. otalgia.

Benign tumours

Benign tumours or swellings are not uncommon in the larynx and most of them are not truly neoplastic.

Neoplastic		Non-neoplastic	
Papillomas	11 %	Vocal cord polyps/nodules	75%
Adenoma	1%	Retention cysts	5%
Chondroma	0.2%	Tuberculous granuloma	3%
Miscellaneous	1%	Other granulomas	2.4%
	13.2%	Amyloid deposit	0.8%
		Miscellaneous	0.6%
			86.8%

Neoplastic benign tumours

Papilloma

Juvenile papillomas, which comprise up to one quarter of all papillomas, occur mainly on the true and false cords and the anterior commissure but often extend into the subglottic space, trachea, bronchi and epiglottis. These papillomas may be caused by a viral infection. They may commence in infancy but the peak incidence is between the ages of 5 and 15 years. They tend to recur but after puberty there may be a tendency to regress spontaneously. Histologically they resemble squamous papillomas elsewhere. Malignant transformation is exceptionally rare unless the larynx has been irradiated.

Solitary squamous papillomas usually grow from the edge of the vocal cord and in its outer two thirds but they may also arise from the ventricular band or subglottic region. They are twice as common in males and most frequent in the fourth and fifth decades. There is a definite tendency for up to 3–4% of these tumours to become malignant. Routine histological scrutiny may reveal gradations of cell atypia.

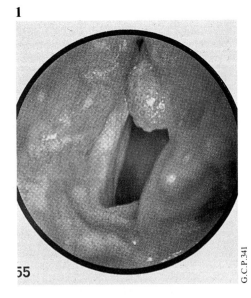

1 Solitary papilloma of larynx on right true and false cord.

Adenoma

These rare tumours are found throughout the respiratory tract mucosa, more commonly below the larynx. Within the larynx the commonest site is in the supraglottic region, frequently in the ventricle where mucous gland aggregates are most numerous. Growth is slow and symptoms are those of mechanical interference. They are sessile with a well-defined margin. Histologically they range from a typically solid variety resembling a benign 'mixed salivary' tumour to an extremely cystic tumour. Another type is the eosinophilic glandular cell cyst adenoma.

Chondroma

There is no clear cut histological distinction between chondromas and chondrosarcomas. Up to one fifth may be malignant and there is a male predominance, mainly in the fifth and sixth decades. Chondrosarcomas are locally aggressive and this behaviour confirms the diagnosis. Most of these tumours arise from the cricoid (70%) and the thyroid cartilege (20%) and the remainder from the arytenoid. Clinically they are smooth and encapsulated but may show mottled calcification on X-ray. Malignant tumours grow with local spread and metastases are rare irrespective of histological appearances. Enormous growth may lead to respiratory embarrassment and a tracheostomy may become urgently necessary.

Other tumours

Other even less common tumours include granular cell myoblastomas of the vocal cords. Schwannomas and neurofibromas of the aryepiglottic fold also occur although involvement of the larynx by multiple neurofibromatosis is uncommon.

Plasmacytoma

Plasmacytomas occur very rarely in the larynx and they are usually single and may be polypoidal or sessile. This site accounts for 25% of the extramedullary plasmacytoma. Lymph node metastases can occur and in a small proportion there may be disseminated disease.

Non-neoplastic benign swellings

Vocal cord polyps

Non-neoplastic polyps of the vocal cord may present as 'true' polyps, Reinke's oedema, or vocal nodules. Prolonged voice strain often precedes the polypoid lesion.

Polyps

2 Polyps are more common in males with a peak age incidence at 40—50 years. They arise from the sub-glottic aspect of the vocal cord close to the anterior commissure; 20% are bilateral.

They are sessile, translucent, with a gelatinous consistence.

Histologically they show traumatic oedema of the connective tissue with vascular engorgement. Small haemorrhages may occur and may lead to fibrosis, hyalinisation and formation of haemosiderin. In such a case the polyp changes in appearance and may be mistaken for a fibroma, angioma or myxoma.

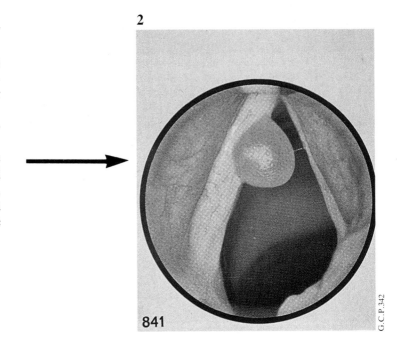

2

841

G.C.P.342

Reinke's oedema

3 Polypoid degeneration of the vocal cords (Reinke's oedema) is characterised by bilateral symmetrical poly-poidal swelling of the whole length of the membranous part of the vocal cords. The aetiology is unknown but may be related to voice abuse. The subepithelial plane on the vocal cords, which is limited by the superior and inferior arcuate lines on the superior and inferior surfaces of the cords and by the anterior commissure in front and the vocal processes posteriorly, fills with a fluid exudate. Clinically the diagnosis is obvious and histology is unremarkable.

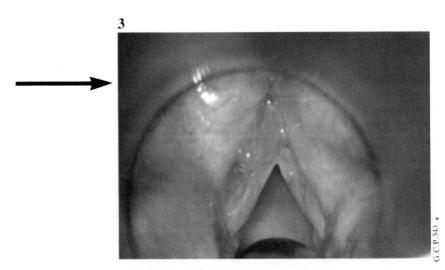

3

G.C.P.343

Vocal nodules

Vocal nodules have many synonyms which indicate those people most commonly affected. They occur at any age and begin during periods of excessive voice strain. Clinically nodules are bilaterally symmetric on the medial edge of the middle of the membranous part of the vocal cord. This part of the cord is most likely to be traumatised with loud vocalisation as this is where maximum excursion of the cord occurs. They rarely exceed 4mm in size and histologically there is marked hyperplasia of the squamous epithelium and hyperkeratosis. Subepithelially there is initially vascular engorgement and oedema which develops in time to fibrosis and hyalinisation.

4

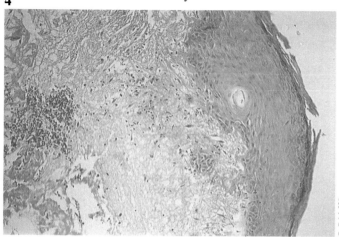

4 Vocal cord – singer's node. In this condition the appearances vary greatly from one case to another. Here, slightly thickened squamous epithelium covers a thick layer of relatively acellular fibrous tissue lightly infiltrated by inflammatory cells. Deep to this there is a small haemorrhage and a network of eosinophilic hyaline material. (*H&E × 100*)

Granulomas

Localised trauma to the larynx may lead to the benign non-neoplastic intubation granuloma and contact ulcer granuloma. In the former the initiating agent is a roughly sited endotracheal tube which rubs off the epithelium from the vocal process and sets up a localised perichondritic granulomatous reaction and the formation of the characteristic swelling. The latter presumably results again from voice abuse when the cords meet each other with considerable force and the small bilateral ulcers are situated in the posterior half of the membranous vocal cord. There is considerable overlap with the condition of contact pachydermia which anatomically also covers the vocal processes of the arytenoids. Epithelial dysplasia and keratinisation are present. Interarytenoid pachydermia is characterised by reactive hyperplasia with pronounced swelling and may be a result of gastric acid reflux.

5

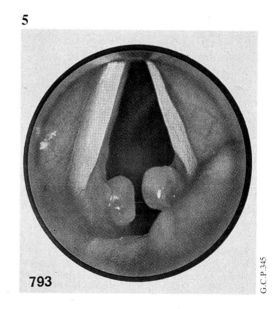

793

5 Intubation granulomas on arytenoids.

Leucoplakia

White patches varying in size may appear on the normally non-keratinising squamous epithelium of the membranous vocal cords. They are composed of keratinising epithelium covered by a thick layer of keratin (keratosis). A small proportion may show a degree of dysplasia with cellular and nuclear atypia which may be difficult to distinguish from carcinoma *in situ*.

Carcinoma *in situ*

In this condition there is intraepithelial malignant change with atypia, bizarre cells and increased mitotic activity. There is usually no rapid progression to invasive carcinoma and the condition may be treated conservatively over many years. If untreated, however, a large proportion ultimately become frankly invasive.

Malignant tumours

Malignant disease of the larynx is relatively uncommon and almost all tumours are squamous carcinomas.

Incidence

Laryngeal cancer occurs more often in men than in women with a peak incidence between 60 and 70 years of age. There are, however, geographical variations in age and sex incidence.

In England and Wales the age adjusted mortality rates have fallen from a peak in 1925 but in women there has been a small upward trend in recent years.

Aetiology

Non-smokers have a low incidence of cancer of the larynx, but the reduction in male mortality rates in England and Wales since 1925 has occurred despite the rise in cigarette smoking in the first half of this century.
   In several other countries a recent increase in male mortality from laryngeal cancer has been linked with urban living and high alcohol and cigarette consumption. Other possible aetiological factors include exposure to wood dust, asbestos, other irritant substances and low dietary levels of vitamins A and C.

6

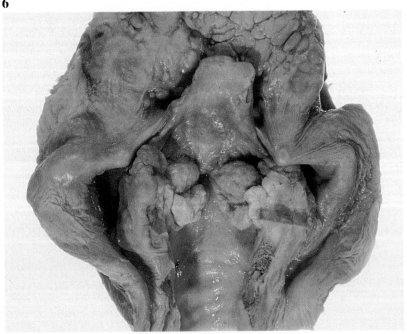

G.C.8756

6 A man of 45 years had suffered from hoarseness for 2 years. He had had neither a laryngeal examination nor treatment. He died suddenly from asphyxia.
   A warty, grey tumour involves the vocal folds, the ventricles and the ventricular folds, and extends to the subglottic and arytenoid areas. A section of the right arytenoid shows the deeper infiltration of the growth.

Histogenesis

The vocal cords are covered by non-keratinising squamous epithelium. Elsewhere the larynx is covered by pseudostratified columnar epithelium. 85% of malignant laryngeal tumours are, however, squamous carcinomas which indicates that squamous metaplasia has occurred either before or during the development of the carcinoma.

Frankly invasive squamous carcinoma is usually moderately to well differentiated and the incidence of lymph node metastases and survival depend on this degree of differentiation.

The larynx is anatomically divided into 3 areas as in (7). About 35% of the tumours originate in the supraglottis, 55% in the glottis and 10% in the subglottic area.

7

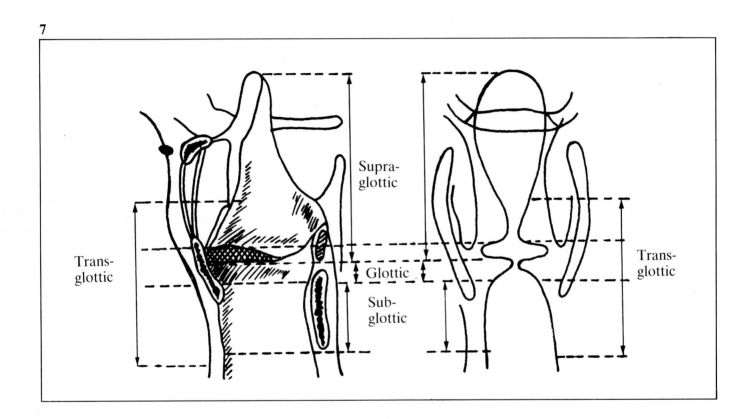

Supraglottic tumours

Supraglottic tumours present late as they do not cause hoarseness or stridor until they are advanced. The commonest tumour arises on the infrahyoid epiglottis and its local spread is to the thyroid cartilage and the pre-epiglottic space. Carcinoma of the ventricular bands is much less common and spreads superficially to the epiglottis, the aryepiglottic fold and the paraglottic space.

Malignant tumours (*Continued*)

Glottic carcinoma

Glottic carcinoma may remain a small localised tumour on one cord or involve a large part of the laryngeal surface crossing the vocal cord. Local spread occurs to surrounding cartilages and to the supra and subglottis. There are two separate types of tumour which do not represent different stages of the same tumour. Tumours limited to the glottis rarely transgress the conus elasticus. The transglottic tumour is aggressive and often invades the paraglottic space.

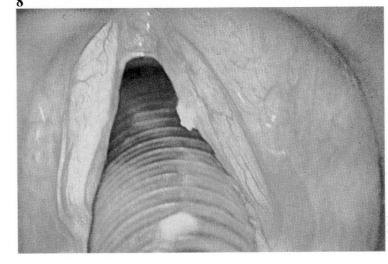

8

8 A very small right glottic tumour.

True subglottic carcinoma

True subglottic carcinoma is usually unilateral and early invasion of the perichondrium of the thyroid and cricoid cartilages and extension through the cricothyroid membrane is common. These tumours often spread through the conus elasticus to the glottis. True subglottic carcinoma presents with stridor, whereas subglottic spread from a glottic carcinoma is associated with hoarseness.

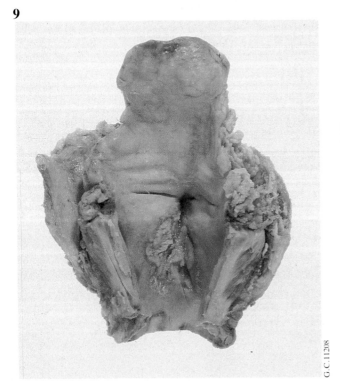

9

9 A man aged 66 developed a squamous carcinoma of the right vocal cord. This tumour disappeared following radiotherapy but three weeks later there was a suspicious area in the subglottic region and a recurrence appeared at this site and the left cervical lymph nodes became enlarged. Laryngectomy and radical excision of the left side of the neck were carried out.

In the subglottic region there is an irregular plaque of carcinoma below the site of the former carcinoma of the right vocal cord. Its surface is partly necrotic and is in places ulcerated.

G.C.11208

TMN Classification

Adequate staging of these tumours (TMN classification) is necesssary for an intelligent approach to management. This requires a full radiological examination and, if necessary, computerised tomography with endoscopy and biopsy to assess the extent of the tumour.

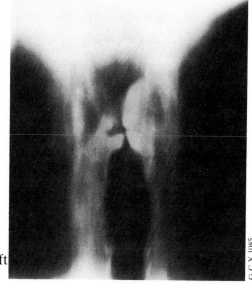

10

10   Laryngeal tomogram showing a left transglottic tumour.

Verrucous carcinoma

Verrucous carcinoma is a rare non-aggressive tumour and seldom metastasises. The tumour has a warty papillary surface which is unusually well differentiated keratinising squamous epithelium. These should be removed surgically as there is a propensity to anaplastic change following radiotherapy.

Adenocarcinoma

Adenocarcinoma is very uncommon in the larynx and the possibility of the tumour being a secondary with the primary in the kidney or GI tract should be considered.

Lymphatic spread

Nodal spread of carcinoma is to the adjacent lymph nodes in the deep cervical chain. Pretreatment clinical staging of these tumours is mandatory but cognisance must be taken of the possibility of supra-added infection or clinical error which is in the region of 20%.

Other malignant tumours

Spindle cell carcinoma

This is a polypoidal tumour with a stroma of dysplastic spindle cells covered by squamous cell carcinomatous elements. About one fifth of these tumours metastasise to the cervical nodes.

Sarcoma

Of these uncommon tumours the most frequent is the fibrosarcoma. This is predominantly a male disease and spread is blood borne or locally along muscle and fascial planes.

Laryngocoeles

These are developmental neck masses caused by entrapment of air in the ventricle of the larynx. Internal laryngocoeles are contained within the larynx, whereas external laryngocoeles have spread out through the thyrohyoid membrane. It is of importance to exclude an associated laryngeal tumour which may give rise to the ball-valve effect causing the laryngocoele. If infection supervenes they are called pyocoeles.

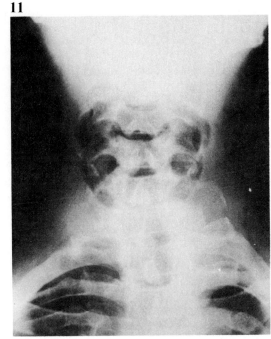

11 A laryngocoele is demonstrated radiologically when the patient does the Valsalva manoeuvre.

Infections

Diphtheria

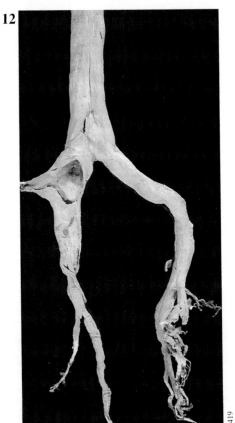

Diphtheria was a common disease and frequently fatal prior to the introduction of immunisation in infancy. The causal organism is Corynebacterium diphtheriae which is spread by droplet infection. It was particularly common in childhood. The acute lesion consisted of a pharyngeal inflammation associated with the formation of a greyish membrane adherent principally to the tonsil and fauces. There was considerable toxaemia and this was associated with both cardiac irregularity, sometimes progressing to failure, and evidence of palsies frequently first noted in the palate. The infection, while primarily in the nasopharynx, can spread downwards into the larynx causing respiratory distress. Occasionally the membrane becomes detached and is expectorated.

12 A diphtheritic membranous cast.

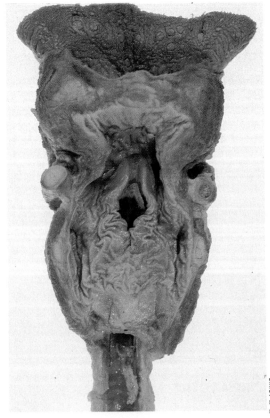

13 Laryngeal diphtheria.

Tuberculosis

Tuberculosis of the larynx is always secondary to pulmonary disease and the causal bacteria are carried to the larynx in the sputum.

In the Western World the disease, as a result of early diagnosis and successful treatment, is now comparatively rare. The disease occurs equally in the two sexes and the majority of cases occur between the ages of 20 and 40 years.

The initial lesion is the formation of small tubercles in the submucosa which may coalesce. Later the overlying epithelium is involved with the formation of shallow ulcers. This is associated with congestion of the surrounding mucosa and some degree of oedema. The commonest affected areas are over the vocal cords and in relation to the arytenoid cartilages and the posterior laryngeal wall.

Oedema, which shows as pallid areas, is commonly found in the epiglottis and the posterior ends of the aryepiglottic folds. The appearances may be in association with a known tuberculous pulmonary infection in which case the diagnosis is readily made. Differentiation from chronic laryngitis, syphilis and carcinoma has to be made.

14

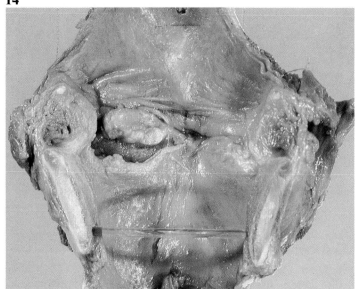

G.C.10137

14 A man of 68 years had suffered from increasingly severe hoarseness for 2 years.

Advanced laryngeal tuberculosis. There is deep ulceration of the left ventricle and the cord is ulcerated, and swollen by tuberculous granulation tissue. The right vocal cord is also swollen but shows only punctate ulceration.

Syphilis

Syphilitic manifestations in the larynx are tertiary and are seldom seen in modern practice. Essentially the lesion is that of a gross ulceration involving the larynx and in addition parts of the pharynx. It has to be differentiated from malignant disease of the larynx.

15

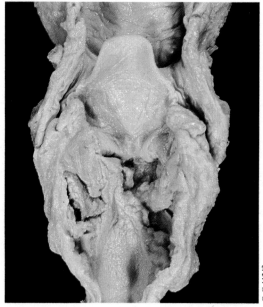

G.C.11242

15 Acquired syphilis. With the exception of the epiglottis the interior of the larynx shows extensive ulceration, the right vocal fold being completely destroyed. The cricoid cartilage is exposed and partly necrosed as is also the proximal cartilage of the trachea.

J.A.M. Murray

External ear

Infections

Acute otitis externa

Acute otitis externa is characterised by inflammation of the meatal skin accompanied by a smelly aural discharge and itching; the hearing may be normal. The disease may be caused by infected water lying in the meatus as after swimming or by repeated attempts to remove wax with, e.g. fingernails, pencils or other sharp objects which damage the meatal skin and allow bacterial invasion. The main organisms found are staphylococcus aureus, pseudomonas, proteus and E. coli. Fungi, particularly aspergillus niger, may also be present, often after antibiotic ear drops. Infection may spread to the conchal cartilage and produce a perichondritis which destroys the normal architecture of the pinna.

'Malignant' otitis externa

'Malignant' otitis externa is not cancerous but is caused by infection in the elderly debilitated patient with pseudomonas. This organism produces exotoxins including a neurotoxin. Multiple cranial neuropathies, necrotising vasculitis and gross tissue destruction may follow. Intracranial spread usually results in death.

Herpes zoster

Herpes zoster may affect the ear and probably the geniculate ganglion in the Ramsay Hunt syndrome. The facial palsy is associated with herpetic vesicles over the pinna, external meatus and tympanic membrane. Spontaneous recovery is the rule but severe pain may be a long-term consequence.

Bell's palsy

The facial nerve may be affected by viral diseases. *Bell's palsy* or idiopathic seventh nerve palsy has been attributed by many to a virus. The nerve is said to swell throughout its intratemporal course from the brainstem to the stylomastoid foramen but the exact pathology is not understood. Almost all (90%) recover spontaneously. Bad prognostic features include severe pain, completeness of the palsy and advanced age of the patient.

Tumours

The incidence is low, 4–8% of all skin cancers. Site – 80% of aural cancers involve the auricle, 12% the external auditory meatus and 8% the middle ear and mastoid.

External meatus cancers are similar to those of the auricle but may present late with pain, otorrhea, a feeling of fullness in the ear and diminished hearing.

Carcinoma of the auricle – The aetiology includes chronic trauma from sun and wind and chronic irritation from a variety of causes.

Squamous cell carcinoma This usually occurs in older males on the postero-superior portion of the pinna but may occur in other sites. Growth is slow and metastases are late. Biopsy is necessary to establish the diagnosis.

Basal cell carcinoma This is commoner in males in the 40s and 50s and is locally aggressive.

Malignant melanoma – This is relatively rare in temperate regions and behaves like other cutaneous melanomas.

Adenocarcinoma arises from the sweat and sebaceous glands and the most noteworthy is the adenoid cystic carcinoma from the ceruminous glands. The average age of presentation is in the fifth decade.

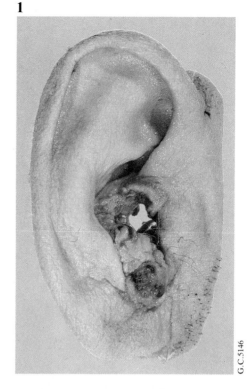

1 An adult right auricula showing a carcinoma.

A nodular warty overgrowth occupies the inferior portion of the cavum conchae, surrounds the external acoustic meatus, and extends for some little distance medially. Microscopically the tumour is a squamous-cell carcinoma.

Miscellaneous lesions

Keratosis obturans – this is a desquamating keratinous mass in the external auditory canal. The aetiology is uncertain but may be related to radiotherapy.

Soft tissue swellings – rheumatoid nodules and gouty tophi may be palpable on the pinna.

Exostosis – these are found deep in bony canal near the tympanic ring. These often occur in swimmers. They are usually asymptomatic unless they block off the meatus causing recurrent otitis externa or deafness.

Chondrodermatitis nodularis chronicis helicis is a small firm nodular benign lesion on the free edge of the pinna which is very painful. It must be distinguished from basal cell carcinoma.

Adenoma

Adenomas are rare, small, painless swellings at the entrance of the meatus. The adenoma of sweat gland origin is termed a ceruminoma. This presents as a small intraverted polypoid swelling in the outer end of the meatus. Local recurrence after excision is common.

Anatomy

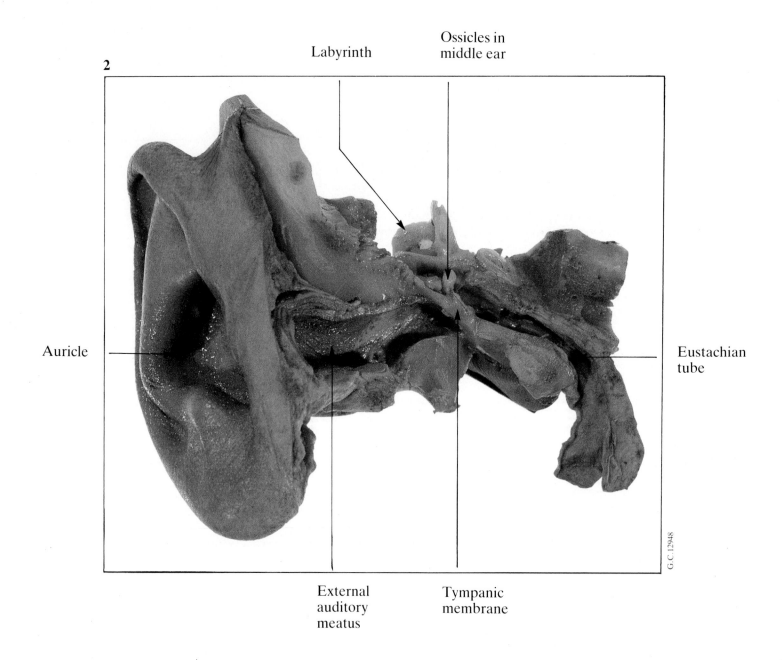

2

Labyrinth

Ossicles in
middle ear

Auricle

Eustachian
tube

External
auditory
meatus

Tympanic
membrane

G.C. 12948

Middle ear

Infections

Acute otitis media

Acute otitis media is an infection of the middle ear which often results initially from a virus complicated by bacterial invasion. The influence of poor Eustachian tube drainage has been suggested.

Incidence

Acute otitis media is extremely common, defying attempts to define a true incidence owing to its frequency. Some attacks of acute otitis media are not even medically treated as there may be many neonates who cannot communicate that their ears are painful.

Aetiology

The winter incidence is high and is presumably associated with the numerous upper respiratory tract infections of the season. In children the short Eustachian tube is thought to allow easy ingress of bacteria. The relative abundance of lymphoid tissue in children and allergic swelling and obstruction may also cause blockage of the lower end of the Eustachian tube. In 50% of cleft palate patients recurrent otitis media is a problem. The commonest pathogens are streptococcus pneumoniae and haemophilus influenzae.

Pathology

Hyperaemia of the middle ear mucosa occludes the Eustachian tube and pressure changes in the middle ear occur. This is followed by exudation from the surrounding blood vessels and goblet cell hyperplasia. The resultant exudate is under pressure and causes severe pain.
    The condition may resolve spontaneously or progress to suppuration.

3

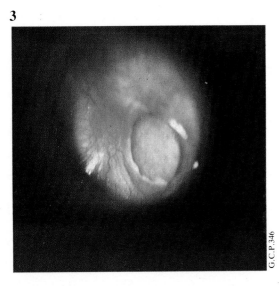

With the advent of suppuration the tympanic membrane perforates spontaneously with dramatic relief of pain. At this stage the majority of patients recover and the condition is self limiting within 6 weeks with healing of the perforation. Up to 5% may progress to the stage of coalescence in which mucosal hyperaemia produces obstruction of drainage of the mucopurulent secretions and again produces pus under pressure.

3 Perforation of left tympanic membrane.

Mastoiditis

Decalcification and osteoclastic resorption of the thin bony septa of the mastoid air cells produce large irregular cavities filled with hypertrophied mucosa, granulations and pus under pressure. Spread through the thin inner table and the thick outer table may produce an abscess. Pain and aural discharge recur and radiography for the first time in the disease shows bony destruction.

Acute mastoiditis is an exceptionally rare occurrence because of antibiotic therapy but chronic otitis media (cholesteatoma) is still a common occurrence.

4

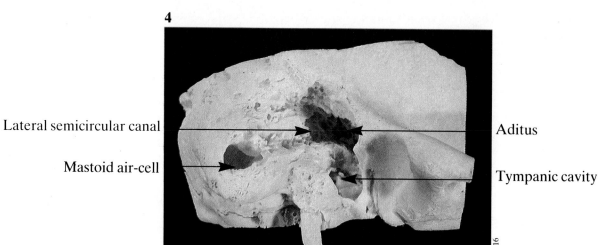

Lateral semicircular canal — Aditus

Mastoid air-cell — Tympanic cavity

G.C.10316

Complications

Extension of bacterial infection outwith the tympanic cavity and mastoid air cells produces complications. These are conveniently listed.

Otogenic

Mastoiditis
Petrositis
Facial nerve palsy
Labyrinthitis
Deafness

Intracranial

Extradural abscess
Subdural abscess
Intracerebral abscess
Cerebellar abscess
Sigmoid sinus thrombosis
Meningitis
Otitic hydrocephalus

These are self explanatory with the exception of otitic hydrocephalus. This condition is thought to result from small infected emboli from a dural sinus lodging in the arachnoid villi of the superior sagittal sinus thus preventing resorption of the CSF.

These complications of acute otitis media may also result from acute exacerbations of chronic otitis media. Their incidence has been greatly reduced since the introduction of antibiotics but they are still not uncommon in some parts of the world.

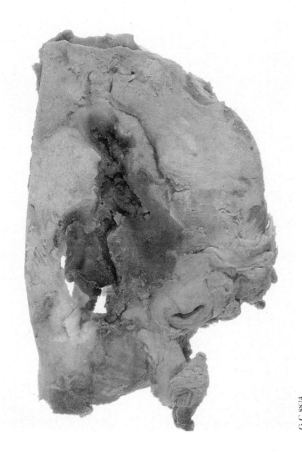

5 From a male aged 55 years who had a left acute otitis media. Local treatment failed to resolve the infection and he subsequently developed unconsciousness. An exploratory operation confirmed a large quantity of extradural pus but he died seven days later.

The specimen shows an intratemporal lobe abscess.

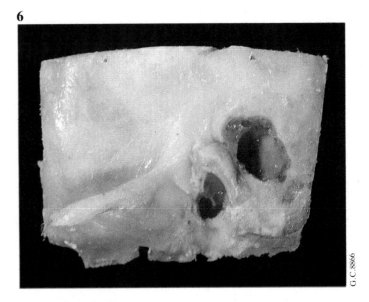

6 From a six year old male following acute otitis media.

Pus was evacuated by a simple mastoidectomy but death ensued from cerebral oedema seven days later.

Chronic otitis media

Chronic otitis media may follow recurrent attacks of otitis media but more commonly the onset of chronic middle ear disease is insidious and a patient may not consult an otologist until a complication occurs. The mucous membrane may be oedematous with submucosal fibrosis and infiltration of chronic inflammatory cells. The formation of polyps or granulation tissue signifies infection of the bone. Progression of inflammation destroys the middle ear. Eventually fistula formation, invasion and destruction of the inner ear dural plates and the facial canal occur and the disease extends outwith the temporal bone.

The term chronic otitis media spans 2 essentially separate disease entities.
1   The progressive dangerous condition of cholesteatoma is attico-antral in site.
2   The benign safe tubotympanic disease involving essentially the pars tensa. This form is further subdivided into the permanent perforation type and the persistent tubotympanic mucosal infection type.

Infections (*Continued*)

Cholesteatoma

Cholesteatoma is an accumulation of exfoliated keratin in the middle ear cleft which arises from keratinising squamous epithelium that has invaded the cleft from the external auditory canal. Primary acquired cholesteatomas arise spontaneously without preceding acute otitis media. The keratin accumulates in concentric onion-like layers which contain cholesterol crystals and the whole secretes bone-eroding enzymes.

Ingress of the cholesteatoma is by a perforation which is initially limited to the pars flaccida and may be the only clinical sign. Usually, however, there is a superimposed infection which produces a constant discharge with the characteristic odour of dead infected squamous cells. Extension of the cholesteatoma into the attic and through the aditus to the mastoid antrum leads to bony erosion and involvement of nearby structures with the complications previously noted in acute otitis media.

7

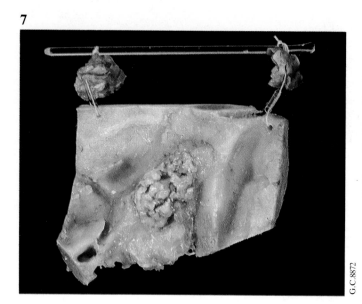

G.C.8872

7 This specimen is from an adolescent who had a cholesteatoma.

The cholesteatoma occupies the middle ear and has destroyed the anterior wall of the external auditory meatus.

The roof of the middle ear is decalcified and the cholesteatoma projects through the posterior surface of the petrous temporal bone.

8

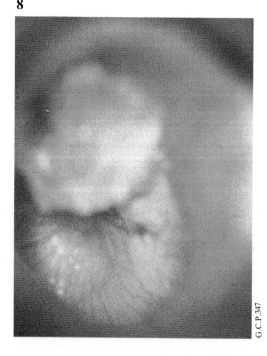

G.C.P.347

8 This picture of the tympanic membrane shows an attic cholesteatoma in a right ear.

9

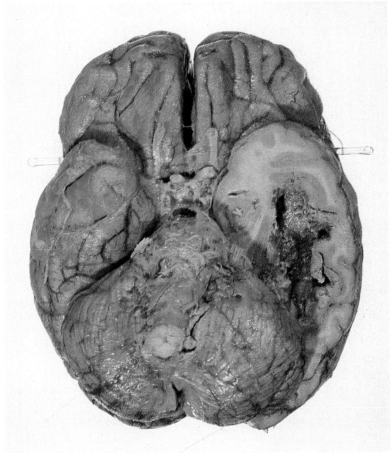

G.C.5123

9 From a patient with chronic otitis media.

The specimen is of the brain showing an extensive oval abscess in the left temporal lobe. There is also a widespread meningitis present.

10

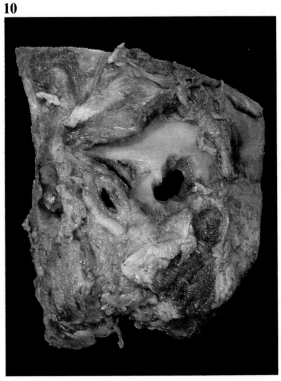

G.C.5124

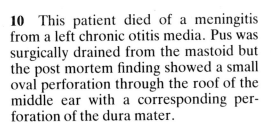

10 This patient died of a meningitis from a left chronic otitis media. Pus was surgically drained from the mastoid but the post mortem finding showed a small oval perforation through the roof of the middle ear with a corresponding perforation of the dura mater.

A rare form of cholesteatoma is encountered in the middle ear with no evidence of migration of squamous cells from the external auditory canal. It probably originates from the ectoderm that forms the notochord.

Secondary acquired cholesteatoma arises from ingrowth of keratinising squamous cells into the middle ear through a long-standing perforation of the tympanic membrane.

Infections (*Continued*)

Tubotympanic disease

Persistent perforation of the tympanic membrane involves the pars tensa. The margins of the perforation are covered with a healed epithelium. The ear discharges intermittently or not at all. In the dry state the middle ear mucosa looks healthy, but when wet the mucosa is red and oedematous; the secretions are profuse and may be mucopurulent and may pulsate. The degree of hearing loss depends on the size of perforation and the amount of fluid present. The chronic tubotympanic infection type may have a considerably larger perforation with a mucoid or mucopurulent profuse discharge associated with upper respiratory tract infections. The middle ear mucosa is grossly oedematous and may be polypoidal.

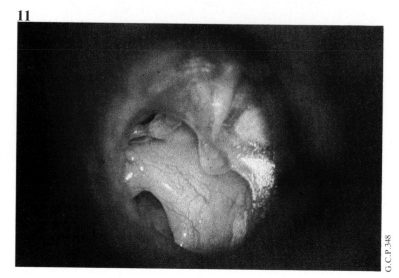

11 Chronic tubotympanic perforation with a dry middle ear mucosa. The long process of the incus and the round window can be seen through the perforation.

Cholesterol granuloma

Cholesterol granuloma occurs in any type of chronic otitis media in which there is stasis with mucosal oedema, exudation and haemorrhage. The middle ear cleft contains granulomatous tissue which contains cholesterol crystals surrounded by foreign body giant cells.

Tympanosclerosis

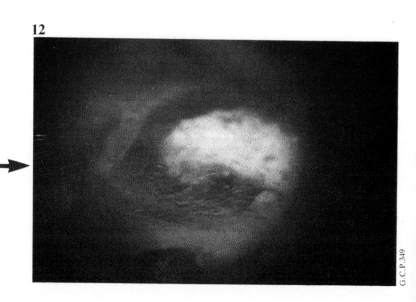

12 Tympanosclerosis is the result of acute recurrent or prolonged otitis media. There is fibroblastic invasion of the subepithelial tunica propria with hyalin degeneration in a thick white submucosal plaque. There is no mucosal or bony destruction. There is no particular site of predilection within the middle ear for this condition but it is most easily seen on the tympanic membrane.

A conductive hearing loss may result from ossicular fixation in this condition.

Serous otitis media

Serous otitis media is a collection of fluid in the middle ear cleft. It is the commonest cause of deafness in young children and has a peak incidence at 5–7 years. After puberty it is usually associated with infection or some other pathology, e.g. nasopharyngeal carcinoma. Various causes have been postulated including an incomplete resolution of acute otitis media, transudation associated with a negative middle ear pressure caused by Eustachean tube blockage, or allergy.

Four types of middle ear fluid are found; serous, mucoid, bloody and purulent. On this basis middle ear effusions have been reclassified as:

1   Acute purulent otitis media (mentioned above).
2   Serous otitis media.
3   Mucoid secretory otitis media.

The latter 2 headings attempt to distinguish between a transudative and secretory activity. Bloody effusions may be the result of trauma, tumour or bleeding dyscrasias.

Middle ear effusions are commoner in children with a cleft palate, atopy and enlarged adenoids.

Clinically the tympanic membrane and middle ear may appear normal or yellowish fluid may be seen with or without bubbles in the tympanic cavity. Apparent shortening of the malleus handle probably reflects negative middle ear pressure. A conductive hearing loss is present and tympanometry confirms the negative middle ear pressure or an immobile drumhead due to fluid in the middle ear. There is growing evidence of a bacterial association with this condition and the middle ear mucosa undergoes metaplasia to produce goblet cells and mucous glands.

Adhesive otitis media

Adhesive otitis media results from inadequately treated acute suppurative otitis media. The conductive hearing loss is progressive from its onset in childhood. The diagnosis of this condition is one of exclusion of the other causes of deafness and by direct inspection at tympanotomy. The incidence apparently varies considerably from author to author as there may be overlap in classification with other inflammatory conditions of the middle ear.

Tuberculosis

Tuberculosis is an uncommon infection of the ear and probably is secondary to disease of the nose or throat. Bony destruction and fistulae are a feature and the presence of a number of small perforations of the tympanic membrane which later coalesce to form a large perforation is characteristic. Further extension of the infection destroys the temporal bone including the petrous part. Pain is notable by its absence.

Infections (*Continued*)

Otosclerosis

Otosclerosis is a primary disease of the osseous labyrinthine capsule characterised by repeated resorption of bone. The most common location for a focus is anterior to the oval window with gradual invasion of the annular ligament and stapes causing bony ankylosis of the stapes and a conductive hearing loss.

13

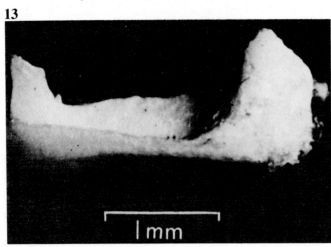

13 The thickened footplate removed during the operation of stapedectomy in a patient with otosclerosis.

Aetiology

The age of onset is usually between 10 and 30 years with little sex differentiation. About 0.5−1% of the population is affected and usually it is bilateral. The disease is hereditary, probably a dominant gene. Pregnancy appears to have little effect on the course of the disease.

Otosclerosis is a slow and irregularly progressive disease where normal bone is at first absorbed and replaced by vascular spongy osteoid tissue. Later the new bone becomes thicker and less vascular. Of great histopathologic importance are the blue mantles which are processes of bone deposited in canals formed by absorption of the normal bone of the otic capsule. Each mantle surrounds a small vascular space. They stain blue with haematoxylin and eosin. Progression of the disease increases the conductive hearing loss. Involvement of the cochlea by this condition results in sensorineural hearing loss. Although pure cochlear otosclerosis has never been found post-mortem, deposits of otosclerosis have been demonstrated in the cochlea with involvement of the oval window.

Histiocytosis X

Histiocytosis X may present in the ear. A fuller explanation of the behaviour of this condition may be seen on p. 66.

Carcinoma

Carcinoma of the middle ear and mastoid has been described but is very rare.

J.A.M. Murray

Part II – Endocrine System

Glossary of abbreviations

ACTH	–	Adrenocorticotrophic hormone
ADH	–	Anti-diuretic hormone
APUD	–	Amine Precursor Uptake Decarboxylase (APUD System)
AT II	–	Angiotensin II
AT III	–	Angiotensin III
ATP	–	Adenosine triphosphate
cAMP	–	Cyclic adenosine monophosphate
CD	–	Collecting ducts
CLIP	–	Corticotrophin-like intermediate lobe peptide
COMT	–	Catechol O-methyl transferase
CRH	–	Corticotrophic hormone releasing hormone
DCT	–	Distal convoluted tubule
DHASO$_4$	–	Dehydroepiandrosterone sulphate
DM	–	Dexamethasone
DPG	–	Diphosphoglycerate
FRH	–	Follicle stimulating hormone releasing hormone
FSH	–	Follicle stimulating hormone
GH	–	Growth hormone
GIF	–	Growth hormone inhibitory factor
GIH	–	Growth inhibitory hormone
GnRH	–	Gonadotrophin releasing hormone
5–HT	–	5–hydroxytryptamine (serotonin)
JGA	–	Juxtaglomerular apparatus
17 KS	–	17 ketosteroids
LATS	–	Long acting thyroid stimulating antibody
LH	–	Luteinising hormone
LPH	–	Lipotrophin hormone
LRH	–	Luteinising hormone releasing hormone
MEN	–	Multiple endocrine neoplasia
MSH	–	Melanocyte stimulating hormone
PCT	–	Proximal convoluted tubule
PIF	–	Prolactin inhibitory factor
PIH	–	Prolactin inhibitory hormone
PNMT	–	Phenyl ethanolamine N methyl transferase
PRH	–	Prolactin releasing hormone
PRL	–	Prolactin
PTH	–	Parathyroid hormone
PVN	–	Paraventricular nucleus
RIA	–	Radio-immunoassay
rT$_3$	–	Reverse tri-iodothyronine
SON	–	Supra-optic nucleus
T$_3$	–	Tri-iodothyronine
T$_4$	–	Thyroxine
TBG	–	Thyroid binding globulin
TBPA	–	Thyroid binding prealbumin
TRH	–	Thyrotrophic hormone releasing hormone
TSAb	–	Thyroid stimulating antibody
TSH	–	Thyroid stimulating hormone
TSI	–	Thyroid stimulating immunoglobulins
$\propto$–LPH	–	$\propto$–lipotrophin
$\propto$–MSH	–	$\propto$–melanocyte stimulating hormone
ß LPH	–	ß Lipotrophin
ß MSH	–	ß Melanocyte stimulating hormone

165

The pituitary gland (hypophysis) has a dual development.

1   From the ventral wall of the diencephalon a diverticulum projects forwards towards the primitive foregut. From this diverticulum develop:

> neurohypophysis from the ventral portion
> infundibulum from the intermediate portion, and
> tuber cinereum from the base.

2   Rathke's pouch, an upgrowth from the nasopharynx, gives rise to the anterior part of the pituitary gland.

In the fully developed nasopharynx the site of Rathke's pouch lies in relation to the nasal septum and roof of the pharynx and may be identified by a small invagination of the mucosa.

1

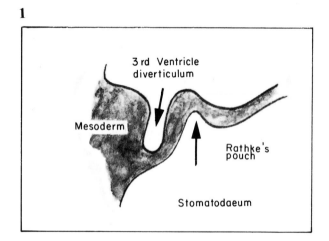

1a

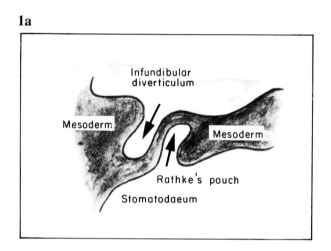

1b

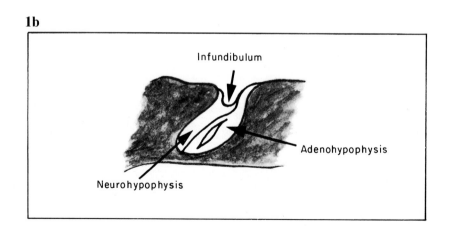

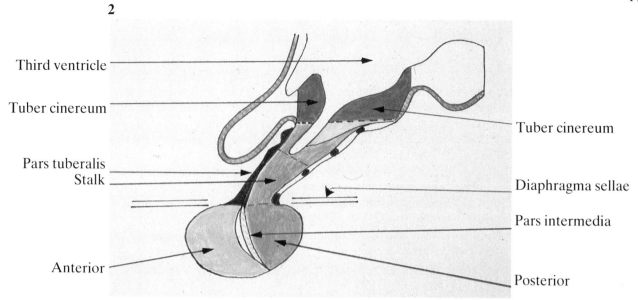

Third ventricle

Tuber cinereum

Pars tuberalis
Stalk

Tuber cinereum

Diaphragma sellae

Pars intermedia

Anterior

Posterior

Neurohypophysis

The neurohypophysis consists of three parts:

(a) median eminence of the tuber cinereum
(b) stem of the infundibulum
(c) pars posterior (neural lobe)

The pars posterior maintains neural connections with the supra-optic and para-ventricular nuclei of the hypothalamus via the hypothalamo-hypophyseal tract, which passes down the infundibulum. It contains thin non-myelinated nerve fibres which are the nerve terminals of the axons of the hypothalamo-hypophyseal tract. These fibres lie in close proximity to blood vessels. Star-shaped cells called pituicytes with long processes extending from their cell bodies are also present. These cells are thought to be modified astroglia.

Rathke's pouch

The cranial end of the foregut terminates at the same level as the cephalic end of the notochord. Immediately beyond this point Rathke's pouch develops as a diverticulum from the stomatodaeum and growing upwards to the ventral aspect of the forebrain, it extends towards the neural plate where it comes in contact with the infundibulum.

In the mesenchyme from which the basal plate of the skull forms, are four centres of chondrification. Between these, in the median plane, lies the primitive craniopharyngeal duct along which Rathke's pouch extends upwards. Later these centres of chondrification fuse, obliterating the craniopharyngeal duct thus separating the apex of Rathke's pouch from which are formed the anterior and the intermediate lobes of the pituitary, and also the pars tuberalis partially covering the infundibulum. The cleft in the intermediate part of the pituitary is a residuum of Rathke's pouch. The more proximal part of Rathke's pouch which communicates with the pharynx is usually obliterated but exceptionally persists as the craniopharyngeal canal. When epithelial remnants of the original Rathke's pouch persist this may give rise to cysts and tumours exhibiting features comparable to adamantinomas. When these arise in the skull they present as suprasellar cysts or craniopharyngiomas which are considered with other lesions of the pituitary.
  Epithelial cells may also persist in the more proximal and generally obliterated part of the tract and give rise to cysts which are palpable in the pharynx. Structurally they may simulate adamantinoma or squamous epithelioma.

Anatomy

The pituitary gland is an ovoid structure usually measuring about 12mm in maximum transverse diameter and weighing about 0.5gm but there is considerable variation, and in post-partum women a 50% increase in size is quite common.

It lies in the hypophyseal fossa of the sphenoid bone, the sella turcica, and is attached to the floor of the third ventricle by the pituitary stalk (infundibulum). The fossa forms a cup-shaped space lying above the sphenoidal sinus and at the margins of this fossa are the anterior and posterior clinoid processes. The roof of the fossa is formed by a double layer of the dura mater, the diaphragma sellae, in the centre of which is an aperture through which the stalk of the pituitary passes.

Many of the important clinical and pathological features resulting from enlargement of the pituitary gland depend upon the anatomical relationships.

3

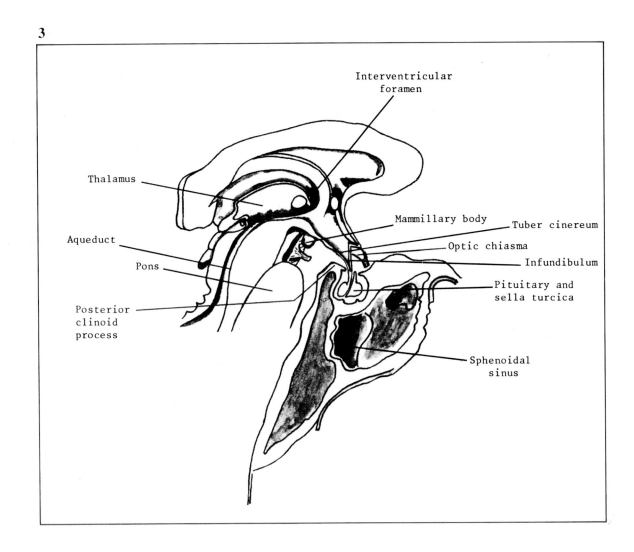

The gland is surrounded by important blood channels. On either side of the pituitary fossa is the cavernous sinus and there are intercavernous sinuses both anterior and posterior to the gland. In the lateral wall of the cavernous sinus run the third, fourth and sixth nerves. The internal carotid artery also lies nearby. Superior to the gland there are the hypothalamus and the corpora mammillaria, while above and in front of the hypophysis lies the optic chiasma.

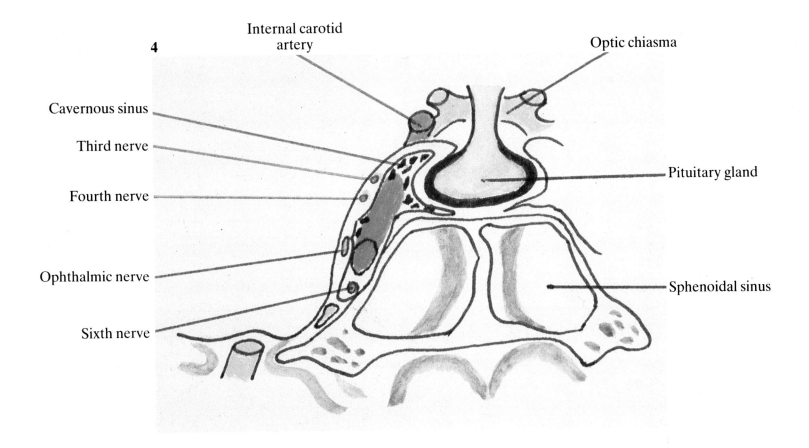

Applied anatomy

Irrespective of the nature of the lesion, enlargement of the pituitary is accompanied by a variety of manifestations due to pressure on individual anatomical structures.

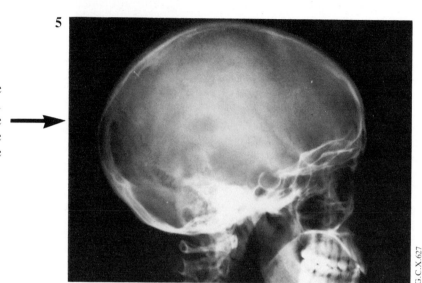

5 When a swelling occurs within the sella turcica the walls of the sella are ballooned outwards by pressure. Where the neoplasm is malignant the base may also be destroyed by infiltration. A further early pressure feature recognised radiologically is the disappearance of the posterior clinoid processes.

Pituitary tumour – upward extension

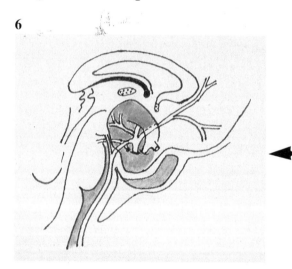

6 Upward growth of the tumour causes tension and later rupture or destruction of the diaphragma sellae and is responsible for intense headaches. Further expansion compresses the hypothalamus which may cause diabetes insipidus. Compression of the aqueduct or foramen of Monro may lead to hydrocephalus. Grosser expansion may involve the frontal lobes or the basal ganglia. Lateral expansion involves the temporal lobes.

Pituitary tumour – downward extension

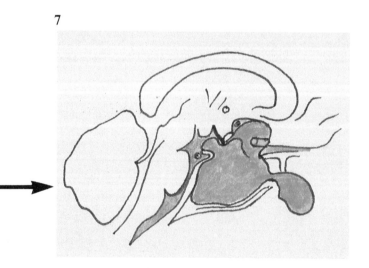

7 Downward expansion of the tumour may occur through the roof of the sphenoidal sinus and the tumour, expanding in the median raphe of the sinus, may reach the posterior pharyngeal wall.

Pituitary tumour – forward and upward extension

Forward and upward expansion compresses the optic chiasma in the mid-line causing bitemporal hemianopia. When the pressure is not central other types of disturbed vision arise as shown in the accompanying diagrams.

8

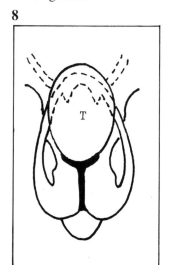

8 Upward growing tumour pressing forward on chiasma.

8a

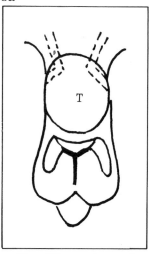

8a Upward growing tumour pressing backward on chiasma.

8b

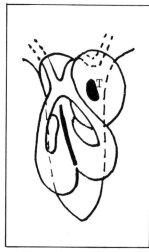

8b Upward growing tumour pressing lateral on chiasma.

Optic nerves

9

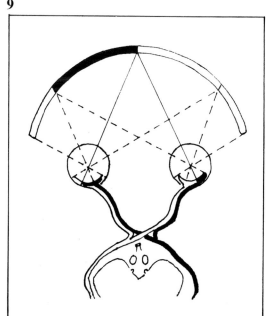

9 Diagram showing how the nerve fibres from the nasal portions of both retinae cross in the chiasma. Pressure here causes temporal defects of vision.

10

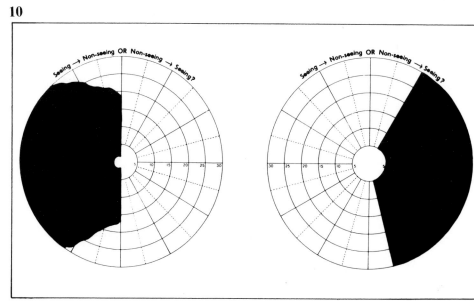

10 Retinal chart – bitemporal hemianopia.

After Cunningham.

Adenohypophysis

The adenohypophysis contains epithelial cells arranged either randomly or in follicles or cords. These cells lie in close proximity to capillary networks and are supported by reticular tissue. On the basis of staining techniques the cells can be divided into two groups:

1   The chromophobes which show little affinity for stains.
2   The chromophils which stain strongly with dyes.

This group can be divided into the acidophils which stain with acid dyes and the basophils which stain with basic dyes. Both can be further subdivided by immunocytochemical methods and ultramicroscopy.

The proportion of these cells varies from one part of the gland to another and in different states of pituitary activity.

11

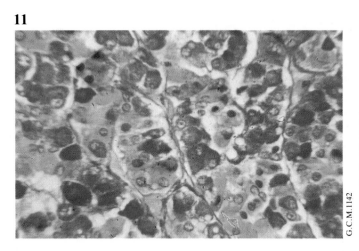

11 Pituitary. Acidophil cells (yellow) and basophil cells (purple) predominate in this field. A few pale chromophobe cells can also be seen. Slidders' pituitary stain. *(×500)*

The adenohypophysis consists of the pars tuberalis
the pars intermedia
the pars distalis (anterior lobe).

The pars tuberalis is an extension of the adenohypophysis which surrounds much of the neural part of the infundibulum. It contains chromophobe cells and small acidophil and basophil cells.

The pars intermedia is poorly developed in man, containing mainly basophil cells. In foetal life it is separated from the anterior lobe by the hypophyseal cleft (remnants of the cavity in Rathke's pouch). In adult life the cleft is represented by a few minute cysts lined by columnar epithelium, sometimes ciliated.

12

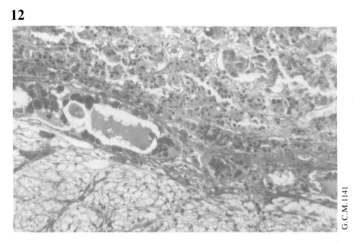

12 Pituitary. Pars intermedia and adjoining portions of the adenohypophysis and neurohypophysis. Basophil predominate in the pars intermedia. They may enclose microcysts, and extend slightly into the neurohypophysis. *Slidders' (×125)*

The anterior lobe forms the main bulk of the adenohypophysis. Chromophil and chromophobe cells are present throughout the lobe but their proportion and distribution vary in different parts. Often the acidophils are most numerous in the two lateral portions (wings), while basophils tend to lie in greater numbers along the vascular stroma, in the anterior portion of the gland and near the pars intermedia.

13

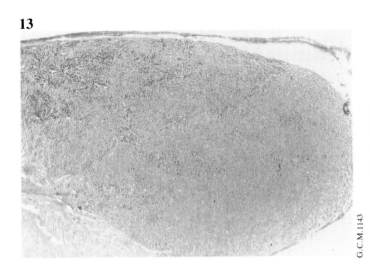

13 Approximately half of an anterior lobe of the adenohypophysis is shown. The yellow acidophils tend to concentrate in the lateral wings while the reddish basophils are more numerous anterocentrally. *Slidders' (×12.5)*

Blood supply

The blood supply is via the superior and inferior hypophyseal arteries on each side.

The superior hypophyseal arteries (of which there are several on each side) are derived from the internal carotid and from the anterior and middle cerebral arteries. They supply the median eminence and the upper part of the infundibulum and anastomose with branches of the inferior hypophyseal arteries over the lower part of the infundibulum.

Over the median eminence the superior hypophyseal arteries end in a capillary network which lies in close proximity to many nerve terminals. From these capillaries arise long portal vessels which pass down the infundibulum to the pars anterior (the hypothalamo-hypophyseal portal vessels). In the anterior lobe these portal vessels open up into vascular sinusoids surrounding the secretory cells.

The inferior hypophyseal arteries arise from the cavernous portion of the internal carotid, and divide into medial and lateral branches which anastomose with the corresponding branches of the inferior hypophyseal artery of the opposite side. They form an arterial circle around the lower portion of the infundibulum and anastomose with branches of the superior hypophyseal artery. Other branches of the inferior hypophyseal artery penetrate the posterior pituitary and break up into capillary networks which lie in close proximity to the nerve terminals in the posterior lobe.

The venous drainage is via vessels which emerge from the gland and drain into the nearby dural sinuses.

Physiology

Hormones of the adenohypophysis

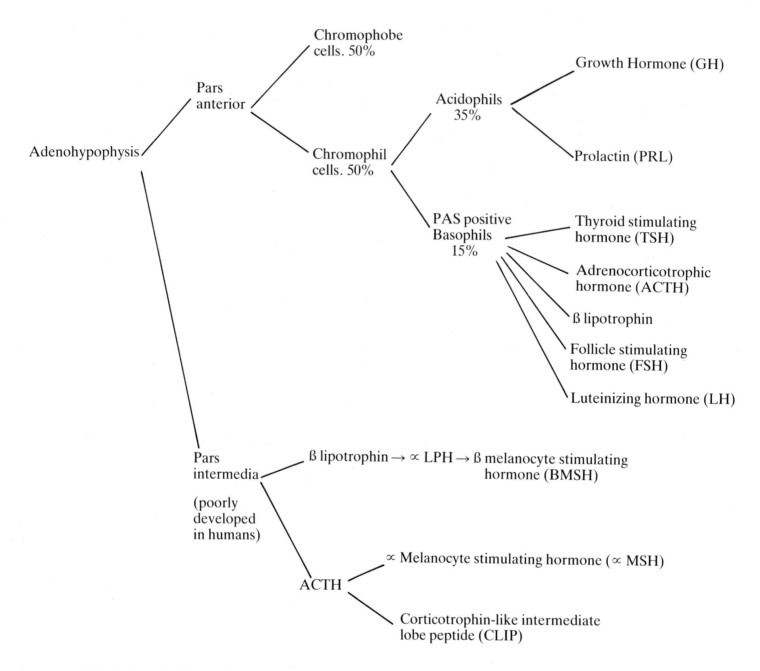

FSH, LH and TSH are glycoproteins which have ∝ and ß sub units. The ∝ sub unit is the same in all; the ß sub units differ in structure and give the hormone its specific characteristics.

FSH, LH and TSH are all trophic hormones which act on other endocrine glands to cause release of hormones.

ACTH, a polypeptide acts in a similar fashion.

GH and prolactin, both proteins, are non-trophic hormones.

Hormone control

Secretion of hormones by the adenohypophysis is controlled by releasing and inhibitory hormones synthesised by the hypothalamus.

14

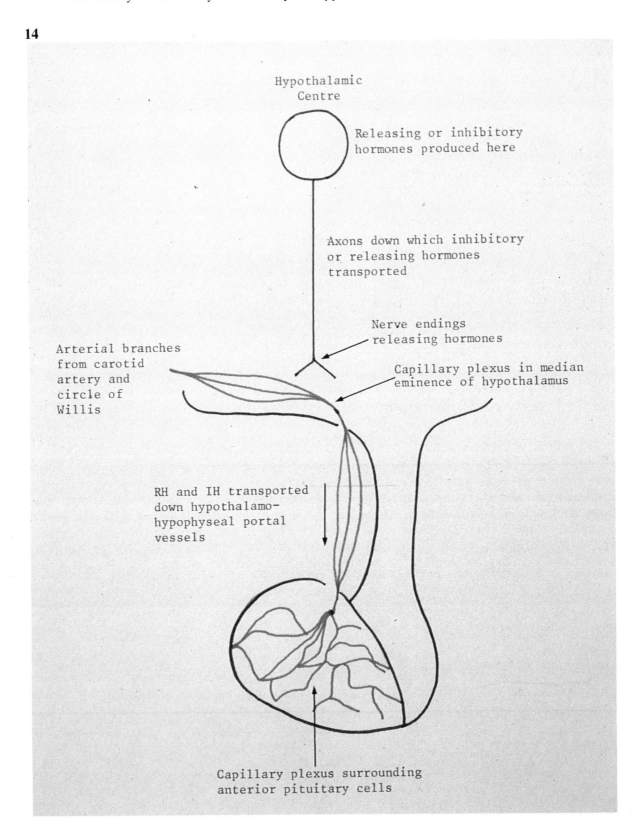

Hypothalamic
Centre

Releasing or inhibitory
hormones produced here

Axons down which inhibitory
or releasing hormones
transported

Nerve endings
releasing hormones

Arterial branches
from carotid
artery and
circle of
Willis

Capillary plexus in median
eminence of hypothalamus

RH and IH transported
down hypothalamo-
hypophyseal portal
vessels

Capillary plexus surrounding
anterior pituitary cells

Hormone control *(Continued)*

Centres from which some of the releasing or inhibitory hormones are produced are given in the following table.

	Hormone	Controlling centre
GRH	Growth hormone releasing hormone	Postulated, not identified
GIH	Growth hormone inhibitory hormone	Anterior hypothalamus
PIH	Prolactin inhibitory hormone (Dopamine)	Arcuate nucleus
PRH	Prolactin releasing hormone	Postulated, not identified
GnRH	Gonadotrophin releasing hormone which acts both as:	Pre-optic area
FRH	Follicle stimulating hormone releasing hormone and as	
LRH	Luteinizing hormone releasing hormone	
TRH	Thyrotrophic hormone releasing hormone	Dorsomedial nucleus
CRH	Corticotrophic hormone releasing hormone	Paraventricular nucleus

After synthesis in the cell bodies of the neurones of these 'centres' the releasing hormones are transported down the axons of the neurones. On depolarisation of the nerve terminals the hormones are secreted from them and pass into a capillary plexus which lies in close proximity to the nerve terminals. Once into the blood stream they pass in the hypothalamo-hypophyseal portal vessels from the hypothalamus to the anterior pituitary where they influence the secretion of a particular hormone (stimulation or inhibition of release). The area of the hypothalamus which contains the nerve terminals from which the hormones are secreted into the capillary plexus is called the median eminence. Releasing hormones act on the anterior pituitary via the adenyl cyclase, cAMP system; hormone release is also calcium dependent.

Long feedback loop control of secretion of trophic hormones

The secretion of the trophic hormones (TSH, ACTH, FSH, and LH) known to be controlled by hypothalamic releasing hormones is also influenced in a negative feedback manner (long feedback loop) by the hormones from the trophic glands. When the plasma concentration of free trophic hormone is low, there is secretion of releasing hormones which in turn causes secretion of the particular anterior pituitary hormone.

In a similar manner some hormones, e.g. tri-iodothyronine (T_3) and thyroxine (T_4) act directly on the anterior pituitary in a negative feedback manner regulating the release of the corresponding hormone (TSH).

Other control mechanisms

Secretion of the non-trophic hormones by the anterior pituitary (growth hormone and prolactin) is controlled by the secretion of inhibitory (and possibly releasing) hormones by the hypothalamus.

Short feedback loop

There is some evidence that some anterior pituitary hormones on release feedback to inhibit the secretion of their releasing hormones (short feedback loop).

In addition to feedback loops controlling the secretion of these hypothalamic hormones, other influences such as stress, heat, cold, and 'biological clocks' causing diurnal variations in hormone release, affect the hypothalamic 'centres'. Some hypothalamic hormones have mutliple actions on the anterior pituitary: e.g. TRH can stimulate the secretion of TSH, prolactin and growth hormone; GnRH stimulates the release of FSH and LH; and GIH (somatostatin) can inhibit the secretion of GH, TSH and PRL.

Hormone control *(Continued)*

Hormones secreted by acidophil cells of the adenohypophysis

Although growth hormone and prolactin are similar in structure the acidophil cells which produce them can be distinguished by immunoperoxidase staining methods and by the size of their secretory granules seen by electron microscopy.

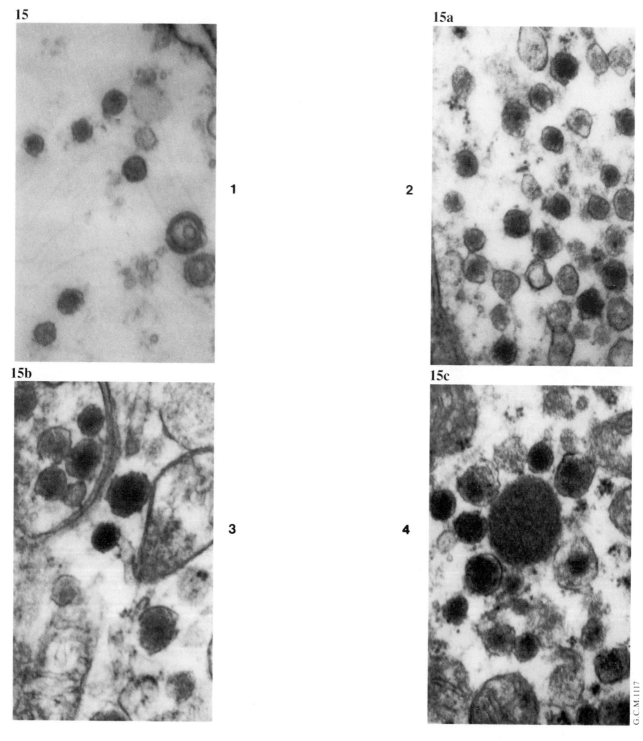

These electronmicrographs show the variable size of the hormone product in anterior pituitary cells. In increasing size, the granules range from the small, TSH variety (1) through ACTH (2), GH (3) to the large prolactin granules (4). *(Lead citrate and uranyl acetate × 40 000.)*

By courtesy of
Dr. K. M. McLaren

16

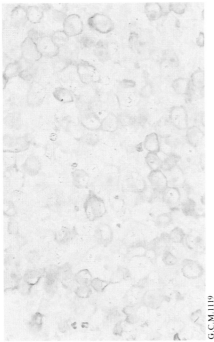

The eosinophil wings of the anterior pituitary comprise cells of both prolactin and growth hormone-producing type. This illustration shows localisation of prolactin using an anti-human prolactin antiserum. Antibody localisation is reflected by a brown-staining product. A similar picture would be produced using antisera to human growth hormone. (×62)

17

18

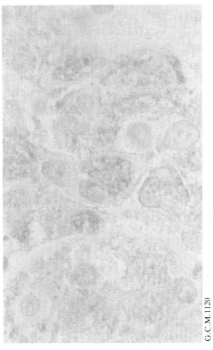

This monomorphic cell population represents a growth hormone secreting adenoma. Histochemistry would show an eosinophil-appearing cell but immunohistochemistry is required in order to establish the hormone product of the neoplastic cells. This illustration uses an antibody to human growth hormone, the antibody binding reflected by a brown-staining product. (×625)

This illustration of an ACTH secreting adenoma of pituitary shows the cytoplasmic granularity of antibody localisation. The technique uses an anti-human ACTH antibody, the binding reflected by a brown-staining product. (×1000)

Growth hormone

The effects of GH on the body are complex and vary according to the age of the individual. Some of the actions are mediated by GH itself, others via somatomedins (substances produced in the liver as a result of stimulation by GH).

1   During growth, chondrogenesis is stimulated (via somatomedins) and cartilage is laid down at the ends of the long bones. The epiphyseal plates widen and bone matrix is laid down and an increase in bone length is achieved. The presence of excess GH leads to gigantism.

2   There is increased protein synthesis and a positive nitrogen balance. This is produced by GH itself and by somatomedins and insulin released as a result of GH stimulation. There is increased transport of neutral and basic amino acids into the cells and stimulation of the ribosomes.

3   Transport of phosphate, calcium, sodium and potassium ions into cells is increased. Increased calcium uptake from the gastro-intestinal tract.

4   Metabolic effects:
   (a)   increased output of glucose from the liver
   (b)   decreased glucose uptake by cells
   (c)   decreased insulin binding to tissues
   (d)   increased lipolysis in adipose tissue by activation of hormone sensitive lipase. Increased levels of free fatty acids in the plasma may give rise to ketosis.
   (e)   in large amounts it is diabetogenic.

The metabolic effects mediated by GH are complex for, in addition to the actions mediated by itself, it causes the release of insulin from the pancreas, which opposes many of the effects, and of somatomedins from the liver which increase glucose oxidation and decrease fat breakdown.

5   It stimulates erythropoiesis.

6   It stimulates milk production because of its similar structure to prolactin.

Factors affecting the output of growth hormone from the anterior pituitary

The output is controlled by hypothalamic factors of which growth hormone inhibitory hormone (somatostatin) has been isolated and synthesized. It contains 14 amino acids and is released from the anterior region of the hypothalamus. The existence of growth hormone releasing hormone has been postulated but it has not yet been isolated. A synthetic preparation, human pancreatic growth hormone releasing factor, simulates its action.

Factors which may influence growth hormone secretion

Increase	Decrease
Deep sleep	Chlorpromazine
Hypoglycaemia	Hyperglycaemia
A protein meal or intravenous amino acids	
Glucagon Oestrogens	Large doses of glucocorticoids
Exercise Stress	Emotional deprivation in childhood
∝ adrenergic stimulation	ß adrenergic stimulation
ß endorphin L-Dopa	Negative feedback of GH
TRH	Hypothyroidism
Androgens during puberty	Third trimester of pregnancy
Malnutrition	Obesity

Thyroid hormones are necessary for the secretion of GH and potentiate its effects on bone.

Tests of growth hormone secretion

The normal value of plasma growth hormone is 0 to 3ng/ml in normal children and adults.

In suspected growth hormone deficiency tests are made to see if plasma GH levels can be elevated.

Tests for growth hormone deficiency

1   Insulin tolerance test.
This test should be conducted with care since it involves induction of hypoglycaemia. Hypoglycaemia stimulates the release of GH and normally the intravenous administration of 0.1 unit of soluble insulin/Kg body weight will cause an increase in plasma GH to more than 8ng/ml at 30–60 minutes after injection.

2   Exercise increases GH output.

3   Arginine infusion which increases GH secretion.

4   L-Dopa. 500mg causes an increase in plasma GH within 30–60 minutes of administration.

Tests for growth hormone excess

1   Estimation of plasma GH.

2   Glucose tolerance test.
The hyperglycaemia will cause a fall in the plasma growth hormone levels to less than 5ng/ml in normal subjects, but not in patients with pituitary gigantism or acromegaly.

Disturbances of growth hormone may be due to a physiological disorder or consequent upon tumour growth.

Growth hormone – gigantism

19

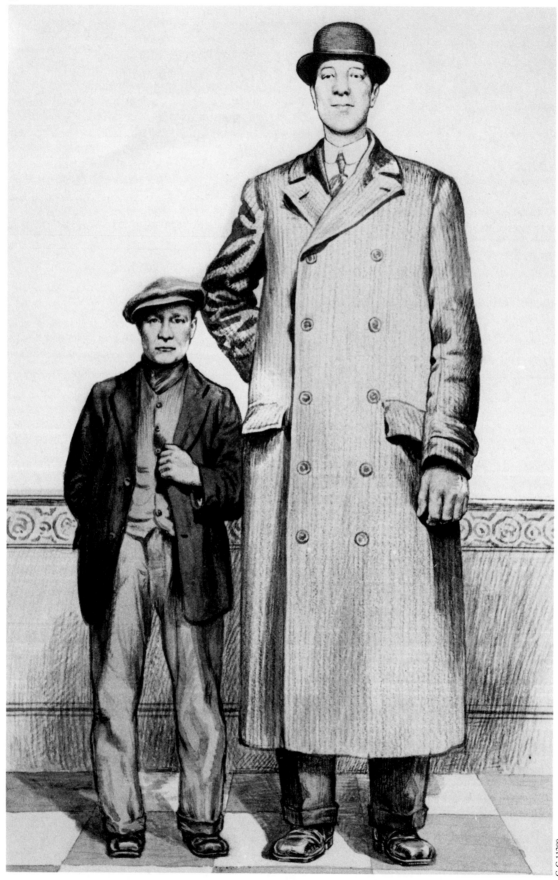

G.C.11280

The effects of hormone overproduction prior to epiphyseal fusion were recorded by Mohr in 1840 and named Gigantism.

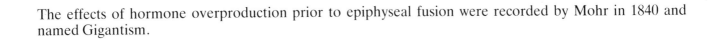

This patient was seen at the age of 20 and it was noted that growth was continuing. He was 7 feet 8 inches tall and weighed over 22 stone. Radiological examination demonstrated failure of fusion of the radius and ulna, and ballooning of the sella turcica, thickening of the vault and enlargement of the lower jaw. His visual acuity was normal. The hands were very large. From the wrist to the tip of the middle finger measured 11½ inches. X-ray showed that there was delay of ossification. The heads of the metacarpals and the base of the thumb metacarpal were fused as they should be at the age of 20.

The illustration shows the comparison of the patient with a man of 5 feet 2 inches.

Atrophy of the gonads with loss of sex hormone secretion occurs. Hypertension and cardiac failure develop at a relatively early age.

This original sketch was presented to the College by Mr. William Robinson in 1920 and was reported in the British Medical Journal in 1921.

Growth hormone – acromegaly

Excessive secretion of GH by an acidophil tumour of the anterior lobe after epiphyseal fusion gives rise to acromegaly. The association of the gross and grotesque deformities of this condition with a tumour of the pituitary was first recognised by Pierre Marie in 1886.

In 1912, Harvey Cushing in his classical dissertation on 'The Pituitary Body and its Disorders' described the hormonal disturbances of acromegaly and also the clinical syndrome which is now associated with his name – Cushing's disease.

Signs of Acromegaly

1 Facial features coarsen. Nose, ears and lips are large and lower jaw protrudes (prognathism). Supra-orbital ridges more marked.

2 Increased size of hands and feet. Hands spade-like. Thickening of soft-tissues leads to carpal tunnel syndrome.

3 Headache and visual field disturbances, bitemporal hemianopia, from pressure by pituitary tumour.

4 Tongue, heart, thyroid and liver enlarge. Hypertension in 35% of patients with acromegaly. Cardiomyopathy.

5 Gynaecomastia and lactation.

6 Abnormal glucose tolerance tests due to the diabetogenic effects of GH.

20

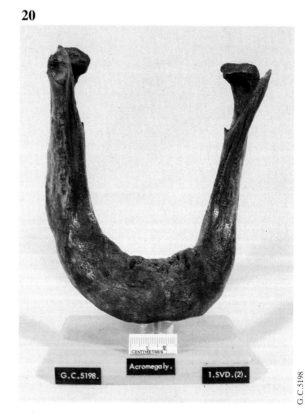

20 Mandible showing the changes associated with acromegaly. The whole of the mandible shares the enlargement. This is especially marked in the anterior part. The alveolar process has undergone great change with loss of the teeth. The mental protuberance is particularly enlarged. The rami are increased in height.

Course of disease

21

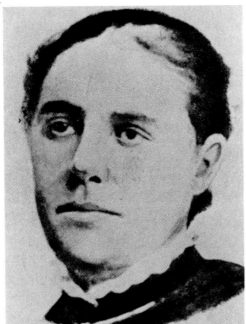

21 Aged 25 years.

21a

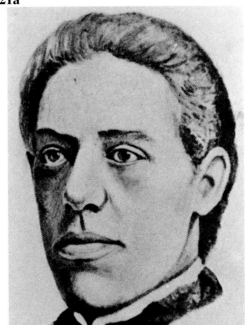

21a Aged 26 years.

21b

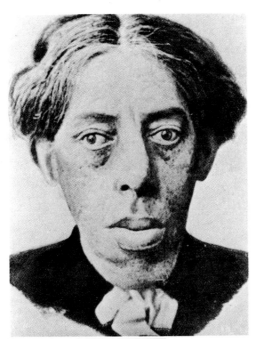

21b Aged 42 years.

21c

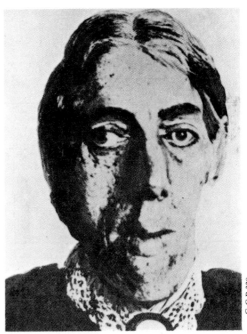

21c Aged 49 years.

This patient, who died at the age of 50, had suffered from evidence of acromegaly for 25 years. Her hands and feet showed the typical deformities of acromegaly and she suffered from loss of vision of the right eye. At post mortem examination there was distension of the sella turcica but no note was recorded of the pituitary tumour which obviously was present.

Growth hormone – tumours

Excessive GH secretion usually results from the presence of an acidophil adenoma of the anterior lobe of the pituitary. Such tumours may be composed mainly of strongly acidophilic cells or may contain poorly granulated cells or a variable admixture with chromophobes.

The tumours vary in size from those which measure only a few mm in diameter to those which expand beyond the pituitary fossa and compress the adjacent structures. Even the small tumours may produce marked hormonal effects.

22

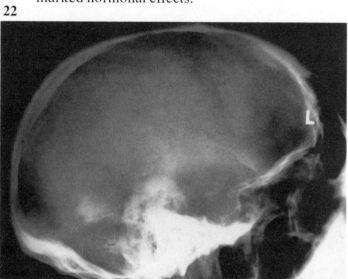

22 From an adult male. The X-ray shows typical enlargement of the pituitary fossa secondary to the adenoma, with very large paranasal sinuses which reflect the generalised bony overgrowth in such cases.

Histology

Acidophil adenomas are usually composed of closely packed rounded or polygonal cells with fairly abundant cytoplasm full of acidophilic granules. Nuclei are generally regular and mitotic activity is low. The cells are usually arranged in solid masses but occasionally some attempt at a columnar or papillary arrangement can be seen.

23

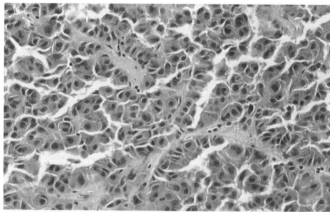

23 Pituitary. An acidophil adenoma composed of large, fairly regular eosinophilic cells supported by delicate stroma. There is some variation in nuclear size but no mitotic activity can be seen. *(H&E ×312)*

Dwarfism

Hyposecretion of GH is one of the causes of dwarfism. Other causes are absence of somatomedin and diminished response to GH or somatomedin by the target tissues, e.g. Turner's syndrome. GH hyposecretion also occurs in Simmonds' disease.

Prolactin

Prolactin is produced by the acidophil cells of the anterior pituitary. It has a similar structure to growth hormone and human placental lactogen (HPL). In females the plasma level is 8 ng/ml and in males 5 ng/ml.

Functions

In female

1   It causes milk secretion from the breast after oestrogen and progesterone have caused lobulo-alveolar development. During pregnancy the plasma prolactin rises steadily, reaching a peak of 10–20 times the non-pregnant value at term. During pregnancy lactation is inhibited by high circulating levels of oestrogen and progesterone, but when these decline post partum, prolactin causes milk secretion. Prolactin levels fall to normal about one week after childbirth but rise on each occasion of breast feeding.

2   It prevents ovulation in lactating women by
   (a)   inhibiting GnRH secretion
   (b)   inhibiting the action of GnRH on the anterior pituitary and
   (c)   inhibiting the action of FSH and LH on the ovary and thus inhibiting ovulation.

3   It has also been suggested that prolactin is involved in the handling of sodium, potassium and water by the kidney.

In male

In the male, prolactin secreted by the pituitary binds to receptors on the Leydig cell and facilitates the action of LH in causing the release of testosterone. Testosterone facilitates the release of prolactin from the anterior pituitary.

Regulation of prolactin secretion in the female

The hormonal control of prolactin secretion is mainly inhibitory, caused by a prolactin inhibitory hormone (dopamine) produced by the arcuate nucleus of the hypothalamus (**24**). It has also been postulated that there is a prolactin releasing hormone although this has not been isolated.

Prolactin *(Continued)*

Factors which may affect prolactin secretion

Increase		Decrease
Nipple stimulation – suckling		L dopa
Oestrogens	Pregnancy	Bromocriptine
TRH	Exercise	Negative feedback
Hypoglycaemia	Stress	i.e. prolactin stimulates
Sleep	Chlorpromazine	hypothalamic neurones to
Renal failure		secrete dopamine and thus inhibit
		further release

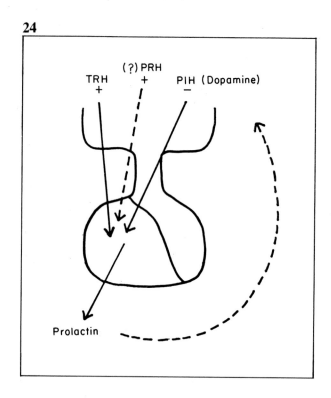

24

Causes of severe hyperprolactinaemia

Acidophil adenomas (prolactinomas) of the pituitary. Dopamine receptor blocking drugs, e.g. chlorpromazine. Lesions, e.g. trauma, sarcoidosis that damage the infundibulum thus impairing the inhibitory influence of the hypothalamus on the pituitary.

Clinical effects of hypersecretion of prolactin

As a result of hyperprolactinaemia the following effects may be observed. Bilateral gynaecomastia (if oestrogens increased or androgens reduced). Galactorrhoea. Impotence. Infertility. Menstrual disturbances. Moderate obesity.

Prolactin function tests

Tests	Responses		
	Normal	Hyperprolactinaemia	Hypopituitarism
Radio-immunoassay of plasma PRL	Female 8ng/ml Male 5ng/ml	Increase	Decrease
Chlorpromazine stimulation	Increase		No increase
Insulin-induced hypoglycaemia	Increase		
Bromocriptine and L dopa	Decrease	Decrease	

Hormones secreted by the basophil cells of the pituitary

ACTH

The ACTH secreting cell (corticotroph) is an APUD cell. In this cell the precursor molecule for ACTH is pro-opiomelanocortin, which within the cell is cleaved into ACTH and ß lipotrophin (ß LPH). On stimulation, both of these substances are secreted. Small amounts of ß endorphin and ∝MSH are also secreted. Both ACTH and ß LPH have MSH activity within their molecules. The function of ß LPH is at present unknown; it is known to contain the amino acid sequence of ß endorphin within the molecule.

ACTH stimulates the secretion of glucocorticoids from the zona fasciculata and androgens from the zona reticularis of the adrenal cortex. In large amounts, e.g. following trauma or surgery, ACTH will increase the secretion of aldosterone from the zona glomerulosa.

25

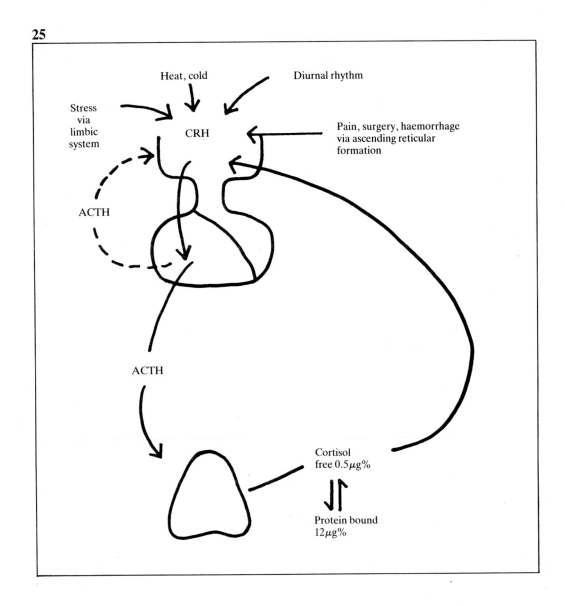

ACTH *(Continued)*

Control of release

1 Feedback mechanisms

Cortisol secreted by the z. fasciculata is carried in the blood both attached to protein and in free form. It is the free form which feeds back to the hypothalamus to regulate the release of corticotrophin releasing hormone (CRH).

Long feedbacks

(a)   When the free cortisol level is high, this inhibits the release of CRH and therefore ACTH (negative feedback). When the free cortisol level falls, CRH output and consequently ACTH output rises.

(b)   Cortisol may also feedback on to the corticotrophic cells of the anterior pituitary to inhibit ACTH release directly.

Short feedbacks

ACTH itself also feeds back onto the hypothalamic centre which mediates CRH release to control its activity (the short feedback loop).

2 Diurnal rhythm

Output of ACTH and consequently cortisol shows a diurnal variation. Output of these hormones starts to rise at about 6 a.m. reaching a peak at around 10 a.m. The lowest secretion rate for ACTH occurs at approximately 12 midnight. The 'clock' regulating the diurnal rhythm for ACTH is situated in the hypothalamus – possibly in the suprachiasmatic nucleus.

3 Stress

Stress can increase CRH and therefore ACTH secretion via two pathways
(a)   via the limbic system in the case of fear and anxiety.
(b)   via the ascending reticular formation in the case of trauma, surgery and haemorrhage. Excessive cold and heat (thermal stress) can also cause the release of CRH.

Clinical effects of excessive production of hormones by basophil cells

Excessive ACTH production from either hyperplasis of the basophil cells or from basophil microadenomas which may be multiple causes Cushing's disease. The clinical features are due to adrenal cortical hyperfunction. (See page 273.)

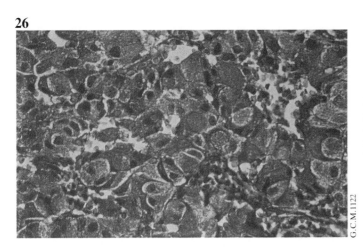

26 Pituitary. A vascular basophil adenoma composed of cells filled with purple-staining granules. There is no nuclear pleomorphism or mitotic activity. *(Slidders' ×625)*

Lipotrophin (LPH)

Primary disorders of LPH hypersecretion or hyposecretion have not been recognised, but LPH levels commonly parallel ACTH levels and account for the pigmentation found in such conditions as Addison's disease and Nelson's syndrome.

In Addison's disease the destruction of adrenal tissue and hence lack of negative feedback lead to excessive production of these hormones.

A similar mechanism operates in Nelson's syndrome where grossly excessive skin pigmentation may follow some years after adrenalectomy for Cushing's disease.

Thyrotrophin (TSH)

TSH is a glycoprotein (½ life approximately 1 hour), containing $\propto$ and ß chains. T_3 and T_4 are carried in the blood mainly bound to protein, but a very small percentage (0.02%) in the case of T_4 is free. The secretion of TSH is controlled by a negative feedback mainly to the anterior pituitary, high levels of free T_4 inhibiting the release of TSH.

27

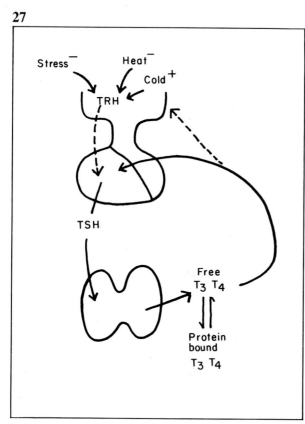

27 There is also a minor feedback of T_3 and T_4 to the hypothalamus. The hypothalamus produces a tripeptide thyroid releasing hormone (TRH) possibly in the dorso-medial nucleus of the hypothalamus, which increases the secretion of TSH. TRH regulates secretion of TSH in special situations, e.g. increased TSH secretion following prolonged exposure to cold, and decreased TSH secretion on exposure to a hot environment. Stress tends to decrease TSH secretion via glucocorticoids inhibiting TRH production.

Effects of TSH on the thyroid

TSH stimulates the thyroid acinar cells. It increases:
1. iodide uptake.
2. the synthesis of mono- and di-iodotyrosine, and of tri-iodothyronine (T_3) and thyroxine (T_4).
3. the proteolysis of colloid.
4. the secretion of T_3 and T_4.
5. thyroid gland blood flow.

Abnormalities of TSH secretion

Hypersecretion is found in primary hypothyroidism. Hyposecretion is found in hypothyroidism secondary to pituitary lesions. In this situation the clinical picture depends on the degree of pituitary hypofunction.

Hypothalamo-pituitary-gonadal interdependence

FSH and LH in the female

Both are concerned in the development of ovarian follicles.

FSH stimulates the initial growth of the ovarian (Graafian) follicle.

LH causes the final maturation of the ovarian follicle, ovulation, the formation of the corpus luteum and its secretion of progesterone.

The secretion of FSH and LH is under the control of a single releasing hormone, gonadotrophin releasing hormone (GnRH), produced in the medial pre-optic area of the hypothalamus. It is a peptide containing 10 amino acids.

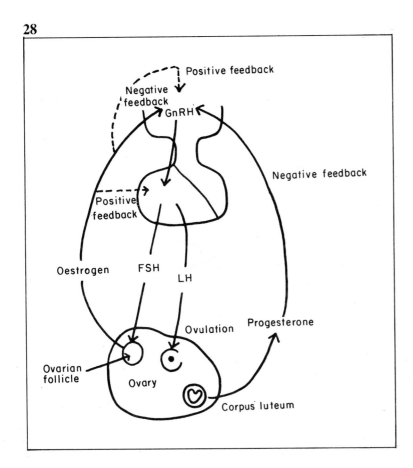

28

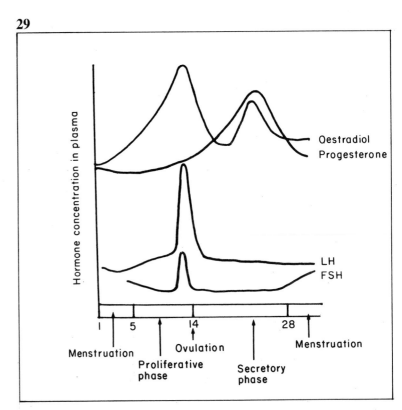

29

Menstrual cycle

The standard menstruation cycle is of 28 days duration, menstruation occurring from day one to day five and ovulation at day 14.

At day 26 to 28 of the cycle preceding the one under consideration, luteolysis of the corpus luteum occurs, with a resultant fall in oestrogen and progesterone secretion. The endometrium is shed and menstruation follows. The fall in the plasma levels of oestrogen and progesterone reduces the negative feedback on the hypothalamus and this in turn leads to the release of gonadotrophin releasing hormone and consequently a small rise in the plasma levels of FSH (especially) and LH.

Under the influence of FSH, 10 to 12 ovarian follicles begin to develop and oestrogen is secreted by them. One of the follicles which has developed faster than the rest secretes a significantly higher quantity of oestrogen which exerts a negative feedback on the hypothalamus to shut off GnRH and thus FSH. The development of this follicle is now independent of FSH, but when FSH secretion declines the other less mature follicles regress. The remaining follicle continues its development to become a mature Graafian follicle, secreting large amounts of oestrogen reaching a peak just prior to ovulation (secretion of 200–300ug/day; plasma oestradiol 200pg/ml). This peak of oestrogen secretion induces the secretion of GnRH and LH activity by positive feedback. The mechanism by which oestradiol acts on the hypothalamo-pituitary axis to induce GnRH and subsequently LH (and FSH) from the anterior pituitary is not fully understood.

At about day 13 of the cycle, there is a spike of LH secretion from the anterior pituitary. There is also a smaller spike of FSH secretion. These peaks are only of short duration but they cause changes in the follicle leading to ovulation which occurs 6–18 hours after the surge of LH. LH is also responsible for the formation of the corpus luteum and the secretion of progesterone. The oocyte recommences meiosis proceeding from the diplotene phase where it has been halted since foetal life to metaphase two of the second meiotic division.

Between days 14 and 20 of the cycle, the corpus luteum matures, and increasing secretion by it of oestrogen and progesterone causes a negative feedback at hypothalamic level on the release of GnRH. Its output falls and with it the outputs of FSH and LH. The corpus luteum is fully mature at about day 21 and is maintained until about day 26. The presence of prolactin does not appear to be essential for the maintenance of the corpus luteum.

Around days 26 to 28 of the cycle, luteolysis of the corpus luteum occurs, but the cause of this regression is not known. If the ovum is fertilised, the implanting blastocyst produces human chorionic gonadotrophin and this rescues the corpus luteum from luteolysis. However, in the absence of pregnancy luteolysis results in a fall in oestrogen and progesterone secretion. This leads to menstruation and the secretion of FSH and LH and hence commencement of a new menstrual cycle.

Tests of hypothalamo – pituitary – ovarian function

1   Measurement of gonadotrophin either in plasma or 24 hour urine sample. If a daily estimation of the plasma levels of gonadotrophins is performed, a pre-ovulatory surge in LH should be observed.

2   Gonadotrophin hormone releasing test. Plasma levels of FSH and LH are estimated six to eight hours after administration of synthetic GnRH subcutaneously.

3   Clomiphene test. If clomiphene is given orally for five days and if the hypothalamo-pituitary axis is intact, there should be a rise in the plasma levels of the gonadotrophins LH and FSH. Clomiphene, by blocking the effect of oestrogen at receptor sites in the hypothalamus, stimulates the release of GnRH and therefore LH and FSH.

4   Ovarian hormones.
   (a)   Urinary oestrogen in 24 hour urine sample. Peak urine output 24 hours prior to ovulation.

   (b)   Plasma oestradiol shows two peaks
      i.   24 hours prior to ovulation
      ii.   also in the luteal phase

   (c)   Plasma progesterone – low values pre-ovulatory, but increased values in the luteal phase.

   (d)   Urinary pregnanediol excretion. Low values before ovulation but increased excretion in the luteal phase.

5   Prolactin. See section on prolactin.

FSH and LH in males

Luteinizing hormone. LH stimulates the Leydig cells of the testis to produce testosterone. Testosterone in the plasma feeds back to the hypothalamus where it influences the release of gonadotrophic hormone releasing hormone and hence LH. A reduction in the circulating level of testosterone will cause an increased output of GnRH and LH. This in turn will stimulate the Leydig cells of the testis to increase testosterone output (negative feedback control mechanism).

Follicle stimulating hormone. FSH stimulates spermatogenesis in the testicular seminiferous tubules.

30

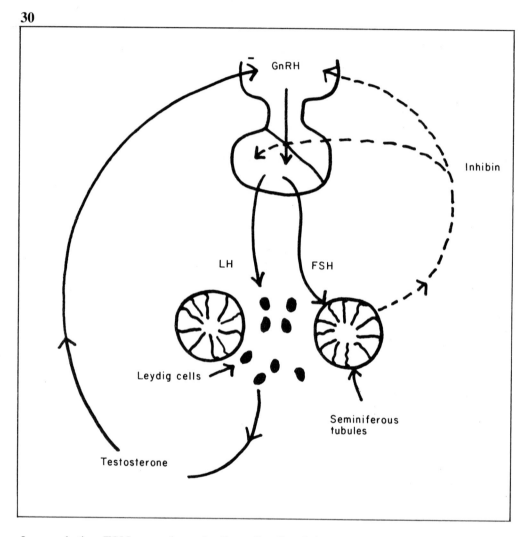

In regulating FSH secretion, the Sertoli cells of the seminiferous tubules produce a protein called Inhibin, which feeds back:
1 to the anterior pituitary to reduce the quantity of FSH released when the FSH containing cells are exposed to GnRH and
2 to the hypothalamus to reduce its GnRH output.

Tests of gonadotrophin production

1   Radio immunoassay of plasma FSH and LH.

2   Gonadotrophic hormone releasing hormone stimulation test. Following the administration of synthetic GnRH there is a rise in the output of FSH and LH and testosterone if the anterior pituitary is functioning normally. In primary hypogonadism, the basal secretion of FSH and LH is increased. In secondary hypogonadism, the rise in plasma FSH, LH and testosterone on GnRH stimulation is reduced or absent.

3   Clomiphene stimulation test. Clomiphene causes the release of GnRH and this in turn stimulates the secretion of FSH and LH and testosterone. This is a test of the hypothalamo-pituitary axis. In hypopituitarism the response is absent or reduced.

4   Radioimmunoassay or competitive protein binding assay for testosterone. Plasma testosterone varies irregularly throughout the day between 4 and 10ng/ml in males between the age of 20 and 50 years. In both primary and secondary hypogonadism, the plasma level of testosterone is low; in primary hypogonadism the plasma levels of FSH and LH are elevated, whereas in secondary hypogonadism they are reduced.

The posterior pituitary

Contains two hormones:

(a) ADH. Anti-diuretic hormone (vasopressin)

(b) Oxytocin

31

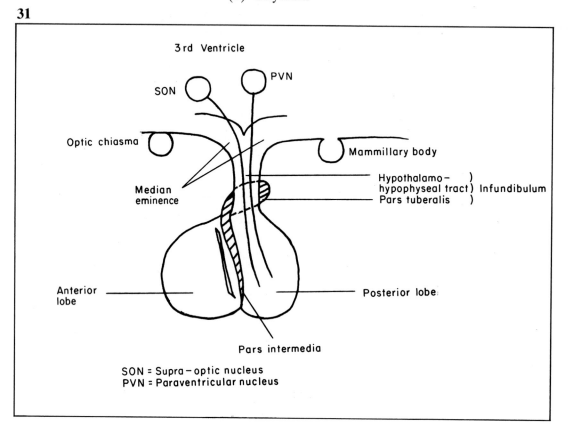

SON = Supra – optic nucleus
PVN = Paraventricular nucleus

Synthesis of posterior pituitary hormones

The two hormones of the posterior pituitary gland are synthesized in the endoplasmic reticulum of cell bodies of the neurones in the Supra-Optic and Paraventricular nuclei of the hypothalamus. After synthesis, they are packaged into granular vesicles and transported down the axons of these neurones, which make up the hypothalamo-hypophyseal tract, and are stored in nerve terminals in the posterior pituitary. ADH is mainly synthesized in the supra-optic nucleus and oxytocin in the paraventricular nucleus.

On synthesis, the hormones are contained within a larger prohormone molecule, that for ADH called pre-propressophysin and that for oxytocin called preprooxyphysin. During axonal transport, the prohormone is cleaved into the hormone and its respective neurophysin.

Release of posterior pituitary hormones

Calcium is necessary for the release of the hormones.

On activation of the particular nucleus action potentials pass down the axons connected to the cell bodies of this nucleus. The permeability of the nerve terminal to calcium is increased and as a result both the hormone and its associated neurophysin are released into the blood stream.

Actions of antidiuretic hormone (ADH)

ADH increases the permeability of the distal convoluted tubules (DCT) and collecting ducts (CD) to water so that water passes from the distal nephron into the hypertonic medullary interstitium. ADH works via activation of adenyl cyclase and cyclic adenosine monophosphate (cAMP); cAMP activates a kinase which phosphorylates a component of the membrane of cells lining the collecting duct, leading to an increased permeability of the membrane to water. Prostaglandin E modulates the effects of ADH. In large amounts ADH is a powerful vasoconstrictor.

Normally 75% of the glomerular filtrate (GF) is absorbed in the PCT and 5% in the loop of Henle.

In the absence of ADH 8% is absorbed in the DCT and CD and 12% of the GF is excreted in the urine (15ml/min: osmolarity – 50mosmoles/L).

By contrast in the presence of maximum ADH secretion 19.7% of the GF is absorbed in DCT and CD and only 0.3% appears in the urine (0.375ml/min: osmolarity – 1300mosmoles/L).

Increased ADH secretion	**Decreased ADH secretion**
Raised osmotic pressure of plasma	Lowered OP of plasma
Decreased extracellular fluid (ECF) volume	Increased ECF volume
Pain, surgery and trauma (via ß endorphin)	Alcohol
Exercise, pulmonary infection and congestive heart failure.	
Head injury	

Drugs: Morphine, Nicotine, Barbiturates, clofibrate, chlorpropamide, carbamezapine.

Syndrome of inappropriate ADH secretion.

Influence of plasma osmotic pressure

A rise in the osmotic pressure of the plasma increases the discharge from osmoreceptor cells in the supra-optic nucleus of the hypothalamus and increases ADH release from the posterior pituitary. There is also stimulation of neurones in the lateral hypothalamus (the thirst centre) and this causes the sensation of thirst.

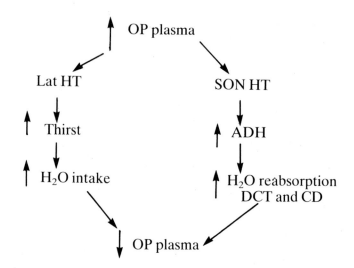

A decrease in the osmotic pressure of the plasma results in decreased stimulation of osmoreceptors in the supra-optic nucleus, leading to decreased ADH output. At the same time a reduction in stimulation of osmoreceptor cells in the lateral hypothalamus reduces the sensation of thirst. The osmolarity of the plasma is maintained at 280mosmoles/L.

Influence of ECF volume

The extracellular fluid (ECF) volume also affects ADH secretion. Sensors of circulating blood volume (part of the ECF volume) are present in the great veins and in the right and left atria, the volume receptors. ADH is released even though the plasma osmolarity is normal. It is seen especially after haemorrhage.

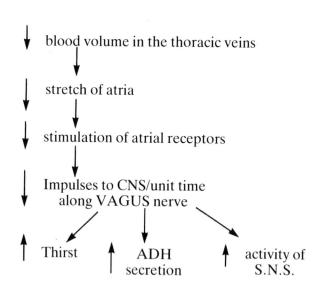

Inappropriate secretion of ADH

In this condition the secretion of ADH is not under normal control. The syndrome can be produced by:

Ectopic production of ADH by carcinoma of ── bronchus (particularly oat cell)
                                            ╲ pancreas etc.

Effects of abnormal secretion of ADH

ADH insufficiency (diabetes insipidus).

Cranial diabetes insipidus is characterised by polyuria and secondary polydipsia. It may be idiopathic and familial but more commonly results from lesions such as tumour, granuloma or trauma damaging the hypothalamus, the pituitary stalk or the posterior pituitary. It has been shown recently that a degree of diabetes insipidus is common in Sheehan's syndrome.

ADH hypersecretion

Excess secretion leads to hyponatraemia and water intoxication. These effects may be brought about by intra or extracranial disease causing excessive release of ADH from the pituitary, or by a variety of drugs which have a similar action or cause increased sensitivity to normal amounts of ADH. They may also be caused by abnormal secretion of a tumour such as bronchial carcinoma.

Oxytocin

The function of oxytocin in males is not known.

Effects of oxytocin secretion in females.

Oxytocin secretion enhances milk ejection in the lactating breast, and contraction of the uterus. ·

Breast

It contracts the myoepithelial cells around the alveoli and lining the small ducts of the breast. This leads to milk let down and increased milk ejection into the large ducts and the nipple. The receptors mediating the response are touch receptors situated around the nipple. Impulses pass along fibres connected to these touch receptors and enter the posterior nerve roots of the spinal cord and ascend in the posterior columns. After traversing synapses in the dorsal column nuclei and the postero-ventral nucleus of the thalamus, impulses are relayed to the post-central gyrus and to the paraventricular nucleus of the hypothalamus stimulating oxytocin release. In lactating women, emotional stimuli also cause oxytocin release via the limbic system and hypothalamus. Oxytocin release is part of the suckling response.

Uterus

The response of contraction of uterine muscle to oxytocin is increased by oestrogens and decreased by progesterone. As pregnancy nears term, the uterus becomes more sensitive to oxytocin and oxytocin release may play some part in the complex process of initiation of labour.

During labour, oxytocin secretion is markedly increased; dilatation of the cervix and vagina consequent upon descent of the head leads, via neural afferent pathways, to stimulation of the paraventricular nucleus and increased release of oxytocin from the posterior pituitary.

Oxytocin released during coitus may, by increasing uterine contractions, aid the passage of sperm into the Fallopian tubes.

Effects of abnormal secretion of oxytocin.

Apart from an otherwise unexplained failure of suckling due to deficiency, the effects of abnormal secretion of this hormone are not known.

Pituitary insufficiency

Hypopituitarism may be acute or chronic and may have a variety of causes.

Acute hypopituitarism

In the *female* when obstetric services are inadequate, necrosis of the adenohypophysis resulting from post-partum haemorrhage is the usual cause (Sheehan's syndrome). Hypotensive shock precipitates thrombosis of vessels in the involuting pituitary producing a disastrous infarction which may prove fatal. In less severe cases varying degrees of chronic hypopituitarism persist.

In the *male* rarely acute hypopituitarism results from head injury and fracture of the skull.

In *both sexes* surgical or radiation treatment of the pituitary may result in acute hypopituitarism.

Chronic hypopituitarism

(Simmonds' disease)

Usual causes: Post-partum infarction of adenohypophysis, or chromophobe adenoma of pituitary

Other causes: Impaired function resulting from pituitary surgery or radiotherapy.
Infective granulomas of pituitary.
Pressure by cyst and non-functioning tumour.
Tumour metastases in the pituitary.
Head injury involving skull fracture.

32

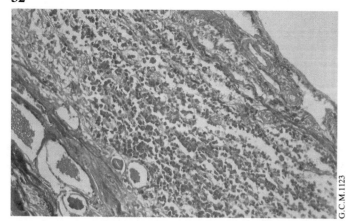

32 Pituitary atrophy. The adeno-hypophysis has been reduced to a thin strand of tissue which is virtually devoid of acidophil cells. *(Slidders' ×50)*

Effects of hypopituitarism

1   Deficiency of ACTH. As a result adrenal zonae fasciculata and reticularis atrophy early leading to decreased glucocorticoids and sex hormones. Basal secretion of aldosterone is satisfactory for some time but there is no stress-induced aldosterone secretion.

2   Deficiency of ACTH and MSH – melanin deficiency – pallor of skin.

3   Growth hormone deficiency – dwarfism in children.

4   Deficiency of TSH – thyroid function depressed – cold is poorly tolerated.

5   Deficiency of gonadotrophic hormones – gonads atrophy and sex cycles stop – some secondary sex characteristics disappear – loss of pubic and facial hair.

6   Tendency to hypoglycaemia when fasted due to deficiency of GH and ACTH.

7   Tendency to stress-induced coma – adrenal and thyroid insufficiency – hypoglycaemia and hypothermia.

8   In cases of pituitary ablation – loss of ADH – transient polyuria.

33

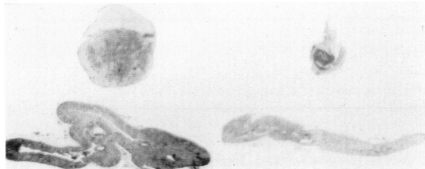

G.C.M.1124

33   Hypopituitarism. The atrophic pituitary and adrenal contrast with the more normal glands on the left.

Hypopituitarism may be of varying degree. It may be limited to congenital deficiency of one or more hormones resulting from pituitary or hypothalamic abnormality. On the other hand the effects of a large tumour may impair virtually all of the functions of the anterior or of the posterior lobe and affect the hypothalamus. The hypothalamus may also be damaged as a result of radiotherapy for such a tumour.

The degree of hypopituitarism and the rapidity of its onset will obviously depend upon the nature and extent of the disease causing it. For example, in post-partum necrosis virtually all the anterior pituitary functions are affected and the disease starts abruptly. By contrast non-specific pressure effects of tumours resulting in hypopituitarism are usually of gradual onset but may eventually result in panhypopituitarism and hypothalamic abnormalities.

The clinical effects of hypopituitarism also depend upon the age and development of the patient at its onset and this is particularly important in the case of growth hormone.

Non-functioning cysts and tumours affecting the pituitary

These include, chromophobe adenomas and carcinomas, cysts of Rathke pouch remnants and cranio-pharyngiomas, epidermoid cysts, suprasellar meningiomas and tumours of the sphenoid.

Chromophobe tumours and craniopharyngiomas are those which occur most frequently.

The pituitary may also be the site of metastatic carcinoma.

Chromophobe adenoma

These tumours were formerly considered to constitute about two thirds of all pituitary adenomas. However, some adenomas which appear chromophobe by conventional staining methods produce hypersecretory hormonal effects and can be shown by ultramicroscopy to have secretory granules of somatotrophic or galactotrophic nature. Other secretory cells may be identified by immunoperoxidase staining.

Nevertheless many chromophobe tumours exert their clinical effects not by hypersecretion but by destroying adjacent tissues as they grow. A small proportion of such tumours are locally malignant either ab initio or from carcinomatous change in an adenoma.

Pathology

Chromophobe adenomas are usually soft and vary in colour from grey-white to red depending on their vascularity. In the larger tumours necrosis, haemorrhage and cyst formation may occur.

34

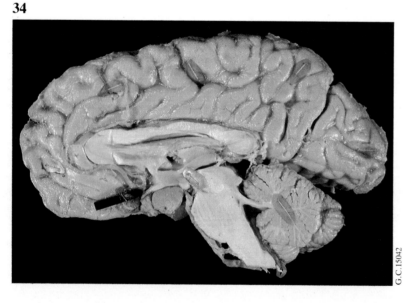

G.C.15042

34 Adenoma of the pituitary. Note its relationship to the optic chiasma (black pointer) and the hypothalamus.

As pituitary tumours expand they balloon the sella turcica and cause pressure effects on adjoining structures.

35

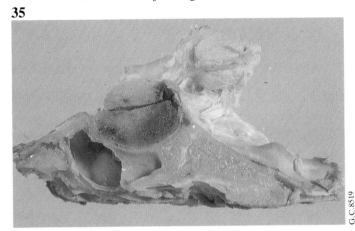

G.C.8519

35 A pituitary adenoma in a male aged 26 years. The tumour had expanded the sella turcica and had caused hypo-thalamic pressure effects including hypogonadism.

36

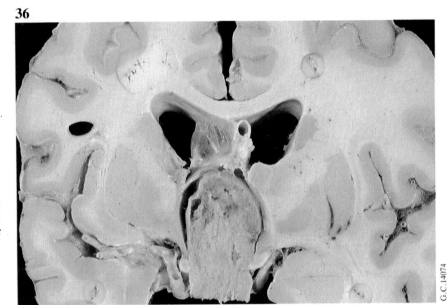

G.C.14074

36 Chromophobe adenoma in a male aged 50 years. Symptoms of a thalamic disturbance had been present for 15 years and there was radiological evidence of a filling defect in the third ventricle, but the outline of the sella turcica was normal. In this unusual case the enlargement was suprasellar. The tumour which shows slight cystic change has filled the third ventricle and caused some obstruction of the foramen of Monro.

Tomography

37

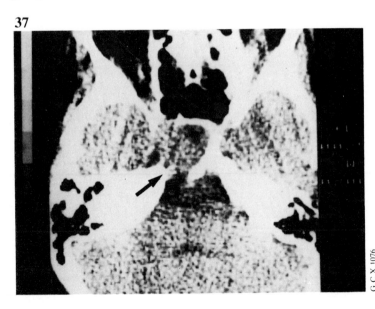

G.C.X.1076

37 Computerised tomography with or without contrast enhancement can give additional information in the diagnosis of pituitary tumours. Transverse section viewed from above showing erosion of the left side of the dorsum sellae by the tumour.

Chromophobe adenoma *(Continued)*

Histology

It is conventional to divide chromophobe adenomas into three histological types.

1 Diffuse   2 Sinusoidal   3 Papillary

Whilst recognition of these patterns is useful to avoid confusion with other intracranial tumours there may be transition between them and even multiplicity of patterns in the one tumour.

Diffuse tumours are composed of rounded or polygonal cells with prominent nuclei and chromophobe agranular cytoplasm irregularly supported by vascular stroma. The nuclei may be regular or show variation in size and density according to the rapidity of growth. If carcinomatous change is present the irregularity becomes more pronounced and mitotic figures appear.

In sinusoidal and papillary tumours the arrangement of cells and blood vessels is more regular, and the cells and their nuclei, particularly in the papillary form, are enlongated.

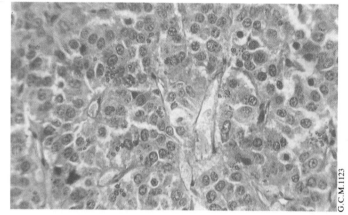

38 Pituitary. A chromophobe adenoma composed of fairly uniform cells showing no mitotic activity. *(Slidders' ×375)*

Parapituitary cysts and craniopharyngiomas

Intrasellar cyst

Intrasellar cysts, usually small, are believed to develop from remnants of Rathke's pouch. They are lined by columnar epithelium, sometimes ciliated.

Suprasellar cyst

These are sometimes solitary cysts lined by squamous epithelium. They cannot be sharply divided from those cystic tumours which are partly solid – the craniopharyngiomas.

Craniopharyngioma

It is believed that these tumours and suprasellar cysts originate in remnants of Rathke's pouch or from nests of squamous epithelial cells, possibly metaplastic, which may be found on the tuber cinereum and the pituitary stalk.

39

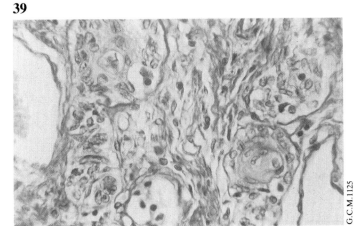

39 Pituitary stalk. Groups of squamoid cells can be seen in the connective tissue of the stalk. *(Slidders' ×500)*

Incidence

They may occur at any age but 50% are met with below the age of 20.

M:F 2:1.

Craniopharyngioma *(Continued)*

Pathology

These tumours are at least partly cystic and commonly vary in size up to 5 cm in diameter. As a result of haemorrhage and of keratinisation calcium may be deposited and foci of ossification may occur and be obvious on radiography.

Most of the tumours are suprasellar. Their growth results in pressure on adjacent structures, and as a result visual disturbance, deficiency of growth hormone and hence dwarfism in children, hypogonadism, and obesity from hypothalamic disturbance may occur.

40

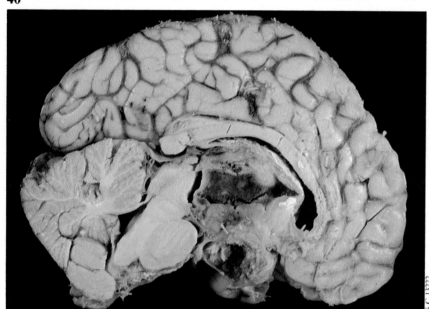

40 From a female aged 16 years. She had headache, vomiting and drowsiness and a right hemiparesis. Radiologically, suprasellar calcification was shown. Ventriculography showed blockage of the foramen of Monro on the right side. At operation a cystic craniopharyngioma was aspirated and partially removed. The patient died two years after operation following recurrence of growth of the tumour and increasing blockage of CSF circulation.

41

41 From a female aged 70. Referred by ophthalmologist who found a pale disc on retinoscopy and diminution in the visual fields.

The skull radiograph shows spotty suprasellar calcification with enlargement of the sella turcica.

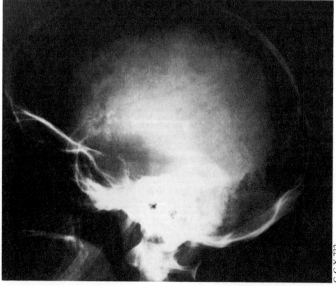

Histology

This may be complex. Features simulating an adamantinoma, basal cell and squamous cell tumours may all be found. The component tissues are well differentiated and there is no malignant tendency.

42

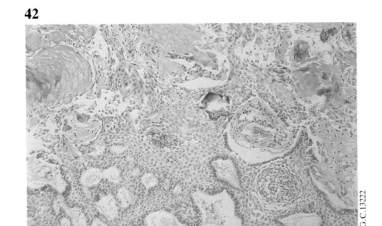

42 Craniopharyngioma. This portion of the tumour includes adamantinomatous-like tissue and masses of pale, degenerating keratinised epithelium. Foci of calcification and multinucleated giant cells can also be seen. *(H&E ×100)*

42a

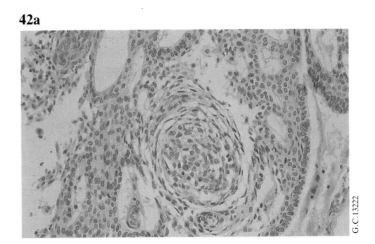

42a Craniopharyngioma. Detail of the epithelium showing palisading of basal cells, microcysts, and epithelial whorls. *(H&E ×250)*

A. D. B. Harrower
M. O. Wright

Development

The development of the thyroid gland commences at the end of the first month of foetal life as a mid-line diverticulum of the anterior wall of the primitive pharynx in the region of the first and second branchial arches. This point in later life corresponds to the foramen caecum at the base of the tongue. The developing thyroid descends over the succeeding weeks to take up its final position in the front of the neck, where it becomes associated with the parathyroid glands and structures arising from the third and fourth arches.

The parafollicular or 'C' cells arise separately from the neural crest.

The anomalies resulting from failure of descent of the thyroglossal duct or from other anomalies of development are considered elsewhere.

Two specimens of the thyroid of normal size and contour. The second specimen shows persistence of the thyroglossal tract at the lower end of which a pyramidal lobe may form.

1a

1

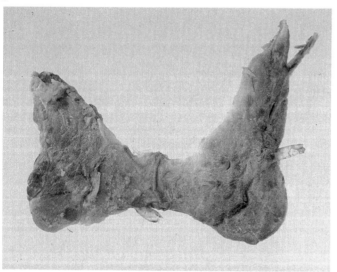

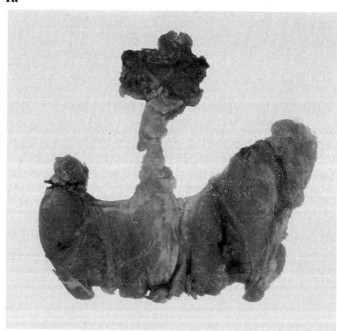

The adult thyroid weighs 20–25 grams and consists of two lateral lobes with a central isthmus which overlies the second, third and fourth rings of the trachea. The lateral lobes closely invest the larynx and trachea and consist of a broad lower pole and a narrow upper pole. In a number of individuals an additional lobe, the pyramidal lobe, arises to the left of the mid-line from the upper border of the isthmus.

Anatomy

The thyroid gland is covered by a true capsule which is a condensation of the fibrous stroma of the gland and is firmly adherent to it. In addition the gland is surrounded by the pretracheal fascia which is attached superiorly to the thyroid cartilage, the cricoid cartilage and the hyoid bone. Between the capsule and the pretracheal fascia is a space which is important because the thyroid vessels cross it as trunks and thereafter ramify on the surface of the gland. The parathyroid glands usually lie in this space on the posterior aspect of the lateral lobes of the thyroid gland, but their number and position are variable.

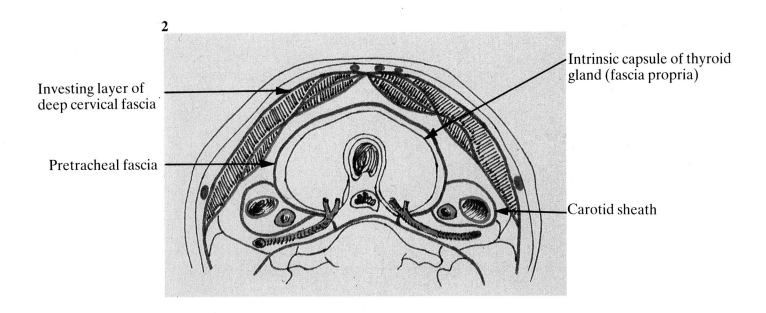

2

Investing layer of deep cervical fascia

Pretracheal fascia

Intrinsic capsule of thyroid gland (fascia propria)

Carotid sheath

Lymphatic drainage

The lymphatics from the thyroid gland mostly drain into the deep cervical lymph nodes along the carotid sheath. In addition there is some drainage to the pretracheal and the brachio-cephalic lymph nodes.

Nerve supply

The nerve supply is entirely autonomic. Non-medullated post ganglionic fibres from the superior and middle cervical sympathetic ganglia enter the thyroid by way of the cardiac nerves, the periarterial plexuses and the superior and recurrent laryngeal nerves. Some of these nerves have a vasomotor function; the majority, however, terminate in close relation to the epithelial cells and have no known function.

Histology

The gland is composed of indistinct lobules separated by connective tissue, each lobule containing 20–40 acini (follicles). The acini are lined by a single layer of cuboidal cells, which rest on a basement membrane and on a rich capillary and lymphatic network. Each acinus contains eosinophilic colloid – a clear, mucoid, iodine containing fluid. The colloid is produced by the cuboidal cells and acts as a store for thyroid hormones, the amount varying inversely with the activity of the gland. The overall histological appearance also varies with the state of activity of the gland but there is a wide variation between different parts of the gland and even in different parts of a single microscope field. In areas of high activity the acini contain little colloid and the lining cells have assumed a large columnar form. Inactivity is associated with involution, 'low' cells and a considerable colloid store.

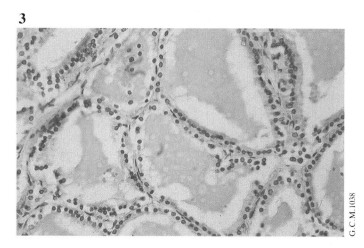

3 Thyroid. A hyperactive portion of a thyroid gland. The epithelium is columnar and the colloid thin and vacuolated. *(H&E ×250)*

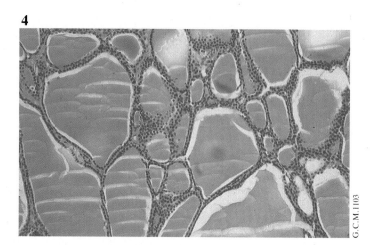

4 Thyroid. Part of a lobule composed of follicles which vary in size. Low cuboidal cells set upon a basement membrane enclose eosinophilic colloid. The appearances in the gland vary according to its activity, and in the lobule illustrated they suggest relative quiescence. *(H&E ×125)*

The parafollicular or 'C' cells, which have the particular property of secreting calcitonin, are scattered diffusely throughout the thyroid and to a less extent within the thymus and elsewhere in the neck. This is in contrast to the situation in reptiles, amphibia, fish and birds where they are concentrated in the ultimobranchial bodies. These parafollicular cells lie close to the acini but are outside the basement membrane. They are larger than the thyroid acinar cells but they stain less densely. They can be identified by immunohistochemical methods (52 U (**13, 14**)) and by electron microscopy (**5**).

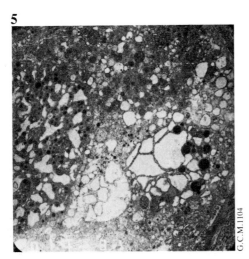

5 This example is derived from a medullary carcinoma but both the neoplastic and the normal 'C' cells show synthesis and storage of small and intermediate-size osmiophilic granules on electronmicroscopy. These are of neuro-endocrine appearance reflecting the neural crest origin of the 'C' cell, a member of the APUD (amine precursor uptake and decarboxylation) series. *(Lead citrate and uranyl acetate ×4000)*

By courtesy of
Dr. K. M. McLaren

Lingual thyroid

Rarely there is a complete failure of descent, the thyroid tissue lying in the base of the tongue (lingual thyroid). Excision of a lingual thyroid may result in the total removal of all thyroid tissue in the body.

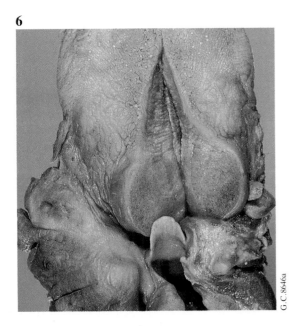

6 Lingual thyroid. The swelling at the base of the tongue was found at necropsy of a woman of 58 years who died from valvular heart disease. There was no history of symptoms arising from the aberrant thyroid tissue. Microscopically the appearances were those of normal thyroid gland.

The swelling has been divided sagittally to reveal glistening thyroid lobules supported by strands of fibrous stroma.

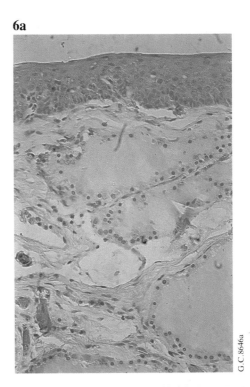

6a Lingual thyroid. Follicles distended by colloid can be seen beneath the squamous epithelium of the tongue. *(H&E ×250)*

Physiology

The function of the thyroid is to produce the iodine containing hormones tetraiodothyronine or thyroxine (T_4) and triiodothyronine (T_3). The first step in this process is the trapping of iodide from the blood by the acinar cells. Iodide absorbed through the stomach and proximal small intestine will provide a plasma concentration of free iodide of less than 1 microgram per 100mls, but by this process of acinar abstraction the local level is raised to 50 times that level. The iodine is bound organically to tyrosine to form monoiodotyrosine and diiodotyrosine. Subsequently, the iodotyrosines are coupled to form triiodothyronine (T_3) and tetraiodothyronine (T_4) – thyroxine, both of which are bound to thyroglobulin and stored in the colloid.

T_3 and T_4 are liberated into the blood stream by proteolytic hydrolysis of thyroglobulin and once liberated 99.98% is bound to the specific carrier protein thyroid binding globulin (TBG) and to a less extent to thyroid binding prealbumin (TBPA) and albumin. All of these plasma proteins have a stronger affinity for T_4 than for T_3 which is not bound to thyroid binding pre-albumin. The protein bound hormones are in equilibrium with the small residual amount of free hormone, which is capable of entering target cells, interacting with specific receptors and thereby influencing intracellular metabolism. Although T_4 comprises 60–90% of the total, T_3 is less firmly bound to protein and is physiologically more active, being more avidly bound by the receptors in the target cell nuclei.

Synthesis and release of hormones by thyroid acinar cell

7

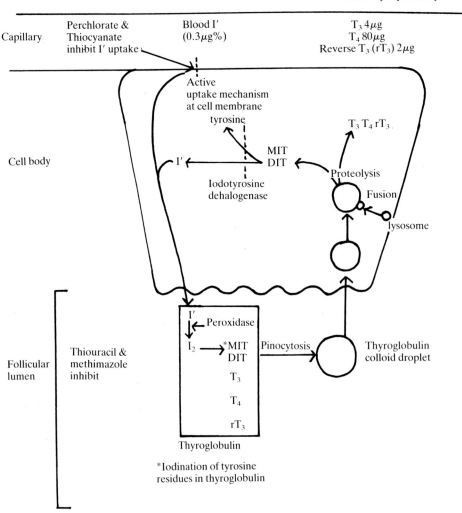

Thyroid hormones in plasma

	T_4	T_3
Total plasma concentration	$8\mu g\%$	$0.15\mu g\%$
Percentage binding to protein	99.98%	99.80%
Percentage binding to TBG	90%	75%
Percentage binding to TBPA	10%	Nil
Percentage binding to albumin	Nil	25%
Free plasma concentration	2ng%	0.3ng%
Half life	6–7 days	2 days

'C' cells of thyroid. C cells produce calcitonin and their function in influencing calcium metabolism is considered on p. 252.

Pituitary and hypothalamic control of thyroid hormone production

Thyroid stimulating hormone (TSH) – thyrotropin – glycoprotein of 25 000 – 30 000 molwt, is secreted by the basophil cells of the anterior pituitary and influences the output of thyroid hormones from the thyroid. It increases the uptake of iodide by the gland, accelerates the synthesis of thyroxine and T_3, and enhances the breakdown of storage thyroglobulin, consequently maintaining the blood T_3 and T_4 levels.

Histologically prolonged TSH stimulation leads to an increase in size and vascularity of the gland with an increase in the number of acini, the height and activity of the follicular epithelium and a reduction in the amount of colloid.

Secretion of TSH by the pituitary is itself controlled by a tripeptide thyrotropin releasing hormone (TRH) which is secreted by the hypothalamus and passes to the pituitary by way of the portal venous system between these organs. The nature of this higher centre control through TRH is largely unknown but stress, emotion and environmental temperatures are all known to affect it. A negative feedback mechanism, by which the blood levels of thyroid hormones influence the activity of TSH, is generally recognised, and is mediated through the effects of thyroid hormones at the pituitary level.

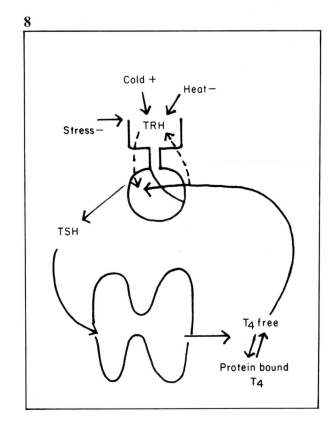

215

Mechanism of action of thyroid hormones

T_3, T_4 enter cells

T_4 converted intracellularly to T_3

T_3 enters nucleus and binds to non-histone proteins in chromatin
$$\downarrow$$
DNA transcription $\rightarrow$ Increased synthesis of mRNA
$$\downarrow$$
Increased protein synthesis in ribosomes
$$\downarrow$$
Production of enzymes which affect cell function and exert actions of thyroid hormones at cellular level.

Hormones – functions

1 Increased oxygen consumption accompanying an increased metabolic rate

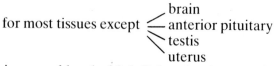

for most tissues except ⟨ brain / anterior pituitary / testis / uterus

An increased level of 2:3 diphosphoglycerate (DPG) in the red cells aids oxygen transfer to the tissues.

2 Small doses of thyroid hormones produce a positive nitrogen balance but larger doses lead to increased loss of nitrogen in the urine as a result of muscle breakdown and loss of protein from bone. Loss of bone protein in this state leads to osteoporosis. Muscle breakdown leads to creatinuria and loss of potassium and a thyrotoxic myopathy.

3 Thyroid hormones are essential for normal brain development and function.

Hypothyroidism

Deficiency of thyroid hormones when the brain is developing causes mental deficiency brought about by decrease in brain weight, in myelination and dendrite branching, and by reduced cholinesterase and succinic dehydrogenase. In the adult hypothyroidism results in slow cerebration and prolongation of reflex times.

Hyperthyroidism

The potentiating effects of thyroid hormones and catecholamines result in restlessness, irritability and acceleration of reflex time.

4 Thyroid hormone is required for normal growth and development. It stimulates the output of growth hormone from the anterior pituitary and potentiates its effects on tissues. In the absence of thyroid hormones bone growth is slowed, and closure of the epiphyses is delayed.

5 Thyroid hormones are required for normal erythropoiesis. In myxoedema anaemia develops, due to a combination of a decreased absorption of vitamin B_{12} and decreased bone marrow metabolism.

6 They are required for breast metabolism and blood flow. There is decreased lactation in hypothyroidism.

7 The thyroid hormones potentiate the effects of the catecholamines on lipolysis, heart, CNS (ascending reticular formation).

8 Lipid metabolism. T_3 and T_4 affect formation of low density lipoprotein receptors. In hypothyroidism the low density lipoprotein receptors are reduced and plasma cholesterol is increased.

9 Carbohydrate metabolism. Thyroid hormones increase:
    glucose uptake from G.I.T.
    glucose utilisation by tissues
    glycogenolysis in liver and muscle
    gluconeogenesis
    insulin breakdown

10 Increased release of glucocorticoids from the adrenal cortex, as a result of increased breakdown and conjugation of glucocorticoids in the liver.

11 Thyroid hormones have an effect on the tissue ground substance. In myxoedema increased amounts of chondroitin sulphate and hyaluronic acid retain water leading to a puffy face.

12 Thyroid hormones affect sexual function.

	Hypothyroidism	Hyperthyroidism
Male	Decreased libido	May cause impotence
Female	Decreased libido menorrhagia and polymenorrhoea	Oligomenorrhoea or amenorrhoea

13 Conversion of carotene to vitamin A in the liver.

Anti-thyroid antibodies

Certain lesions of the thyroid have been found to be attributable to an autoimmune reaction. These are discussed in detail later. In these diseases two main classes of antibodies have been identified.

The first group are readily found in Hashimoto's (chronic lymphocytic) thyroiditis and are particularly directed against either microsomal antigens or thyroglobulin itself. The presence of this group of antibodies is associated with a propensity to progressive thyroid failure, resulting from antibody-mediated thyroid cell destruction.

The second group, which are found in the great majority of patients with Graves' disease (exophthalmic goitre), have the facility to stimulate thyroid cells in a manner analogous to TSH. They are thought to be directed against the TSH receptor in the thyroid cell membrane and are variably called thyroid stimulating immunoglobulins (TSI) or thyroid stimulating antibodies (TSAb).

The first of this class of antibodies was named the long acting thyroid stimulator (LATS). Assays for this compound were found to be laborious and positive results were found only in a minority of hyperthyroid patients. More recent methods of assessing TSAb activity have depended on the measurement of in vitro cyclic AMP production by human thyroid cells maintained in culture.

Disturbances of thyroid function both hyperthyroidism and hypothyroidism can be recognised clinically but an assessment of the degree of activity of the gland depends upon scientific tests.

Tests of thyroid function

Name of test	Nature of test	Method
Direct measurement of circulating thyroid hormones	Thyroxine (T_4) tri-iodothyronine (T_3) blood content either as total (bound and unbound) or free fractions	Radioimmunoassay

Comments – total hormone levels influenced by the levels of thyroid binding globulin.

Thyroid hormone binding capacity	An assessment of the degree of saturation of TGB	By adding excess radioactive T_3 to a serum sample and removing the residue by absorption on resin sponge

Measurements – the amount of the resin uptake expressed as a percentage of the total T_3 is inversely proportional to the available binding sites TGB.

Comments – T_3 resin uptake is always taken in conjunction with serum T_4 levels to confirm an abnormal T_4 measurement and to exclude one which might be due to variations in binding proteins.

Radioactive iodine uptake	Measurement of radioactive iodine entrapment by thyroid	A small tracer dose of I_{131} with a half life of 8 days or of I_{132} with a half life of 2.26 hours is administered by mouth and the rate at which it is cleared from the blood stream relates to the thyroid activity

Measurements – after oral administration of radioactive iodine, measurements are made at 24 and 48 hours (late uptake studies), but 4 or 6 hour levels (early uptake studies) are valuable in hyperfunctioning states.

Radioactive technetium, which is concentrated in the thyroid in the same way as iodine but is not organically bound, is a useful alternative for early uptake studies.

Comments – radioactive iodine tests are safe and useful but there is a fairly wide overlap between normal and abnormal activity. Although in general uptake correlates positively with thyroid activity the values vary with the iodine content of the diet and in certain circumstances the results must be interpreted with caution. Thus in patients with endemic goitre there may be an increased uptake in the absence of hyperthyroidism. By contrast a reduced uptake may occur in the absence of hypothyroidism after partial thyroidectomy, after the administration of thyroxine or antithyroid drugs, or in the early phase of subacute thyroiditis.

Errors may arise from the inherent nature of the test and the lack of patient co-operation. In current practice it is mainly performed to assist in establishing the aetiology of an individual case of hyperthyroidism or in the assessment of a patient's suitability for therapeutic radioiodine administration.

Name of test	Nature of test	Method
Serum thyroid stimulating hormone	Assessment of serum content	Radioimmunoassay

Measurements – normal range 1.0 to 6mU/1. High in hypothyroidism and as a consequence of negative feedback the serum level rises in response to inadequate blood levels of thyroid hormones. In hyperthyroidism it is suppressed and therefore undetectable.

Comments – hyperthyroidism with a detectable serum TSH raises the rare possibility of a TSH – producing anterior pituitary tumour.

Thyroid suppression	By the exogenous administration of T_3 the production of TSH is suppressed	Baseline radioactive iodine uptake is measured, followed by the administration of $25\mu g$ T_3 6 hourly for 7 days. Residual radioactivity is estimated and the radioactive iodine uptake reassessed

Measurement – the uptake is reduced in normals and in endemic goitre. No change in thyrotoxicosis and some non-toxic nodular goitres.

Comments – the extent of the fall that indicates a positive result is uncertain but is usually less than 20% of the administered dose or 40% of the initial level.
   In patients with thyrotoxicosis this test can be dangerous leading to a thyroid crisis especially in elderly patients.

Radioisotope scan	Measurement of the iodine uptake by the thyroid	Injection of radioactive iodine or technetium followed by scanning or Gamma camera

Measurements – outline of gland defined.

Comments – areas of increased uptake, e.g. certain adenomas demonstrate the size and nature of the lesion.

Ultrasound	The size, contour and distribution of the gland and of any abnormalities, e.g. cysts, adenomas, or carcinomas	Ultrasound scanning

Comments – this is a non-invasive method of examination.

Other tests

Tests which have been employed in diagnosis of thyroid disease but are now used infrequently include: assessment of the protein bound iodine of thyroid activity after administration of TSH; estimation of the basal metabolic rate, and klinometry of the Achilles tendon contraction.

Goitre

The term goitre is given to any swelling of the thyroid gland. The lesion may be diffuse or nodular in form, neoplastic or non-neoplastic in nature, and may be unassociated with any hormonal upset (simple), or associated with hyperthyroidism (toxic).

Simple goitre

A diffuse enlargement of the thyroid caused by cellular hyperplasia is thought to be due to an increased sensitivity to pituitary TSH secretion. When low thyroxine levels are found they are usually secondary either to a relative or absolute deficiency of iodine or to a primary enzyme deficiency within the thyroid.

The commonest cause of iodine deficiency goitre is an unusually low level of iodine in the water supply. The deficiency explains the geographical distribution of the disease and the term endemic goitre. In some areas this may be exaggerated by the effects of chronic gastro-intestinal infections or by a diet rich in fat and calcium, both of which impair the intestinal absorption of iodine, or by the presence in the diet of specific goitrogens which reduce thyroid hormone production. Goitrogens of this type are found in soya beans and in brassicas such as cabbage and kale. Some poisons, cobalt, boron and cyanide, are also specific goitrogens.

There is a physiological form of goitre which develops in girls during puberty and lactation in which there is an increased requirement for thyroid hormones. When this is coupled with a marginal iodine deficiency or an increased urinary loss, it is followed by a compensatory diffuse hyperplasia. This usually returns to normal or at the least to a minimal residual swelling. Sporadic goitre may be caused by an inherent lack of one or more of the enzymes concerned with thyroid production (dyshormonogenesis). It usually occurs as a familial disorder.

The histological pattern is heterogeneous with hyperplasia (evolution) and regression (involution) occurring simultaneously in different parts of the gland. The initial change is hyperplastic with a uniform enlargement and an increased number of acini, the height and number of the acinar cells increasing, but with a reduction in colloid. During involution, the acinar cells decrease in height and the colloid accumulates. Later the acini become so enormously distended that they break down to form large pools of colloid and a typical honeycomb appearance in the entire gland (the so-called colloid goitre). With further repeated cycles of hyperplasia and involution nodules resembling adenomas form and the gland becomes replaced by zones or nodules of hyperplasia interspersed with colloid cysts. Haemorrhage and necrosis may result in considerable fibrosis with accumulation of haemosiderin and cholesterol. Fibrous tissue may surround the nodules and sometimes calcification is extensive.

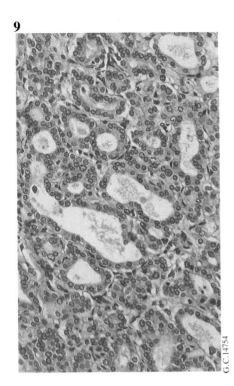

G.C.14754

9 Colloid goitre. A focus of hyperplasia in a large goitre. In this early stage before involution and colloid storage have occurred, the nuclei are large and show some variation in size. *(H&E ×250).*

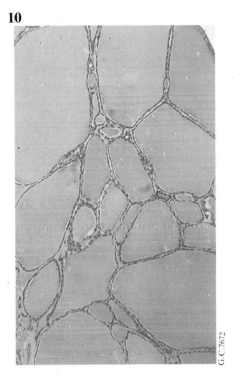

G.C.7672

10 Colloid goitre. Colloid storage is now marked causing great variation in the size of the follicles and attenuation in the enclosing epithelium. *(H&E ×125)*

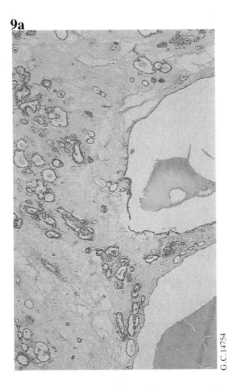

G.C.14754

9a Colloid goitre. Degeneration has resulted in fibrosis and cyst formation. Regenerating follicles are present in the fibrous tissue. *(H&E ×50)*

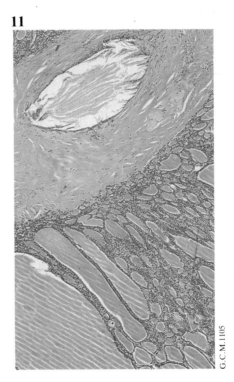

G.C.M.1105

11 Colloid goitre. Degeneration. An area of fibrosis contains an accumulation of cholesterol crystals. *(H&E ×50)*

Simple goitre (Continued)

The histological changes are reflected by the gross pathological changes and show corresponding variations in character and dimension.

A simple goitre may vary in size from a barely detectable swelling to an enormous enlargement which may project forwards from the neck, hang down onto the chest, or may enlarge into the mediastinum (retrosternal goitre). The sex incidence shows a small female preponderance except in the goitre of puberty which is almost exclusively found in girls. The texture may vary from the smooth and firm diffuse goitre to the irregular nodularity characteristic of the nodular colloid goitre.

Colloid goitre represents a later stage and is the result of involution. It may be of long duration and is sometimes very gross.

12

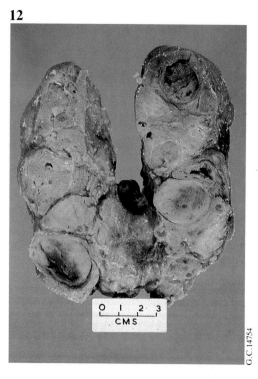

13

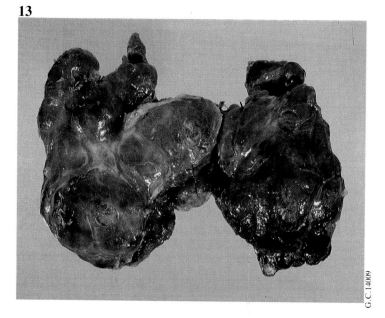

12 Diffuse simple goitre with nodular areas. The specimen includes both lateral lobes, the isthmus, and the pyramidal lobe. All are enlarged. The lateral lobes have been sectioned to show that in addition to generalised enlargement of the gland many nodules have formed. Some appear 'adenomatous', some show degenerative changes with partial liquefaction, and small cysts have also developed. Fibrosis is not marked in this gland.

13 From a male aged 61 years. There had been a massive enlargement of the thyroid of long duration. The illustration is that of the main mass of the thyroid and the colloid character can be seen from its external surface. The weight of the excised thyroid was 1,270gm and the overall measurements of the excised gland were 18.2 × 24.5 × 6.5cm. At operation a large portion of the thyroid lay behind the sternum (retrosternal goitre).

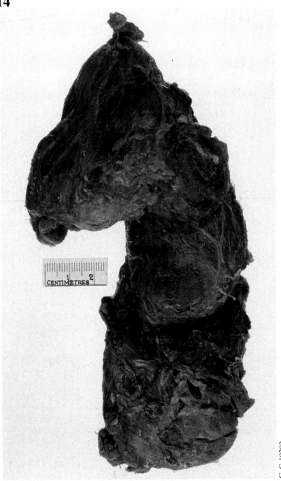

The goitre is from a woman of 60 who had been aware of a neck swelling for 10 years. There was a family history of goitre. Five months before operation she began to have attacks of palpation and breathlessness. A goitre was present in the neck and the X-ray examination suggested that it had extended into the superior and anterior mediastinum. At operation the lower part of the goitre was so firmly adherent to the mediastinum that the upper two inches of the sternum had to be split to dislodge it.

G.C.10282

14 *Specimen*
Upper part The pyramidal-shaped portion of the thyroid consisting of the right lobe, isthmus and part of the left lobe was present in the neck.
Middle third This portion of the greatly enlarged left lobe lay in the superior mediastinum.
Lower third The remainder was in the anterior mediastinum and much of its surface is covered by the divided pericardial adhesions.

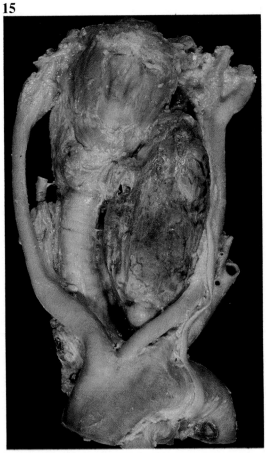

15 This example of a goitre extending into the mediastinum was an incidental finding at necropsy. The right lobe and isthmus of the thyroid show no abnormality of note. By contrast the left lobe is greatly enlarged reaching the arch of the aorta – displacing both trachea and the left common carotid artery and adjoining structures.

Simple goitre *(Continued)*

Cyst formation

Cyst formation in the thyroid usually occurs as a complication of colloid goitre. It results from disruption of attenuated follicular walls especially in nodules which are active and associated with local haemorrhage. As the cyst distends it causes pressure atrophy of the surrounding gland and replacement fibrosis. Haemosiderin pigmentation resulting from haemorrhage is frequent and calcification may occur. Microcysts are common in enzyme-deficient sporadic goitre.

16

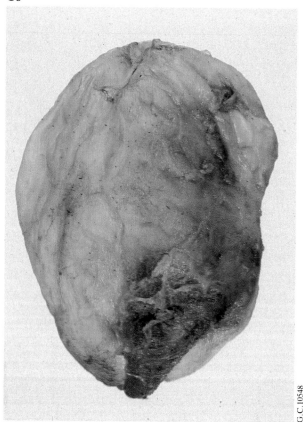

G.C.10548

16 From a female aged 79 with a swelling in her neck for 6 years. She had stridor and dyspnoea.

The large cyst extended from the mandible to the sternum. The cyst was easily enucleated and the patient obtained immediate relief. The cyst measures 12 × 10cm and is unilocular. The contents before fixation were fluid and semi-translucent. A thin layer of thyroid tissue remains attached near the lower part of the preparation.

17

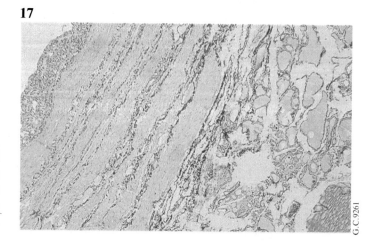

G.C.9261

17 Part of the wall of a thyroid cyst. The inner part of the wall is formed mainly by pale hyaline fibrous tissue arranged in parallel bands. In this case the inner surface is covered by regenerated thyroid epithelium (top left). *(H&E ×40)*

18

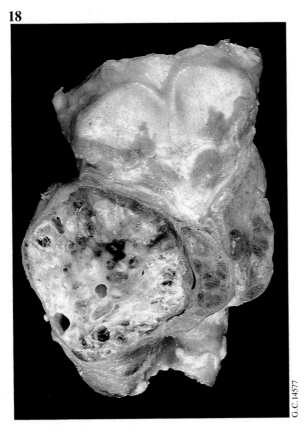

19

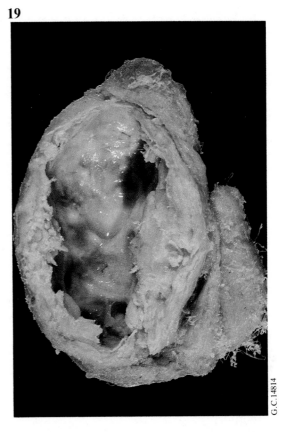

18 In this example of colloid goitre an unusually large solitary nodule has formed in the right lobe. It shows extensive fibrosis and cyst formation and is partially calcified indicating longstanding duration.

19 This thyroid cyst was an incidental finding at necropsy. It measured 6cm in maximum diameter and occupied most of the right lobe. Its heavily calcified wall enclosed the colourless fluid. The left lobe of the gland was normal in size.

Serum total thyroxine levels and thyroid hormone binding (T_3 resin uptake) are usually normal in a simple goitre but may occasionally be borderline or low. Serum TSH can be elevated despite normal serum hormone levels. Radioactive iodine uptake is normal except where the primary defect is an enzyme deficiency.

Primary toxic goitre

This disease was associated with the name of Graves who described the classical features. Many other names are commonly employed including exophthalmic goitre, hyperthyroidism, thyrotoxicosis etc.

Primary toxic goitre occurs almost invariably in women with no history of previous thyroid disease. The primary disability results from excessive circulating Thyroxine (T_4) or Triiodothyronine (T_3) or both. It is known that the stimulus to this hypersecretion is not mediated through the anterior pituitary, the TSH levels being excessively low. TSAb may be present and the measured levels may correlate with the degree of the hyperthyroidism. However, TSAb cannot be totally implicated as the cause of the disease and it may prove to be an epiphenomenon in response to some antecedent factor. Primary toxic goitre is now considered to be an autoimmune disease and this is supported by the characteristic histological appearance of a diffuse or focal lymphocytic collection. The exophthalmos caused by swelling of retro-orbital tissues which often complicates hyperthyroidism has recently been shown to be associated with an immunoglobulin binding to retro-orbital antigens and distinct from thyroid antibodies. Primary toxic goitre has a worldwide incidence and may occur at any age including children though usually in the third, fourth and fifth decades. Although much commoner in women than in men, the incidence is more equal in areas of endemic goitre.

Pathology

The entire thyroid gland is highly vascular, usually with a uniform consistence and appearance. Its cut surface loses the normal glistening appearance imparted by colloid and becomes more fleshy. Although usually showing some enlargement, there is no relation between the size of the gland and the degree of clinical activity.

20

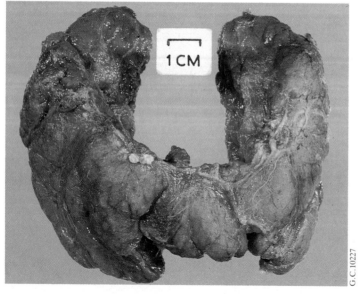

1 CM

G.C.10227

20 Primary toxic goitre. A female of 22 had suffered the symptoms of thyrotoxicosis for 2 years, and for a short time a feeling of oppression in the throat, with difficulty in swallowing and hoarseness. Her thyroid was enlarged, soft and pulsatile and she had slight exophthalmos.

At operation, after a preliminary course of iodine, the gland was found to be about 4 times the normal size and about 5/6 of it was removed. Two years later she was reported to be well with no signs of thyroid dysfunction.

Both lateral lobes, the isthmus and a small pyramidal lobe are shown. Although the gland is considerably enlarged its outline is fairly uniform. The capsule is thin and numerous vessels can be seen running beneath it.

The epithelial cells lining the acini are diffusely hyperplastic, tall columnar in shape and with active mitosis. The increase in cellular volume often produces epithelial infolding thus forming an overall papilliferous appearance. The colloid is reduced in amount and presents with a scalloped edge facing the acinar cells. Lymphocytes and sometimes lymphoid follicles may be scattered throughout the gland. The picture is, however, far from uniform and there may be areas of involution with colloid storage intermingled with the hyperplasia.

Case of untreated thyrotoxicosis

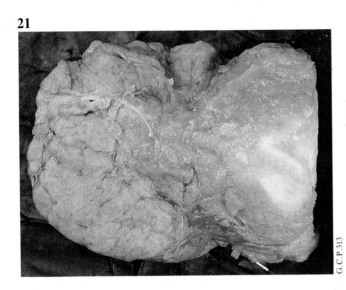

21 A middle-aged woman suffered from the embolic complications of atrial fibrillation and died before a definitive diagnosis was made. At necropsy the thyroid was found to be about twice its normal size and appeared to be deficient in colloid.

Microscopic examination confirmed that it was hyperplastic and hyperactive thus establishing the diagnosis of thyrotoxicosis. Prior to admission to hospital there had been neither a diagnosis nor treatment for thyroid disease.

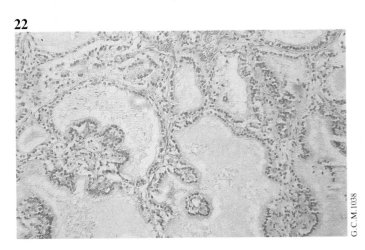

22 Thyrotoxicosis. Hyperplasia has resulted in follicles which are irregular in shape and variable in size. The follicular colloid stains poorly and shows peripheral vacuolation. The epithelium shows a tendency to papillary formation. (H&E ×100)

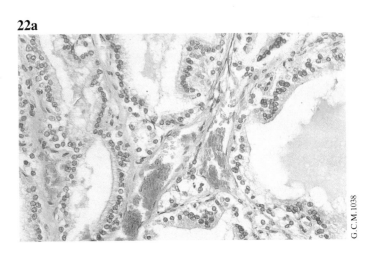

22a Thyrotoxicosis – same case. The epithelium is columnar and is heaped up in places. The interfollicular stroma is highly vascular. (H&E ×250)

Primary toxic goitre *(Continued)*

Course of disease

The onset of thyrotoxicosis may be abrupt following an acute illness or some emotional stress. Alternatively, the syndrome may develop gradually over a period of weeks or months. The progress is unpredictable with frequent relapses and remissions but each episode is progressively more severe, culminating sometimes in a thyroid crisis. This represents a phase of intense thyrotoxicosis especially affecting the cardiac muscle. It may prove fatal. Both the clinical features and histology react to the administration of certain drugs notably thiouracil and iodine. There is diminution of the thyrotoxicosis. The cellular changes are different with the two drugs and are illustrated.

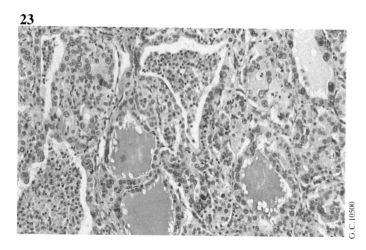

23 Thiouracil hyperplasia. Hyperplastic changes are intense resulting in solid foci of thyroid cells and in exfoliation of cells into follicles. There is marked variation in nuclear size and some mitotic activity. *(H&E ×150)*

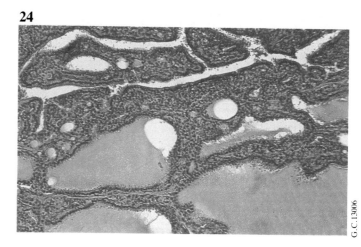

24 Thyrotoxicosis after 14 days preoperative iodine. Hyperplasia and papillary formation are still well marked but colloid is returning to the follicles and is deeper staining. *(H&E ×100)*

Diagnosis

The diagnosis of thyrotoxicosis is initially made on the clinical features. In the fully established case it is obvious, but in the early, the mild and the atypical case there may be difficulties, in particular, in its differentiation from an acute anxiety state. In thyrotoxicosis, however, there is generally an elevation of the serum thyroxine (both total and free) and T_3 levels. The serum TSH is suppressed and cannot be stimulated by intravenous TRH. Microsomal and thyroglobulin antibodies may be detectable but are usually in low titre.

Secondary toxic goitre

(Plummer's Disease)

Toxic nodular goitre commonly occurs in older women who have had a simple goitre for some time. Occasionally, the thyrotoxicosis is associated with hyperactivity in a single hyperplastic nodule (uninodular goitre) but more commonly the whole gland is involved (multinodular goitre). The gland is often quite large and is distorted by numerous smooth round lobules which are composed of solid thyroid tissue, often showing extensive colloid change but sometimes being replaced by cysts. The histological appearance is diverse, with a spectrum ranging from a colloid storage phase in some areas to varying degrees of hyperplasia in others.

In secondary thyrotoxicosis the disease is more uniformly progressive. Phases of remission are much less frequent. As in primary thyrotoxicosis the disease may ultimately regress and may even be followed by a phase of hypothyroidism.

25

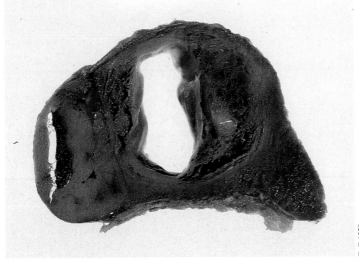

25 The specimen is from a woman aged 32 years who presented the symptoms of toxic goitre, exophthalmos, palpitation and tachycardia. After excision of the nodular portion of the thyroid the symptoms disappeared. Two nodules are present, one mainly cystic and the other consisting of pale hyperplastic thyroid tissue showing minor cystic change. Haemorrhage has occurred in both nodules.

Hypothyroidism

In childhood (crétinism)

Hypothyroidism in the newborn child may be due to a variety of causes. These fall into two groups:

1   When the thyroid gland is atrophic or absent. Most of these cases are due to unexplained agenesis; rarely deficiency of TSH secretion accounts for the hypothyroidism.
2   When the thyroid gland function is impaired by ectopia, or when it is goitrous. The goitre most commonly occurs in areas with a high incidence of endemic goitre. Occasionally administration of anti-thyroid drugs during pregnancy accounts for the goitre. In a proportion familial enzyme deficiency is responsible.

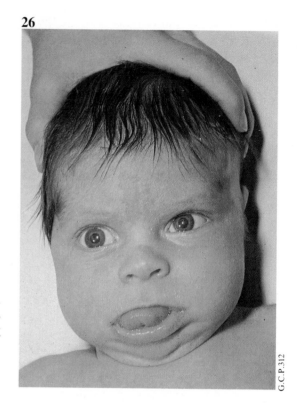

26   In this picture of florid cretinism due to thyroid atrophy the diagnosis should be obvious to all. Screening programmes of the newborn have, however, shown that the diagnosis in many is by no means obvious and entails special investigations to establish.

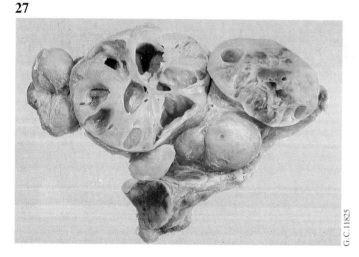

27   This example of nodular goitre is from a man of 31 who had a family history of goitre. He had been born with goitre and cretinism and had been treated with thyroxine throughout his life. The specimen is the enlarged right lobe of the thyroid showing gross lobulation and cyst formation due to colloid goitre. Recent haemorrhage has occurred in some of the lobules.

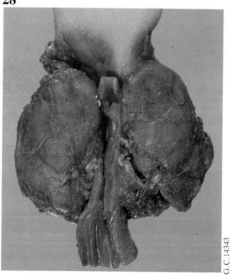

28   In this specimen from a still-born child the thyroid is uniformly greatly enlarged. This neonatal goitre occurred in the offspring of a mother who suffered from thyrotoxicosis and had received thiouracil during pregnancy. The histology in this condition is similar to that of thiouracil hyperplasia in the adult.

In the adult (myxoedema)

Adult hypothyroidism or myxoedema is seven times more common in females than males. Although sometimes spontaneous, it more often occurs either as a consequence of autoimmune destruction or as a sequel to thyroid surgery or the treatment of thyrotoxicosis with radioactive iodine. Temporary hypothyroidism may also occur during treatment with antithyroid drugs. Typically the gland is small and shrunken due to loss of thyroid follicles and is firm, grey and fibrous.

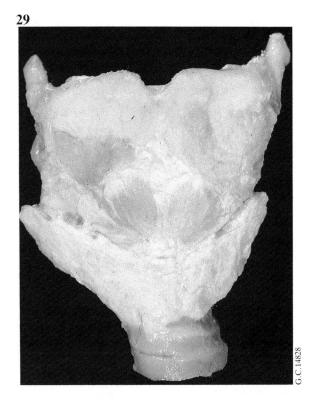

29 From an elderly female who was admitted to hospital following an accident to her chest, fracturing her ninth rib. During the previous 7 months she had become progressively lethargic and dyspnoeic. Her general condition had deteriorated and she was confused. There was gross evidence of myxoedema. The patient died 9 days after admission. At post mortem examination the thyroid showed total atrophy being replaced by fibrous tissue.

Microscopic examination confirms the extensive destruction of follicles and replacement by fibrous tissue. The process is accompanied by lymphocytic and plasma cell infiltrate. Multinucleated cells and Askanazy cells are not uncommon and sometimes squamous metaplasia can be seen.

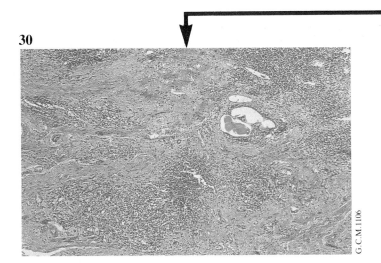

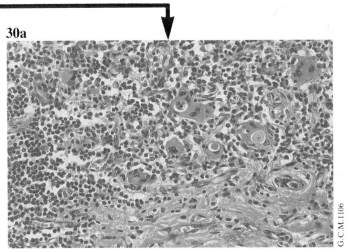

30 Myxoedema. As a result of an autoimmune reaction much of the thyroid tissue has been destroyed and there is considerable fibrosis and chronic inflammatory infiltration. Only two small degenerating thyroid follicles remain. *(H&E ×50)*

30a Same case showing degenerating thyroid epithelium in a field of plasma cells and lymphocytes. Several of the epithelial cells are multinucleated. *(H&E ×250)*

Thyroiditis

The term thyroiditis has been applied to a number of conditions of dissimilar aetiology and character.

Acute pyogenic thyroiditis

Bacterial infections of the thyroid are uncommon, the organisms entering the gland by way of the blood stream, lymphatics or by a direct extension from the larynx.

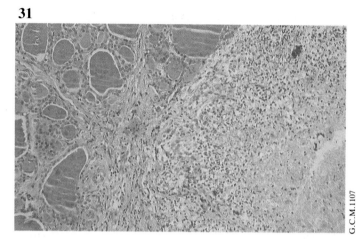

31 Thyroid abscess. A thick layer of granulation tissue infiltrated by inflammatory cells and undergoing fibrosis separates amorphous necrotic debris from the surrounding thyroid tissue. *(PAS ×125)*

Subacute thyroiditis

(De Quervain's Disease)

This is probably caused by a virus and usually follows an acute upper respiratory tract infection, appearing most commonly in women in the 40–50 age group. The gland is diffusely enlarged, may be painful and is sometimes adherent to the surrounding tissues. The earliest histological change is an inflammatory destruction of acinar epithelium which allows the colloid to extrude and to act as a foreign body. There is infiltration with mononuclear cells, giant cells and lymphocytes, but the condition is self-limiting and resolution is complete.

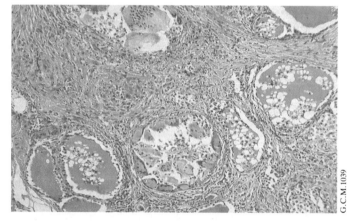

32 De Quervain's thyroiditis. The inflammation has resulted in degeneration of both epithelium and colloid and in disruption of the thyroid follicles. Fibrosis has ensued and multinucleated giant cells have formed. *(H&E ×100)*

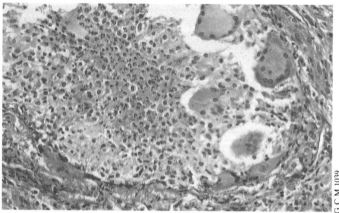

32a Same case. A degenerating thyroid follicle is filled by inflammatory cells including polymorphs and by epithelial and colloid debris. A number of the giant cells appear to be of epithelial origin. *(H&E ×250)*

Invasive fibrous thyroiditis

(Ligneous thyroiditis, Riedel's struma)

Invasive fibrous thyroiditis is a rare condition of unknown aetiology. Although it has been attributed to a late phase of Hashimoto's disease, there is no conclusive evidence to suggest that it is an autoimmune disease. Part or all of the thyroid is enlarged and woody hard. It is firmly adherent to the adjacent structures and may cause severe pressure effects. In about one-third of cases it may be associated with fibrosis elsewhere in the body, such as the mediastinum or the retroperitoneal area. Histologically it is characterised by an extensive inflammatory fibrosclerosis with destruction of the acinar tissue and invasion of surrounding tissue including, e.g. strap muscles of neck.

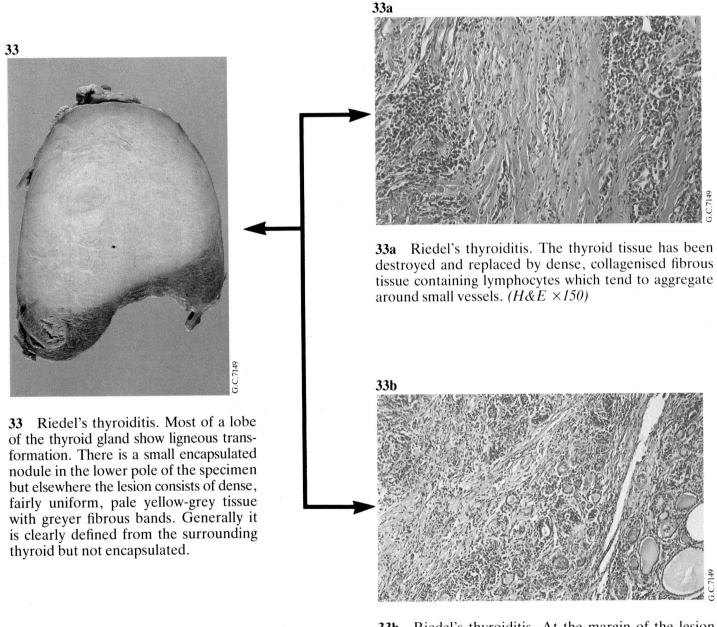

33 Riedel's thyroiditis. Most of a lobe of the thyroid gland show ligneous transformation. There is a small encapsulated nodule in the lower pole of the specimen but elsewhere the lesion consists of dense, fairly uniform, pale yellow-grey tissue with greyer fibrous bands. Generally it is clearly defined from the surrounding thyroid but not encapsulated.

33a Riedel's thyroiditis. The thyroid tissue has been destroyed and replaced by dense, collagenised fibrous tissue containing lymphocytes which tend to aggregate around small vessels. *(H&E ×150)*

33b Riedel's thyroiditis. At the margin of the lesion there is usually a fairly abrupt transition to relatively normal thyroid tissue (right). *(H&E ×100)*

233

Thyroiditis *(Continued)*

Chronic lymphocytic thyroiditis

(Hashimoto's disease)

An autoimmune disease associated with antibodies reactive to thyroglobulin and the microsomal constituents of the acinar cells. Its incidence is virtually restricted to women and it may develop either in previously normal glands or in the presence of a simple or a toxic goitre. The thyroid is uniformly enlarged, with a firm or hard consistence.

Histologically there is a widespread parenchymal atrophy with eosinophilic degeneration of the acinar epithelium and scanty colloid. In addition, the characteristic feature is a diffuse lymphocytic infiltration coupled with numerous lymph follicles, each showing prominent germinal centres. Ultimately, there is progressive fibrosis of the entire gland. Thyroid function is at first normal but it is usual for hypothyroidism to develop after some years. On occasions there may be a period of transient hyperthyroidism in the early stage of the disease, but this seldom persists.

34

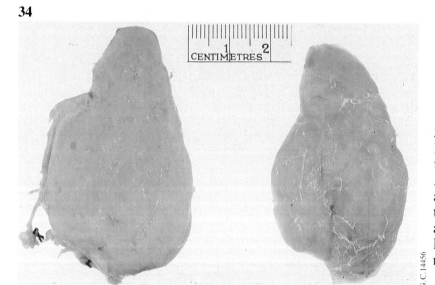

34 The patient was a woman of 68. Her thyroid gland had been enlarged for 2–3 years and she had received treatment by thyroxine and prednisolone because of it. A few weeks before admission to hospital she had noticed an increase in size and tenderness of the gland arousing the suspicion of malignancy. A frozen section taken at operative examination of the gland suggested Hashimoto's disease and both lobes of the gland were resected.

34a The gland is heavily and diffusely infiltrated by chronic inflammatory cells, mainly lymphocytes and plasma cells. A lymphoid follicle with germinal centre has formed. Sparse but recognisable pale thyroid epithelium can be seen in the inflammatory infiltrate. *(H&E ×100)*

34a

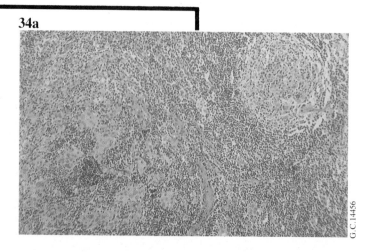

35

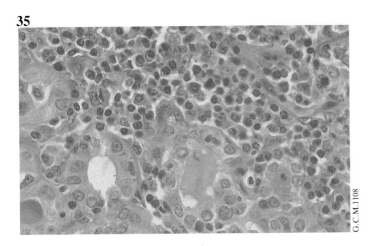

G.C.M.1108

35 Hashimoto's disease showing plasma cells around thyroid follicles. *(H&E ×500)*

36

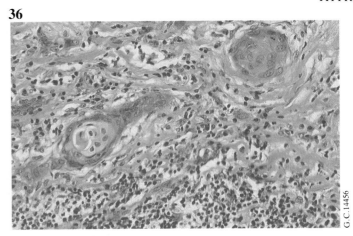

G.C.M.1456

36 Hashimoto's disease. Squamous metaplasia sometimes occurs in foci of thyroid epithelium surviving in fibrous tissue. *(H&E ×250)*

37

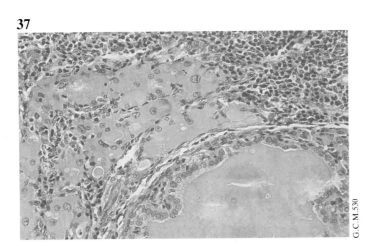

G.C.M.530

37 Hashimoto's disease in a case of 'burnt-out thyrotoxicosis'. Askanazy (Hürthle) cells with abundant eosino-philic cytoplasm are present. Below, poorly staining colloid is enclosed by columnar epithelium showing some tendency to papillary formation. *(H&E ×250)*

38

Askanazy (oxyphil, Hürthle) cell of thyroid. This de-generate change in the thyroid epithelial cells is charac-teristic of Hashimoto's thyroiditis but may be found in other thyroid conditions. The intense pink staining by eosin at histological level is reflected ultrastructurally by diffuse cytoplasmic occupation with mitochondria. Functional activity such as thyroglobulin synthesis is much reduced. *(Lead citrate and uranyl acetate ×25000)*

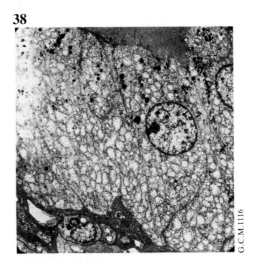

G.C.M.1116

By courtesy of
Dr. K. M. McLaren

Adenoma

On occasions a patient presents with an apparently smooth rounded nodule situated within the thyroid. The differential diagnosis is difficult since it may be either a solitary hyperplastic nodule, a cyst or a benign or malignant tumour and the nature of the lesion is only disclosed by histological examination.

True adenomas of the thyroid are most common in middle-aged women and usually present as slowly growing solitary nodules in an otherwise normal gland.

Histology

Several varieties of adenomas are described, the solid ('foetal'), papillary or follicular. A few are formed mainly by Askanazy (Hürthle) cells. Experience has shown that many papillary tumours of the thyroid prove to be malignant. Most benign adenomas are follicular. Usually well encapsulated, they may rarely assume malignant characteristics. Occasionally thyroid follicular adenomas may develop autonomous function, resulting in clinical hyperthyroidism.

1

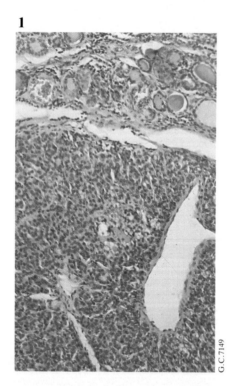

1a

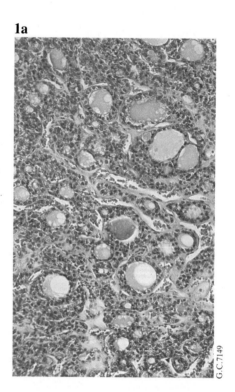

1 Thyroid adenoma. In this field the adenoma consists of a solid mass of epithelial cells separated by a thin fibrous capsule from the thyroid tissue (above). *(H&E ×125)*

1a Another field from the same tumour showing a follicular pattern. *(H&E ×125)*

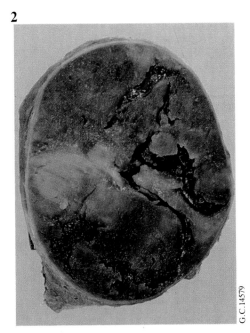

2 A solitary follicular adenoma of thyroid 7cm in diameter. It occupied most of the lobe and only a small portion of thyroid outside its capsule can be seen.

G.C.14579

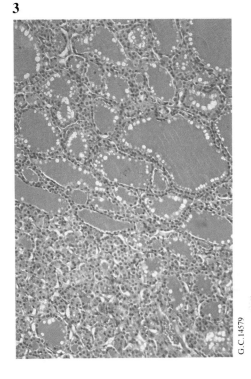

3 Thyroid. Follicular adenoma. A field of the above specimen showing an area of hyperactivity. Peripheral vacuolation appears in the colloid in the affected area. *(H&E ×125)*

G.C.14579

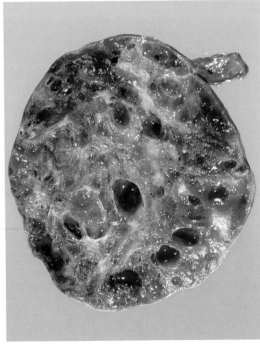

4 A large solitary nodule removed at operation. It measures 10.5cm in maximum diameter and shows considerable cystic change with accumulation of colloid. There is much fibrosis.

G.C.4584

Carcinoma

Carcinoma of the thyroid is an uncommon tumour, of diverse structure and behaviour. Four main types are described.

Unlike most malignant tumours, the prognosis depends more on the microscopic type of tumour than on the extent of the disease. At one time, the incidence was significantly higher in goitrous areas, varying from 4% in such areas to 0.5% elsewhere, but more recently this difference has become less obvious. It occurs predominantly in females with an overall F:M ratio of 2 to 3:1. In younger age groups the ratio may reach as high as 8:1.

There are a number of predisposing factors, apart from the relationship to nodular goitre. Local irradiation is certainly a factor, carcinoma being more common in individuals who have received radiation treatment to the neck, especially in childhood. There is some doubt as to whether treatment with radioactive iodine has a similar predisposition.

Papillary

Papillary tumours are the commonest thyroid cancers particularly in children and young adults. The tumour presents as a greyish mass varying in size and consistence. Many tumours are 2–3cm in diameter when they first attract attention.

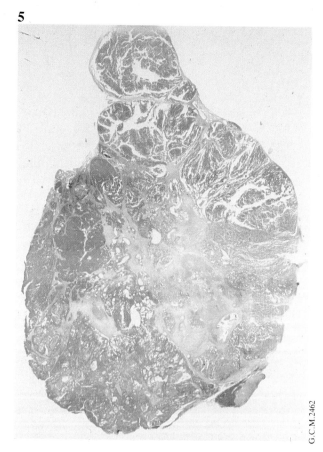

5

5 A whole section of an unusually large papillary carcinoma of the thyroid. Some parts are frankly papillary; others are becoming solid. The degree of fibrosis in a portion of the nodule is suggestive of antecedent disease. *(H&E ×1.5)*

G.C.M.2462

Histology

Well differentiated cells of characteristic appearance with large pale 'ground-glass' nuclei and nucleoli are for the most part arranged in a papillary formation, but often there are areas with a follicular structure and others arranged in solid masses. In spite of this variation, the tumours behave in accordance with their papillary element rather than the apparently more malignant follicular areas. Calcispherules and foci of calcification often occur.

6

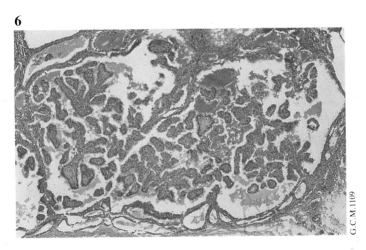

6 Thyroid papillary carcinoma. Part of a well differentiated carcinomatous nodule from one lobe of the thyroid. In addition to the striking papillary formation colloid is present, some of it intrafollicular. *(H&E ×50)*

6a

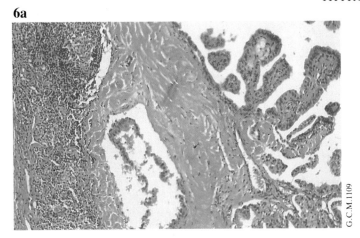

6a Same case. A section of an ipsilateral cervical lymph node showing metastatic papillary carcinoma – still well differentiated. *(H&E ×100)*

7

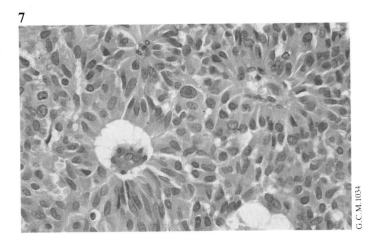

7 Thyroid. A more solid papillary carcinoma showing mantles of columnar cells pallisaded around small blood vessels. There is some variation in cell pattern and nuclear size. *(H&E ×312)*

7a

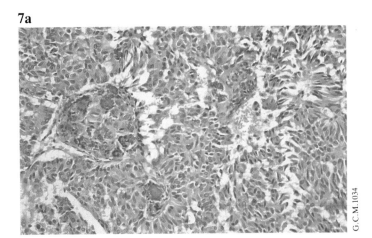

7a Same case. Foci of calcification are present. Multinucleated giant cells tend to form in the larger aggregates. *(H&E ×150)*

Progress

The tumour grows very slowly but there may be multiple foci within one lobe and 10% are bilateral. There is no capsule to the tumour but, although it invades locally, it may remain within the capsule of the thyroid for a long period of time. Spread occurs by lymphatics to the deep cervical lymph glands but only rarely by the blood stream. On occasions, a tumour may present as a lymph node metastasis long before the primary tumour is clinically apparent. The primary tumour may be very small but the metastases will continue to occur until the ipsilateral lobe of the thyroid is removed. The prognosis in papillary carcinoma is very good with a 10 year survival of 80–90% even in children, and even when there is evidence of metastatic deposits the prognosis remains good.

Follicular

Follicular tumours occur in an older age group and are both less common and more malignant than the papillary carcinoma. They are usually solitary and well defined, generally presenting as a solid fleshy nodule.

Progress

Initially circumscribed, they may possess a fairly well defined capsule but later tend to invade the adjacent thyroid tissue and to extend into the surrounding structures of the neck. Involvement of the recurrent laryngeal nerves is an early feature. Distant spread is by the blood stream, usually to the lungs, bone and brain. In some cases the first evidence of the disease may be a distant metastasis. The prognosis is much less favourable than with papillary carcinoma. Extensive metastasis may become evident even when the primary lesion is small.

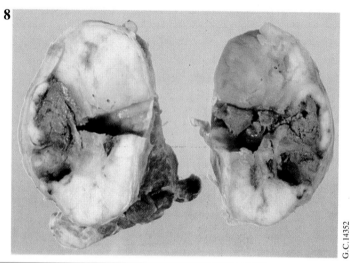

8

G.C.14352

8 The specimen is from a women of 69 who had a tumour on the left lobe of the thyroid gland and pulmonary metastases.

The left lobe has been bisected to show a tumour occupying all of the lobe except for a small portion of normal gland below. Areas of haemorrhage have occurred in the pale grey tumour.

Microscopically the tumour was a poorly differentiated follicular carcinoma with much anaplasia.

Histology

Histologically the tumour shows variation but the characteristic picture is of well differentiated cells arranged in follicles with a variable colloid content.

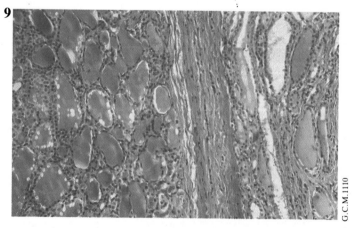

9

G.C.M.1110

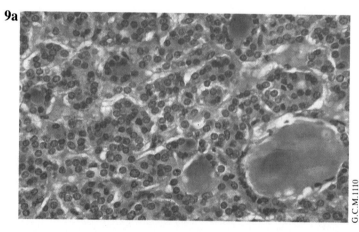

9a

G.C.M.1110

9 Thyroid follicular carcinoma. This well differentiated tumour (left) mimics the normal thyroid tissue lying outside its fibrous capsule. *(H&E ×125)*

9a Thyroid follicular carcinoma. A well differentiated tumour. Although some parts are solid the nuclei are uniform and there are no mitoses in this field. *(H&E ×312)*

10

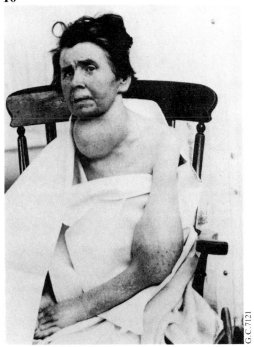

A women of 65 with a large carcinoma of the thyroid developed a pathological fracture of the left arm. The lower end of the left humerus has been sectioned to show the large tumour metastasis.

A small portion of the radius can also be seen. There is extensive necrosis which was associated with liquefaction. Much of the tumour is encapsulated.

10a

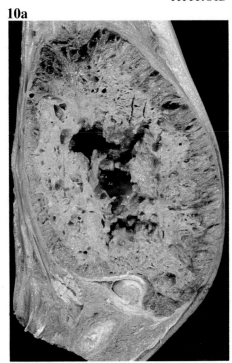

Hürthle tumour

A variant of the follicular carcinoma has been described in which the majority of the cells are large and eosinophilic and certain observers have described these as arising from the interacinar groups of cells as described by Hürthle. The lesion may be simple (adenoma) or malignant (carcinoma) and the tumours retain the eosinophilic characteristics. There is disputation as to whether these should be regarded as variants of the follicular carcinoma or considered a separate identifiable neoplasm.

11

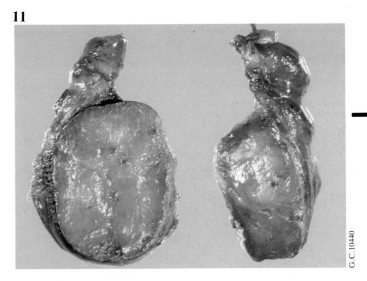

11 A Hürthle cell tumour resected from a woman of 38 who had noticed a neck swelling for 3 months. It is ovoid, 3 × 2.5cm in cross section, and encapsulated. Its pale colour contrasts with that of the surrounding thyroid.

11a

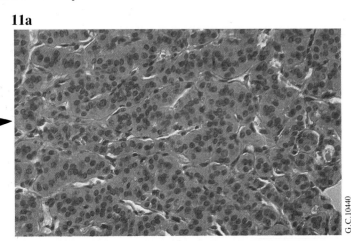

11a The tumour is composed of eosinophilic cells arranged in trabeculae. Nuclei are fairly uniform and there is no mitotic activity. Numerous capillaries run between the columns of Hürthle cells. *(H&E ×250)*

Medullary

An uncommon tumour often bilateral derived from the parafollicular or 'C' cells,
with a very wide age distribution and a slow rate of growth.

It has the particular property of secreting calcitonin and rarely serotonin (5-HT) and prostaglandins.
There is evidence to suggest a genetic basis for some cases of medullary tumour. It is frequently associated
with neural crest tumours in other sites, e.g. the phaeochromocytomas seen in the multiple endocrine
adenomatosis (MEA) type II syndrome, first described by Sipple (*see* p. 306).

Progress

The tumour grows slowly sometimes remaining localised without treatment for up to 20 years. Late spread
occurs to the cervical lymph glands.

12

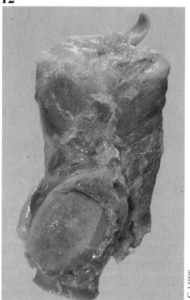

A woman of 68 died suddenly from necrotising enteritis
after hemicolectomy for a carcinoma of the caecum. No
regional metastases were found at necropsy. There was
a tumour nodule in the right lobe of the thyroid gland.

12 The illustration shows a lateral view of the right
lobe of the thyroid gland which has been sectioned to
reveal a discrete tumour nodule. It was firm and
centrally shows grey semi-translucent tissues. It proved
on microscopic examination to be a medullary
carcinoma.

12a

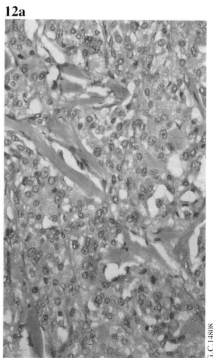

Histology

The tumour is composed of solid sheets of rounded or
polygonal cells set in a fibrous stroma. It is characterised
by the presence of amyloid material within the stroma
and around the malignant cells.

12a Thyroid. Medullary carcinoma.
The tumour is composed of fairly uniform cells in irregular groups set in
abundant eosinophilic and relatively
acellular stroma. (*H&E ×250*)

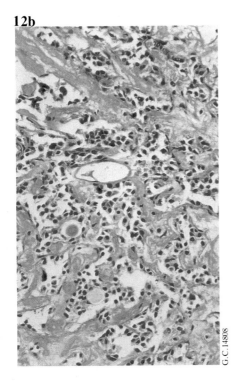

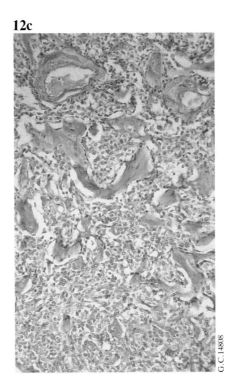

12b Thyroid. Medullary carcinoma. In this section the stroma is very abundant and the tumour cell nuclei are rather pyknotic. *(Congo red ×250)*

12c Same case. The stroma stains orange red indicating the presence of amyloid. *(Congo red ×125)*

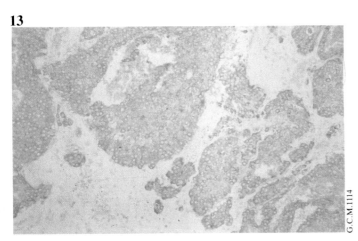

13 Medullary carcinoma of the thyroid: immunohistochemistry.

The derivation of this tumour from 'C' cells can be demonstrated by binding of antiserum to human calcitonin in the tumour cells. Here the resulting intra-cytoplasmic granules are displayed by a red-staining product. *(×25)*

By courtesy of Dr. K. M. McLaren

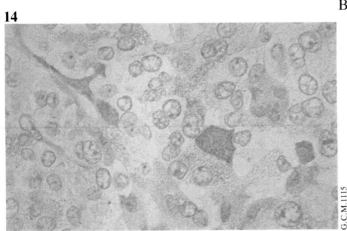

14 Some medullary carcinomas of thyroid are less well differentiated and in this example only occasional cells show obvious staining using an anti-human calcitonin antibody. *(×250)*

Undifferentiated

Undifferentiated carcinomas, the least common of the thyroid cancers, occur usually in older patients, especially women, and often when there has been a preceding history of goitre. The tumours are hard, white and non-encapsulated.

Progress

The tumour grows very rapidly and spreads by direct invasion of the surrounding structures. Death usually results from the local effects of the tumour but in the few patients who survive the tumour may give rise to metastases. The average survival time in anaplastic carcinoma is 6 months and the 5 year survival is less than 5%.

Histology

The tumours consist of primitive undifferentiated cells arranged in compact masses. Small cell varieties may be difficult to differentiate from malignant lymphomas. Pleomorphism is common and mitoses are frequent.

Very rarely tumours may exhibit giant cell and spindle cell characteristics.

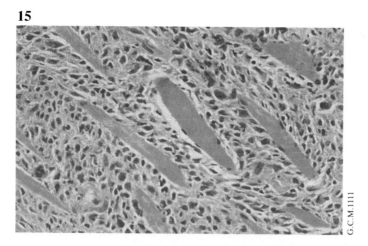

15 Thyroid. Undifferentiated carcinoma. Pleomorphic tumour cells have invaded perithyroid muscle. (H&E ×312)

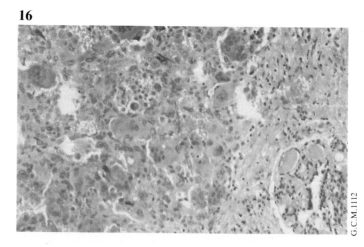

16 Thyroid. Giant cell tumour. The appearance of this unusual tumour contrasts with the focus of surviving thyroid (bottom right). (H&E ×150)

Squamous carcinoma

Rarely thyroid carcinomas show squamous differentiation in some areas. This metaplasia probably originates in the tumour cells themselves.

17

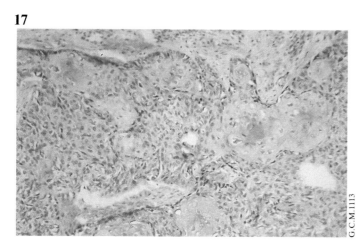

17 Thyroid. Squamous carcinoma. A well differentiated tumour showing pronounced keratinisation. *(H&E ×100)*

Investigation

The differential diagnosis of thyroid lesions especially tumours is facilitated by diagnostic imaging techniques. The radioisotope scan will demonstrate the size, outline and activity of the mass, and an ultrasound scan will distinguish between a cystic and a solid lesion. The examination will also demonstrate any deposit of calcium salts.

By needle biopsy the pathological character of the lesion can be established and may be essential in differentiation.

Malignant lymphoma

The thyroid gland may be invaded in the generalised spread of a malignant lymphoma arising in some other organ. Sometimes, however, the tumour first presents in the thyroid gland – a primary thyroid lymphoma. Such a tumour occurs mainly in elderly women and may be preceded by Hashimoto's disease. In a number of cases the alimentary tract is simultaneously or subsequently involved by malignant lymphoma. In later stages the disease may disseminate widely.

Histology

The tumours are of non-Hodgkin type and are formed predominantly either by small cells of the lymphocyte type or by larger less differentiated cells. Distinction from small cell undifferentiated carcinoma is often difficult.

18

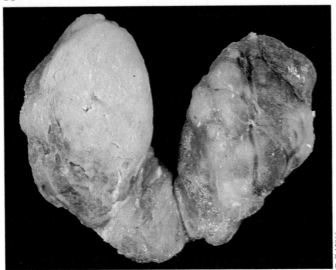

18 A man of 59 developed a mass in his left axillary lymph nodes diagnosed as a reticulum cell sarcoma. He died a year later despite intensive therapy. Widespread dissemination was found at necropsy.

In the specimen a tumour nodule in the right lobe of the thyroid has been sectioned to reveal a pale grey homogeneous surface. Several small nodules can be seen beneath the capsule in the left lobe.

19

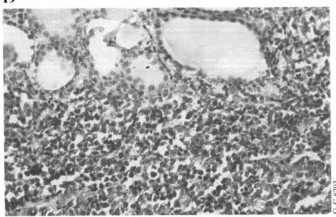

19 From a woman of 73 who had a swelling of the left lobe of the thyroid for 4 months. The left lobe was widely infiltrated by malignant cells of the lymphoid series. *(H&E ×250)*

Thyroid – Tuberculosis

Tuberculosis of the thyroid, never a common disease, is now very rare. It usually presents as a mass resulting from spread of infection from tuberculous cervical lymph nodes or from laryngeal tuberculosis. Haematogenous spread may cause multiple foci.

The gross and microscopic appearances are similar to those of tuberculous lesions elsewhere.

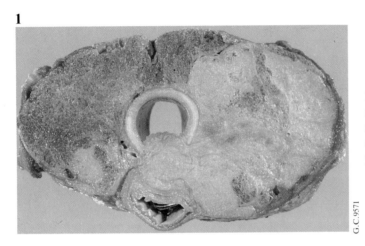

1 A horizontal section of a thyroid gland which shows destruction of virtually the whole of the right lobe by caseous tuberculosis. The disease extends between the oesophagus and trachea and there is also a similar focus in the posterior portion of the left lobe.

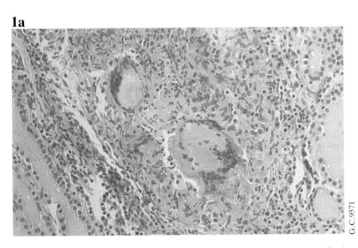

1a A portion of the thyroid gland which surrounded a caseous area showing the characteristic tuberculous giant cells and epithelioid cells. *(H&E ×250)*

James Fraser

M. O. Wright

Abnormalities of function of the parathyroid glands are of significance not because of their frequency but because of their bizarre presentation and the dramatic relief that follows successful management.

Anatomy – development

There are usually four parathyroid glands but the number may vary from two to six. Oval in shape, they are yellow/brown ovoid bodies measuring approximately $3\times6\times2$mm in size and weighing from 30 to 100mgm. Originating in the neural crest they develop from the third and fourth branchial clefts, the upper glands from the fourth and the lower from the third. Ultimately they lie on or are embedded within the posterior aspect of the lateral lobes of the thyroid. The superior pair lie relatively constantly at the junction of the middle and upper thirds of the lobes and on their posterior surface. The inferior pair are less constant, usually being sited either lateral and posterior to the lower poles or at a lower level in relation to the inferior thyroid veins. Less frequently a gland may lie between the oesophagus and trachea or rarely within the mediastinum. One or two glands may be absent, there being no rule as to which site is most commonly affected. These variations in location are of special significance to the surgeon undertaking the operative removal of parathyroid tumours. Frequently it is difficult to identify the site of the lesion.

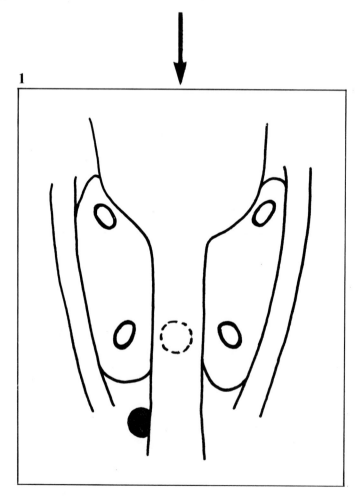

1   Diagram of posterior aspect of the thyroid showing the sites of the parathyroid glands.

Histology

The glands consist of secretory epithelial cells arranged in groups, interspersed with fat cells and separated by a rich sinusoidal network. The fat cells do not normally appear until after puberty but then increase in number up to the age of 40. There are two types of secretory cells: (1) the 'chief' or 'principal' cells which are small with poorly staining vacuolated cytoplasm and vesicular nuclei; (2) the 'oxyphil' cells which are less numerous, larger in size with a granular eosinophilic cytoplasm and deeply staining nuclei. The chief cells secrete parathyroid hormone but the function of the oxyphil cells is not clearly understood. A third cell type, the 'water-clear' cells, has been demonstrated, but they are derived from the 'chief' cells and are mainly a feature of hyperplastic or neoplastic glands.

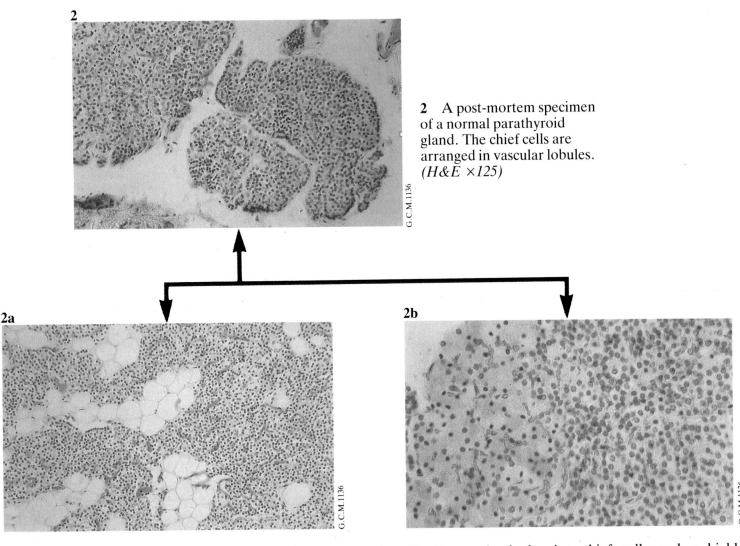

2 A post-mortem specimen of a normal parathyroid gland. The chief cells are arranged in vascular lobules. (*H&E ×125*)

2a Parathyroid – normal. Strands of adipose tissue are present. The parathyroid tissue shown is composed mainly of chief cells. Cell size and nuclear appearance are very regular. (*H&E ×125*)

2b Same gland showing chief cells and a highly vascular focus of oxyphil cells. The oxyphil cell cytoplasm is abundant and eosinophilic and the nuclei tend to be pyknotic. (*H&E ×312*)

Physiology

The parathyroid glands secrete a hormone (parathormone) which plays an important role in regulating calcium and phosphate metabolism. It acts mainly by increasing the excretion of phosphates through the renal tubules thus releasing phosphate and calcium from the skeleton.

Serum phosphate

0.8 – 1.4mM/L

At pH 7.4 the ratio $\dfrac{HPO_4''}{H_2PO_4^-} = \dfrac{4}{1}$

Serum calcium

9.83 $\pm$ 0.12mg per 100mls
2.5mM/L
50% Non-diffusible, non-ionised – attached to protein
45% Diffusible and ionised – the physiologically important fraction
5% Diffusible, non-ionised – calcium citrate, phosphate and bicarbonate

The serum calcium is regulated to keep its level within narrow limits. Two hormones, parathormone and calcitonin, and Vitamin D are involved in this homeostatic process.

Parathyroid hormone (parathormone) is a polypeptide of M.W. 9500 produced by the chief cells of the parathyroid glands. Together with calcitonin and Vitamin D it regulates the distribution of calcium in the body. A decrease in the calcium concentration in the blood perfusing the parathyroid glands causes the release of parathyroid hormone which exerts its effects on bone, kidney and the gastrointestinal tract.

Effects of PTH on bone

PTH causes increased reabsorption of calcium and phosphate from bone
(a)   by a rapid process – within 10 minutes.
(b)   by osteoclastic osteolysis. This is a much slower mechanism.

Parathyroid hormone (PTH) activates osteoclasts to secrete
(a)   proteolytic enzymes which digest the ground substance and collagen (collagenase) and
(b)   citric and lactic acids which render soluble the bone salts.

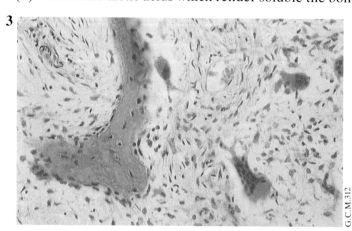

3   Osteitis fibrosa. Osteoblasts can be seen around a spicule of bone and osteoclasts are present in the cellular fibrous tissue. *(H&E ×250)*

Effects of PTH on the kidney

PTH (a) increases renal tubular reabsorption of Ca^{++} Mg^{++} and H^+.
(b) increases excretion of phosphate, sodium, potassium, amino acids and bicarbonate.
(c) stimulates the conversion of Vitamin D (the 25 (OH) D_3 metabolite) to its active form $(1,25 (OH)_2 D_3)$.

Gastrointestinal tract (GIT)

Parathyroid hormone acting via the active form of Vitamin D $(1,25 (OH)_2$ cholecalciferol) increases the absorption of calcium and phosphate from the gastrointestinal tract (GIT).

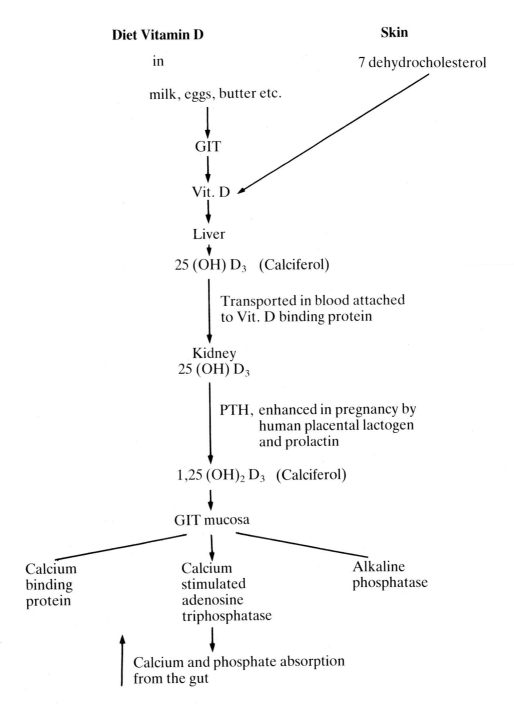

Calcitonin

The effects of parathyroid hormone on the serum calcium level are opposed by the hormone calcitonin produced by the parafollicular or C cells of the thyroid. Its release is stimulated by a rise in the serum (Ca^{++}) perfusing these cells and also by the hormone gastrin.

Calcitonin reduces the serum calcium and phosphate level by acting on bone, kidney and intestine.

It has the opposite effects to parathormone and works more rapidly (one hour compared to several hours for parathormone).

1   It inhibits the osteoclastic reabsorption of bone by:
   (a) decreased formation of osteoclasts
   (b) decreased osteoclastic activity

2   It increases the urinary excretion of calcium and phosphate.

3   It decreases the intestinal absorption of calcium.

Calcitonin is thought to have a weak effect in adults and its importance in the long term regulation of the serum calcium level is uncertain.

Lesions of the parathyroid must be studied both in regard to any hormonal disturbance if present and the structural nature of the causal lesion within the gland.

Classification of parathyroid disease

Pathophysiology	Parathyroid abnormality

1 increased secretion of parathormone	(a) Hyperplasia
	      Primary
	      Secondary
	      Tertiary
	
	(b) Adenoma
	
	(c) Carcinoma

2 decreased secretion of parathormone	(a) Congenital absence
	
	(b) Surgical removal
	
	(c) Pathological destruction
	      Infarction, Haemorrhage
	      Secondary tumours

Hyperparathyroidism

Abnormalities of parathyroid function may be primary or secondary and usually present as hyperparathyroidism. Less commonly clinical disturbances may arise from hyposecretion of parathormone.

Primary hyperparathyroidism occurs when parathormone secretion is increased either by primary hyperplasia of the gland, or more commonly by a parathyroid adenoma.

Secondary hyperparathyroidism develops in response to a persistently lowered serum calcium and an elevated phosphorus. This may result from a variety of causes.

1 Low Ca^{++} diet
2 Pregnancy and Lactation
3 Malabsorption
4 Rickets and Osteomalacia
   (Vitamin D deficiency)
5 Abnormal renal function due to chronic
   renal failure; resulting from
   dialysis after renal transplantation

The term tertiary hyperparathyroidism is used when an autonomous adenoma develops in one or more of the hyperplastic glands of secondary hyperparathyroidism.

Pseudohyperparathyroidism is a term sometimes applied to the hypercalcaemia associated with malignant disease. The hypercalcaemia may develop irrespective of bone metastases and is attributed to ectopic secretion of a PTH-like substance by the tumours, e.g. carcinoma of the lung or breast.

Primary parathyroid hyperplasia

The cause is unknown. All the glands enlarge each showing uniform microscopic evidence of the hyperplasia and of functional hyperactivity.

Histology

4

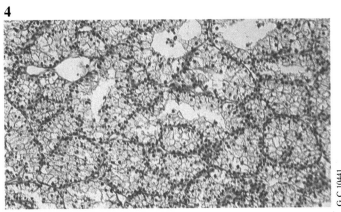

4 The fat lobules of the normal gland are reduced or may disappear altogether to be replaced by sheets of acini of 'chief' cells many of which take on the characteristics of 'water-clear' cells. These cells are of variable size but are usually large with a clear cytoplasm which may contain small eosinophilic granules. The nucleus also varies in size and characteristically is basally orientated.

(H&E ×150)

In secondary hyperparathyroidism the histological findings in the uniformly enlarged glands are similar to those in primary parathyroid hyperplasia.

Parathyroid adenoma

The parathyroid tumour is usually a functioning adenoma composed of cells mainly resembling the chief cells of the normal gland but with a variable pattern and cell type. It occurs at any age and affects women three times more frequently than men. Usually it is small, ovoid with slight lobulation, 1 to 2cm in diameter. Weights ranging from 0.4 to 120gms have been reported. It is soft and varies from orange yellow to chocolate brown in colour, sometimes with haemorrhagic foci and frequently containing cysts. Commonly it originates from one of the inferior parathyroids behind or within the lower lobe of the thyroid, but any one of the glands may be involved and up to 10% may lie in an aberrant site. Rarely there may be more than one tumour.

Pathology

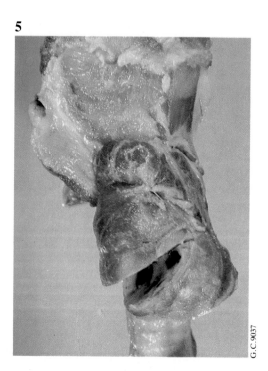

5 A posterolateral view of the neck structures of a man who suffered severe osteitis fibrosa. A parathyroid adenoma 4cm in diameter lies on the thyroid gland. The darkened areas which have been exposed are haemorrhagic cysts.

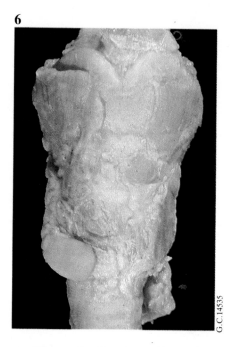

6 The buff-coloured parathyroid adenoma (1.8×1.5cm) shown at the right lower pole of the thyroid was found at necropsy of a woman of 77. It was associated with minimal osteitis fibrosa and impaired renal function with focal deposits of calcium in tubules.

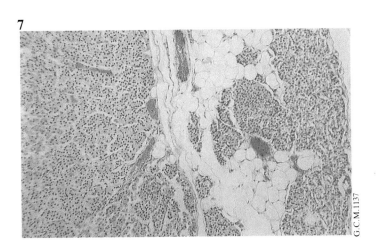

7 Parathyroid adenoma. The adenoma (left) is, in this field, separated by adipose tissue from the normal parathyroid. Note the similarity in cell structure. *(H&E ×100)*

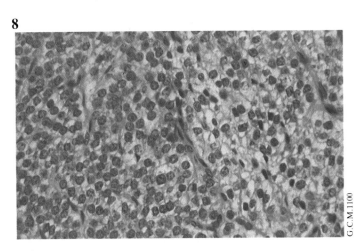

8 A parathyroid adenoma associated with osteitis fibrosa. Chief cells predominated. This field has been chosen to illustrate a focus of clear cells (right). *(H&E ×500)*

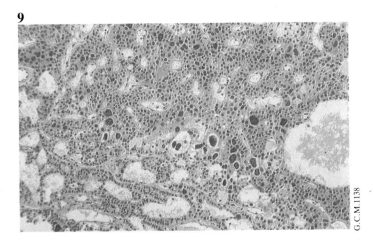

9 Parathyroid adenoma from mediastinum. A variant of the usual pattern showing acinar formation. Some of the cells have single giant nuclei. There is no mitotic activity. *(H&E ×125)*

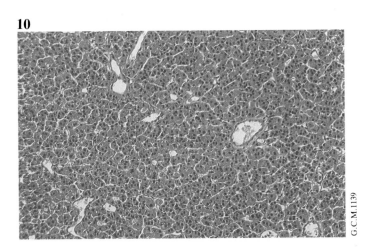

10 Oxyphil parathyroid adenoma. The cytoplasm of the cells is strongly eosinophilic and clearly defined. The nuclei stain densely. *(H&E ×125)*

Primary hyperparathyroidism

Effects

Effects on blood chemistry

Total body calcium level reduced.
Serum calcium level raised 12–15mg % (3–3.75mm/L)
Serum phosphate level reduced.
Increased alkaline phosphatase levels.

Effects on bone

Extreme osteoclastic activity in bones causing bone resorption and fibrous replacement. In advanced disease bone cysts and osteoclastomas may develop. The effects are illustrated in the pathology.

11

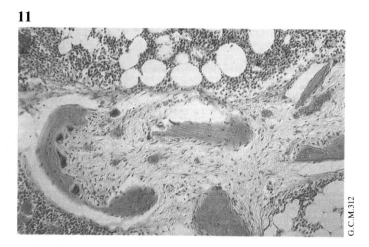

G.C.M.312

11 Osteitis fibrosa – head of humerus. Bone trabeculae are being eroded and replaced by fibrous tissue. *(H&E ×125)*

12

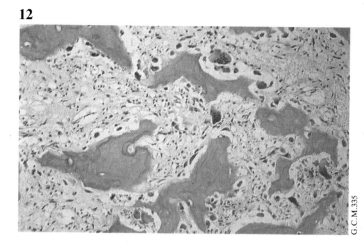

G.C.M.335

12 Osteitis fibrosa of ilium. Very active disease. The fibrous tissue is cellular and contains many osteoblasts and multinucleated osteoclasts. *(H&E ×250)*

A woman of 53 had suffered from pain in the right hip for eight years, followed by pain in both tibia and in the lumbosacral region. Radiology suggested osteitis fibrosa and there were cysts in both humeri, and the left femur. Serum calcium was 14.8mg% and the alkaline phosphatase was raised.

At operation a parathyroid tumour measuring 4.3×2.5×1cm was found lying behind the fascia of the lower pole of the left lobe of the thyroid. The fascia was incised and the tumour was removed without difficulty.

G.C.10318

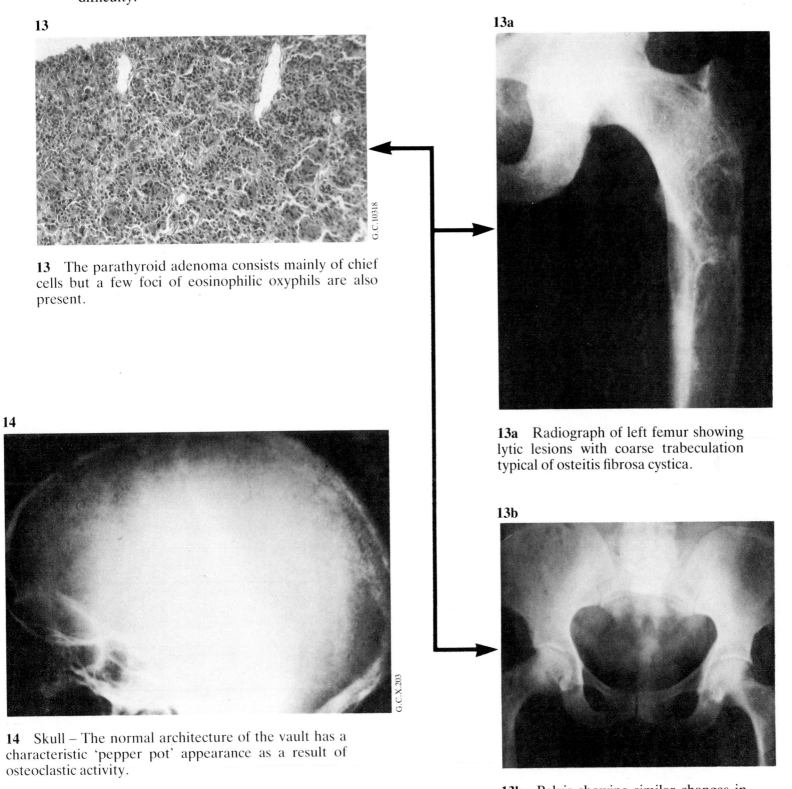

13 The parathyroid adenoma consists mainly of chief cells but a few foci of eosinophilic oxyphils are also present.

13a Radiograph of left femur showing lytic lesions with coarse trabeculation typical of osteitis fibrosa cystica.

13b Pelvis showing similar changes in the right femoral neck.

14 Skull – The normal architecture of the vault has a characteristic 'pepper pot' appearance as a result of osteoclastic activity.

257

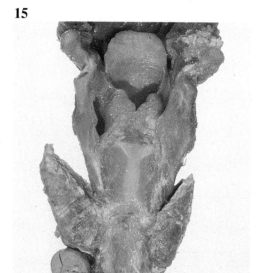

15 Thyroid gland
At the left lower lobe of the thyroid gland there is a pale brown parathyroid adenoma which caused severe osteitis fibrosa.

Osteitis fibrosa and parathyroid adenoma

The photographs illustrate the parathyroid adenoma, the left humerus and the right femur as seen at post-mortem examination on a mason's labourer aged 49. After suffering from aching pains in his limbs for five years, he sustained a stress fracture of the left humerus when lifting a heavy brick. The fracture which was just below the junction of the middle and lower thirds of the bone gradually consolidated but seven months later whilst travelling in a bus his arm was jolted and fractured about 5cm above the former fracture. This again consolidated but he died suddenly six months later from a 'heart attack'. The bone changes are of a severity which fortunately are seldom seen nowadays.

G.C.6256

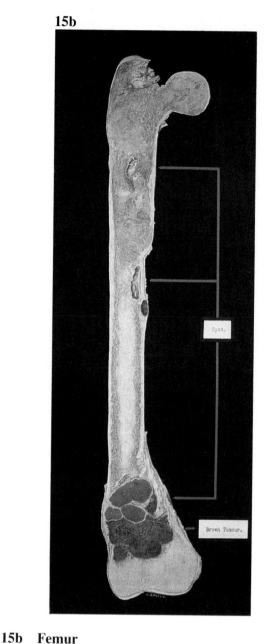

15b Femur
The femur has roughly maintained its normal shape but the upper half is thickened by post-resorption formation of new bone. Several cysts can be seen. The lower end is distorted by them and by the growth of a giant cell sarcoma.

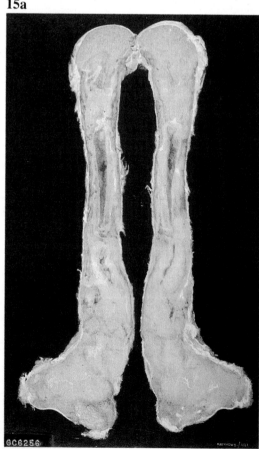

15a Left humerus
The upper half of the bone although affected by osteitis fibrosa has roughly maintained its normal shape. Much bone resorption and replacement by fibro-osteoid tissue has occurred, and there is considerable subperiosteal thickening. The lower half is greatly distorted as a result of the former fractures and the loss of normal bone, and is expanded by fibro-osteoid tissue.

15c

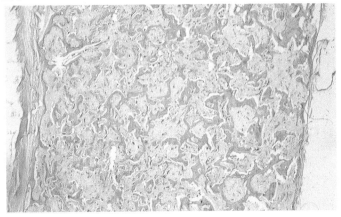

15c A full thickness section of calvarium. The normal cortical and cancellous bone and marrow have been replaced by fibrous tissue and by remodelled trabecula. *(H&E ×10)*

15d

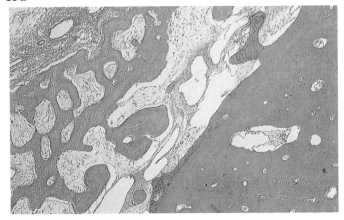

15d Femur. Between the periosteum (top left) and the cortical bone (right) formation of poorly calcified new bone has occurred. Osteoclasts and some osteoblasts are arranged mainly along trabecular borders. The fibrous tissue is cellular and not well collagenised. *(H&E ×40)*

15e

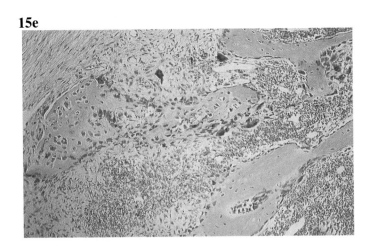

15e Haemorrhage has occurred in the cellular tissue between the particles of woven bone. The osteoclasts and osteoblasts are very numerous and are atypical – probably a pre-malignant change. *(H&E ×100)*

15f

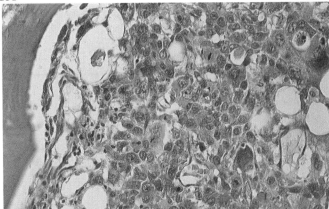

15f The sarcoma of the lower end of the femur is composed of large uninucleated and multinucleated cells. Many mitotic figures are present. *(H&E ×250)*

Other effects of primary hyperparathyroidism

Metastatic calcification

With elevated levels of serum calcium, there may be metastatic calcification especially in lungs, kidneys, thyroid, stomach, arteries and cornea.

Effects upon central nervous system

In hypercalcaemia, central nervous system excitability is depressed, causing mental apathy, drowsiness and muscle weakness.

Calcium ions affect membrane permeability and excitability. They compete with sodium ions for certain sites on the cell membrane. A rise in the extracellular fluid concentration of calcium ions causes a decrease in membrane permeability to sodium ions. An effect of this is to raise the level of depolarisation necessary to cause the explosive increase in membrane permeability to sodium ions associated with the upstroke of the action potential. Membrane excitability is reduced and nerve and muscle cell membranes are more stable. In many of these patients the true nature of the condition is not appreciated and they are treated initially for mental disturbance, sometimes being admitted to mental institutions.

Effects upon kidney

Associated with elevated tubular concentrations of calcium and phosphate there is an increased incidence of renal calculi.

The urine volume is increased due to an inability to concentrate the urine caused by:
- (a) increased osmotic load (calcium)
- (b) renal damage caused by nephrocalcinosis and/or renal calculi.

16

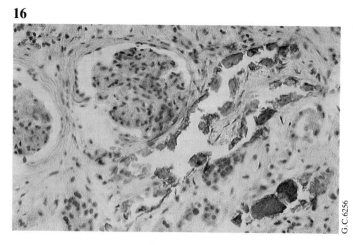

16   Kidney in osteitis fibrosa. The epithelium of one of the tubules is calcified. Particles of calcium are present in another tubule (microlithiasis). *(H&E ×250)*

Parathyroid carcinoma

Carcinoma of the parathyroid is very rare and a diagnosis can only be made on the evidence of local invasion of the capsule and surrounding tissues. The microscopic appearances are often little different from those of an adenoma. Distant metastases are rare.

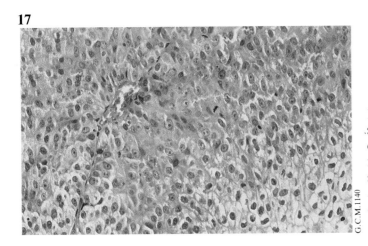

17

17 Parathyroid carcinoma. The tumour shows mitotic activity. The nuclear/cytoplasmic ratio is increased and there is some variation in nuclear size and shape. Some cells are spindle-shaped and their margins are rather poorly defined. *(H&E × 250)*

Hypoparathyroidism

In adults hypoparathyroidism may result from absence or atrophy of the parathyroid glands, or from insensitivity of the target tissues to PTH (pseudohypoparathyroidism). Most cases, however, result from surgery involving the parathyroids, thyroid or larynx.

After parathyroidectomy the osteoclasts are inactive. The serum phosphate rises. The serum (Ca^{++}) falls from 10mg% to 6 to 7mg% in three days (2.5mM/L to 1.6mM/L).

As a result of a decreased level of ionised calcium: the CNS becomes hyper-excitable; there is increased neuronal permeability to sodium; tetany, hyper-reflexia, carpopedal spasm and laryngeal stridor may occur.

Latent tetany can be demonstrated by:
1   Tapping the facial nerve, in front of the lobe of the ear, and observing a brisk contraction of the facial muscles (Chvostek's sign).
2   The application of a blood pressure cuff to the arm; on inflation of this to arterial pressure, carpopedal spasm may be observed (Trousseau's sign).

James Fraser

M. O. Wright

Adrenal 55

Embryology

The adrenal cortex develops during the fourth week of foetal life (6mm) as a series of buds from the coelomic cells between the root of the mesentery and the root of the mesonephros. In the 12mm foetus the cortical mass forms a ridge. Sympathochromaffin tissue develops simultaneously. The primitive medullary tissue migrates from the neural crest and between the 12 and 19mm stage penetrates the cortical tissue from its medial side.

1

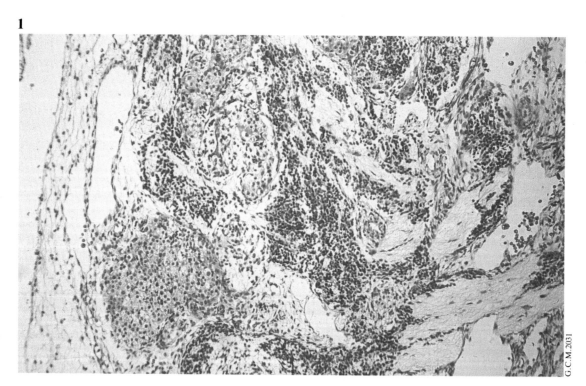

1 Part of the adrenal of a 25mm crown-rump embryo. In the left lateral area clusters of pink cortical cells can be seen. On the right the adrenal is invaded on its medial side by the darkly staining sympathogonia from the neural crest. *(H&E ×320)*

Foetal adrenal

1 Tissue which will ultimately form the three zones of permanent cortex account for only 20% of the foetal cortex.
2 The other 80% is foetal adrenal cortex which produces dehydroepiandrosterone sulphate ($DHASO_4$). This is directly converted in the foetoplacental unit into oestrone and oestradiol, or after $16 \propto$ hydroxylation in the foetal liver into oestriol.

Further development of the cortex

The cortex develops as two separate layers. The outer layer persists as the permanent zona glomerulosa. Immediately after birth there is a dramatic degeneration in the inner layer which commences with the event of birth unrelated to the age of the foetus and extends into the second year of life. During the process of degeneration there is growth and differentiation of the permanent cortex into its three definitive layers. This process of development is usually completed by puberty.

Adrenal rests

Aberrant cortical tissue may occur adjacent to the adrenal, in the spleen, beneath the capsules of the kidneys, in the retroperitoneal space or close to the testes or ovaries.

2

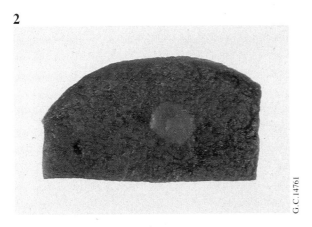

G.C.14761

2 The capsule of the kidney has been stripped revealing a thin plaque of pale adrenal cortical tissue lying on the surface of the kidney.

In addition to their presence in the adrenal medulla, chromaffin tissues are normally found in various sites along the course of the aorta, and in the paraganglia. The longer and more distally located pre- and para-aortic structures form the organ of Zuckerkandl near the root of the inferior mesenteric artery.

The relative importance of the adrenal medulla and organs of Zuckerkandl changes after birth. In early infancy the noradrenaline production is mainly in the organs of Zuckerkandl but later the activity of the adrenal medulla increases and the organs of Zuckerkandl tend to atrophy.

The development of tumours from aberrant cortical tissue or extra-adrenal chromaffin tissue is a well recognised, though uncommon occurrence, and presents many difficulties in clinical diagnosis. These tumours, comparable in all respects to those more normally located, may be associated with hormonal disturbance.

Blood supply

The adrenals are highly vascular organs and the arrangement of their blood supply is complex.

The arterial supply is derived from the inferior phrenic artery, directly from the aorta and the renal artery.

There is, however, no constant order in which these arise and individual vessels are not usually definable, there being multiple small twigs going to the superior, medial and inferior aspects of the gland. The arteries form a free anastomosis on the surface from which vessels pass at right angles into the gland. Branches from the suprarenal may cross to the upper pole of the adjacent kidney and therefore the blood supplies of the adrenal, kidney and sometimes of the testis and ovary cannot be considered as wholly independent.

The venous drainage of the gland is much simpler. All or almost all of the veins channel into one large central adrenal vein. The right vein is very short, travelling transversely from the hilum to the vena cava. The left vein is rather longer also leaving at the hilum but descending to the renal vein opposite the termination of the internal spermatic vein.

The lymphatics of the adrenal communicate freely with the adjacent aortic lymph vessels.

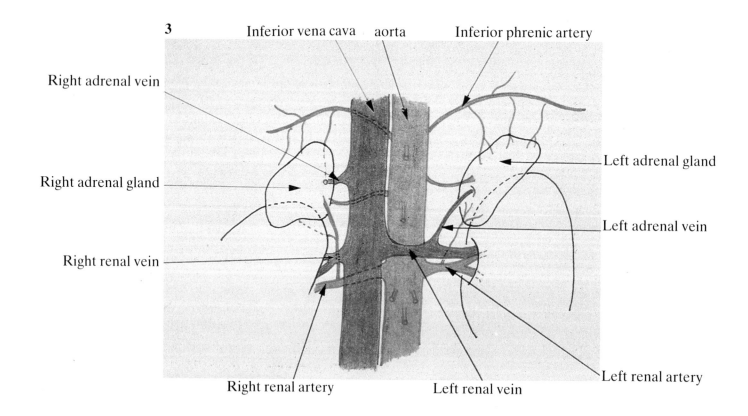

3   Inferior vena cava   aorta   Inferior phrenic artery

Right adrenal vein

Right adrenal gland

Right renal vein

Right renal artery

Left adrenal gland

Left adrenal vein

Left renal artery

Left renal vein

Portal circulation inside adrenal gland

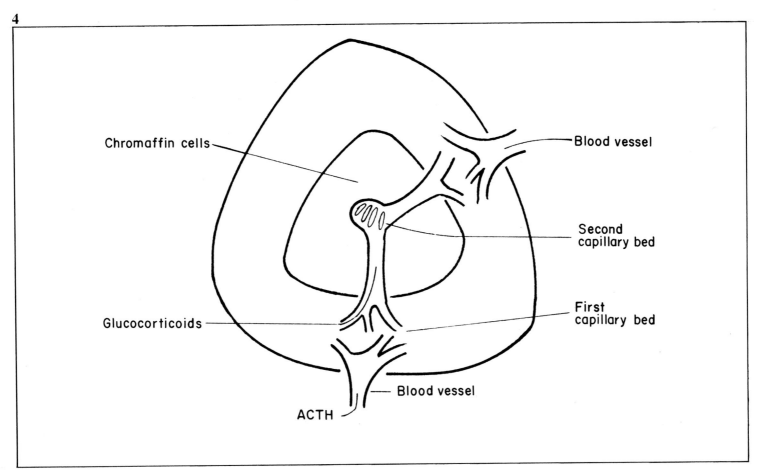

4

Chromaffin cells

Glucocorticoids

Blood vessel

Second capillary bed

First capillary bed

Blood vessel

ACTH

4 Blood with a high cortisol level passes into the medulla from the cortex and influences both the size of chromaffin cells and the synthesis of enzyme PNMT in the medulla.

Nerve supply

There is an extensive sympathetic innervation to the suprarenal but it appears to be restricted to the medulla, there being no detectable supply to the cortex. Efferent fibres leave the spinal cord ipsilaterally and principally between T6 and L3. The majority of these fibres are preganglionic and 50% are myelinated and remain so until they enter the gland substance. They are carried to a plexus in close relation to the main adrenal vessels through the coeliac, the phrenic and renal plexuses and also by direct fibres from the great splanchnic nerve. From their course on the vessels the fibres pass to the medulla where they form small primary plexuses surrounding medullary cell groups. They finally end in close contact with the chromaffin cells though never apparently penetrating them.

Histology

The preponderance of the adult gland is made up of cortex. This can be divided into three layers:

1. The outer zona glomerulosa producing primarily mineralocorticoids
2. The zona fasciculata producing glucocorticoids and
3. The zona reticularis, the source of androgens and oestrogens.

The central glandular tissue is the medulla and is composed of columns of large, irregular polyhedral cells. The cytoplasm is granular and stains brown with chrome salts.

1 *Cortex* – 3 layers. No break in cellular continuity.

Zona glomerulosa – inconspicuous and narrow. Cells – small, scanty cytoplasm, abundant mitochondria, abundant RNA, lipid content small.

Zona fasciculata – the broadest zone. Cells – large with abundant lipid. Mitosis found only in this zone.

Zona reticularis – a narrow zone. Cells – show only scanty eosinophilic cytoplasm, abundant mitochondria and RNA.

2 *Medulla* – large chromaffin cells. Cells in irregular columns forming a lattice-work around sinusoids.

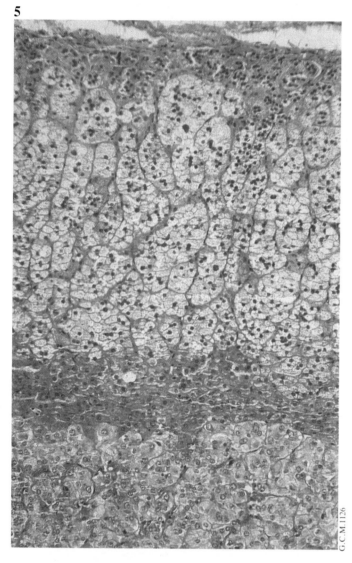

5 Adrenal cortex and outer medulla. *(H&E ×200)*

6 Part of the cortex and medulla of a rabbit adrenal stained to demonstrate cortical lipid in zz. fasciculata and reticularis. *(Oil red 0 ×40)*

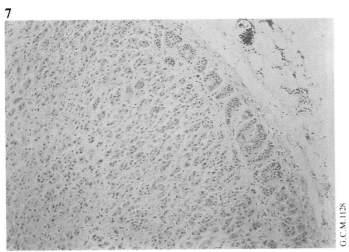

7 Adrenal cortex showing z. fasciculata and well defined z. glomerulosa. *(H&E ×50)*

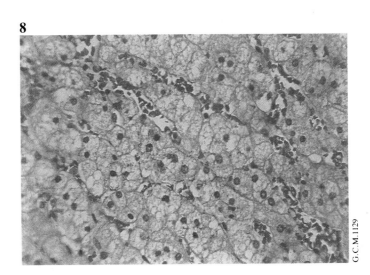

8 z. fasciculata – columns of lipid-rich vacuolated cells. *(H&E ×250)*

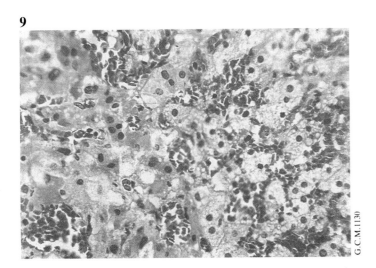

9 Cells of z. reticularis right and of medulla left. *(H&E ×250)*

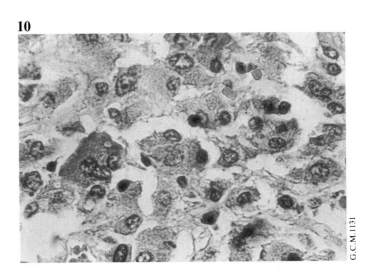

10 Medulla – chromaffin reaction. Brown staining has resulted from fixation in potassium bichromate. *(H&E ×375)*

The adrenal steroids are derivatives of cholesterol and contain the cyclopentanophenanthrene nucleus.

Steroids with 18 carbon atoms have oestrogenic activity, e.g. oestradiol.

Steroids with 19 carbon atoms are androgens, e.g. dehydroepiandrosterone.

Steroids with 21 carbon atoms and ketone at position 20 are glucocorticoids, e.g. cortisol.

Steroids with mineralocorticoids, e.g. aldosterone.

Steroids with progestogens, e.g. progesterone.

Steroid biosynthesis

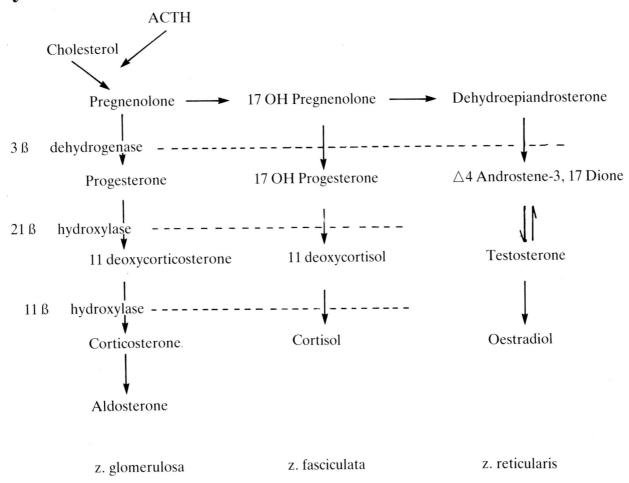

Secreted steroids

Major		Minor	
Mineralocorticoid	Aldosterone	11 deoxycorticosterone	Oestradiol
Glucocorticoid	Cortisol and corticosterone	11 deoxycortisol	
Androgen	Dehydroepiandrosterone		

Daily secretion of major steroids (mg)

Aldosterone	0.15
Cortisol	20
Corticosterone	3
Dehydroepiandrosterone	21 (male) or 16 (female)

Steroid metabolism

Cortisol

In the liver, cortisol is reduced to di- and tetra-hydro-cortisol and conjugated with glucuronic acid. It is rapidly excreted by the kidney. Some cortisol is converted to cortisone. 10% of the secreted cortisol is converted in the liver to 17-ketosteroids which are subsequently conjugated with sulphate and excreted in the urine. The metabolism of corticosterone is similar to that of cortisol, but no 17-ketosteroids are formed.

Aldosterone

Aldosterone is converted in the liver to di- and tetra-hydroaldosterone glucuronides and excreted in the urine.

17-ketosteroids

In the male 70% of urinary ketosteroids are secreted by the adrenal or are formed from the conversion of cortisol in the liver. 30% are derived from testosterone (testis) which is not itself a 17-ketosteroid but gives rise to metabolites which are.

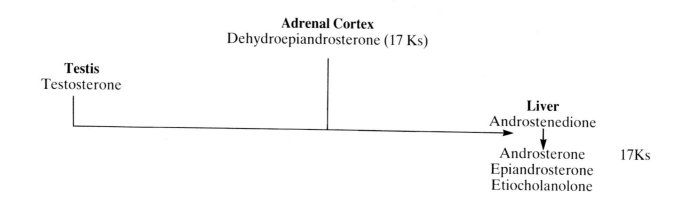

These compounds are conjugated with glucuronic acid or sulphate in the liver and excreted in the urine.

Urinary output per 24 hours		17-ketosteroids	15mg male
Cortisol di- and tetra-glucuronides	5–10mg		10mg female
Aldosterone di- and tetra-glucuronides	20–30µg	17-OH corticosteroids	5–20mg

Control of cortisol secretion

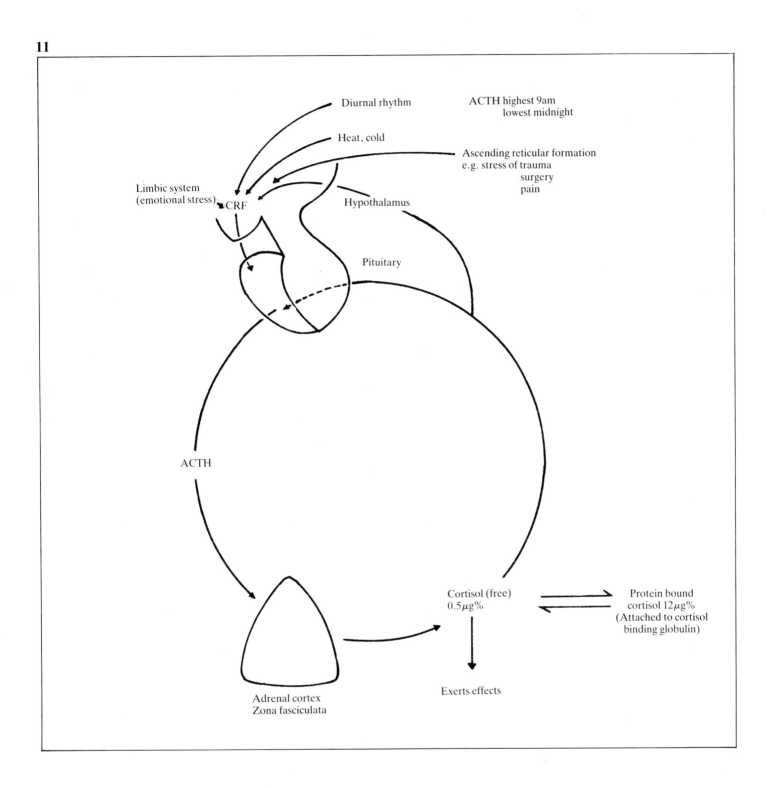

Functions of cortisol

1 Cortisol increases:
   protein breakdown

   amino acid uptake by the liver and deamination and transamination in the liver.

   gluconeogenesis and blood glucose levels.

   lipolysis and plasma levels of free fatty acids.

2 Potentiates the effect of catecholamines on vascular reactivity lipolysis and bronchodilatation.

3 Is concerned in the excretion of a water load.

4 Increases secretion of gastric acid and pepsin. Alters mucosal resistance to irritant action of gastric juice.

5 Cortisol increases the number of circulating RBCs, platelets and neutrophils. It decreases:
   circulating eosinophils and basophils

   circulating lymphocytes by decreasing production and increasing destruction

   the size of lymph nodes and the thymus.

When secreted in increased amounts, glucocorticoids

1 Affect acute inflammation by:
   stabilising lysosomal membranes and decreasing the release of leucocyte endogenous pyrogen.

   By decreasing:
   the effect of bacterial toxins
   the release of kinins and histamine.

   By decreasing fibroblastic activity and the walling off of abscesses.

2 Cause osteoporosis.

3 Inhibit growth by decreasing the secretion of growth hormone.

Cushing's syndrome

Cushing's syndrome refers to a series of clinical signs and symptoms coupled with metabolic abnormalities due to excessive production of glucocorticoids or to steroid therapy. Most cases occur in adults and in females.

The excess of glucocorticoids may be attributable to:
    (a)   stimulation of the adrenal cortex by excessive ACTH or
    (b)   excessive production of adrenal glucocorticoids not dependent on ACTH stimulation.

A.   ACTH-dependent glucocorticoid secretion

   1   Production of ACTH by a basophil adenoma (which may be minute) of the anterior pituitary (Cushing's disease).
             or
     By a non-endocrine tumour (ectopic ACTH), e.g. oat cell carcinoma of the bronchus.

   2   Failure of normal suppression of pituitary ACTH secretion by cortisol feedback mechanism.

B.   Autonomous glucocorticoid secretion

   1   Adrenocortical hyperfunction.

   2   Adrenocortical adenoma or carcinoma.

   3   Secretion of glucocorticoids by other tumours.

In adults, naturally occurring Cushing's syndrome is associated with basophil pituitary adenomas and adrenocortical hyperplasia in about 80% of cases. In children, however, adrenocortical tumours predominate.

12

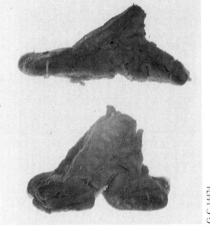

13

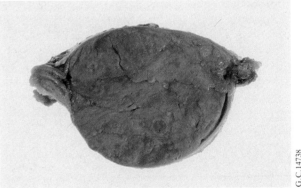

12 From a female aged 42 who suffered from hypertension, glycosuria, weight increase and a Cushingoid appearance for 5 years, and gross obesity for 1–2 years. The adrenals removed at operation weighed right – 8.0g, left – 9.2g, and microscopically showed diffuse and focal hyperplasia.

13 From a female aged 31 years with a history of mitral valvotomy and gastroenterostomy who developed Cushing's disease. At operation the left adrenal contained an adenoma measuring 3.5cm in diameter and was excised.

The histology of these lesions is described later.

Cushing's syndrome *(Continued)*

Clinical manifestations

1 Decreased protein synthesis leading to decreased growth.

2 Thinning and stretching of the skin and subcutaneous tissues. Rupture of the subcutaneous tissues leads to the appearance of red-purple striae.

3 A redistribution of body fat, with increased amounts over the back, interscapular area, the abdomen and face (moonface).

4 Bruising as a result of capillary rupture due to poor connective tissue support.

5 Poor wound healing (protein synthesis).

6 Muscle weakness due to loss of protein, loss of potassium.

7 Alterations in carbohydrate and lipid metabolism leading to insulin resistant diabetes with ketosis in approximately 20% of patients.

8 Sodium and water retention leading to hypertension and oedema. Hypertension can also result from increased levels of glucocorticoids potentiating the catecholamines to cause increased vascular reactivity.

9 Osteoporosis due to the effects of glucocorticoids on bone proteins.

10 Personality changes – emotionally labile, increased $\propto$ rhythm, toxic psychosis.

11 Adrenal androgen secretion may be increased leading in women to amenorrhoea and hirsutism.

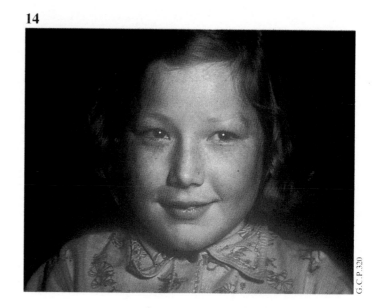

14

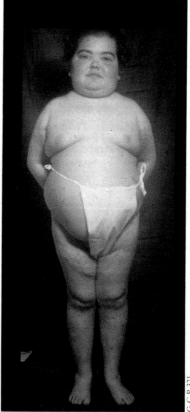

15

Investigation

Constant biochemical findings

Plasma cortisol levels raised.

Diurnal variation in cortisol excretion absent.

Other tests

Dexamethasone suppression test.

Estimation of plasma ACTH levels.

Estimation of urinary 17-ketosteroids (produced by z. reticularis).

Glucose tolerance test.

X-ray of spine for osteoporosis.

The results of these investigations vary according to the cause of Cushing's syndrome.

Cause of Cushing's syndrome	Dexamethasone (DM) test effect on ACTH secretion	Plasma ACTH	Urinary 17-ketosteroids
ACTH-dependent disease			
(a) Pituitary	Low dose DM – no suppression High dose DM – suppression	Increased	Increased
(b) Ectopic	No response	Increased	Increased
Adrenal Adenoma	No response	Reduced	Reduced due to ACTH reduction
Adrenal Carcinoma	No response	Reduced	Increased by autonomous secretion by the tumour

Cushing's syndrome *(Continued)*

Histology

It may not be possible to demonstrate histological abnormalities in either the pituitary or adrenals. Abnormalities which have been reported are:

<table>
<tr><td>Pituitary</td><td>Adrenal</td></tr>
<tr><td>In many cases a basophil adenoma is present but it is often small (microadenoma) and difficult to find.</td><td>Cortical hyperplasia
Cortical adenomas
Cortical carcinomas</td></tr>
<tr><td>Crooke's hyalinisation of the basophils.</td><td></td></tr>
</table>

Adrenocortical hyperplasia

Hyperplasia may result from excessive ACTH stimulation or may be autonomous and then may or may not be associated with overt endocrine disturbances. Hyperplasia can affect the cortex diffusely or may be nodular or show a combination of these features. Frequently when the hyperplasia appears to be autonomous the cortical cells are filled with lipid. Under strong ACTH stimulation, however, their lipid content is discharged. Thus in ACTH-dependent Cushing's disease some of the cells of the z. fasciculata become more solid and eosinophilic, resembling those of the z. reticularis. Correspondingly the gross appearance of the adrenal cortex changes, losing some of its normal yellow colour and becoming more fleshy.

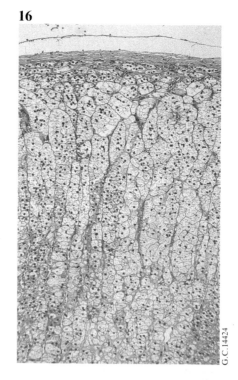

16 Adrenocortical hyperplasia – Cushing's syndrome. The z. fasciculata is increased in depth and its inner layers are depleted of lipid. The z. glomerulosa which is non-ACTH-dependent is thinned by compression. *(H&E ×100)*

Adrenocortical tumours

Larger hyperplastic nodules of the adrenal cortex re-semble adenomas. The term adenoma is usually applied when the lesion is discrete or solitary, when it compresses and thins the surrounding cortex and when it is encapsulated. Larger adenomas in turn may be difficult to distinguish from well differentiated carcinomas. Normal lipid-rich cells predominate. About ⅓–½ of the adrenocortical tumours causing Cushing's syndrome are carcinomas. The cortex of the contralateral adrenal is often hypoplastic unlike that in adrenocortical hyperplasia.

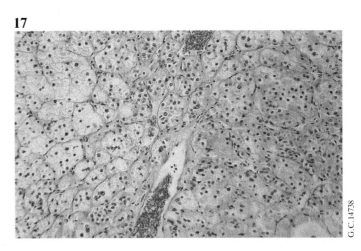

17 Adrenal cortical adenoma associated with Cushing's syndrome. A quite vascular adenoma composed of well differentiated cells of z. fasciculata. Those on the right show lipid depletion. No mitotic activity. *(H&E ×125)*

Pleomorphic adenoma

Many tumours closely simulate the features of an adenoma without evident histological characteristics of malignancy despite their progressive and invasive behaviour. In others, a degree of cellular pleomorphism and irregularity of pattern is evident, with hyperchromatism of the nuclei and, in some instances, the presence of bizarre multinucleated giant cells.

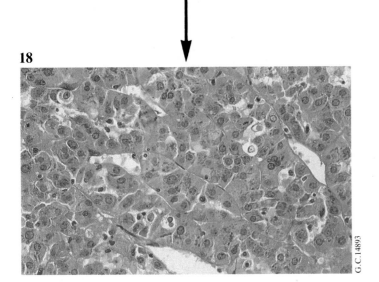

Carcinoma

5% of cortical tumours are carcinomas. Highest incidence between ages 20 to 40 but examples in childhood are well recognised. There is a large female preponderance. The mortality is very high.

In smaller tumours the distinction between adenoma and carcinoma is difficult to recognise, since the lesion appears to be encapsulated and its invasive nature is obscured. Larger bulky tumours, which are highly vascular and show central necrosis, are frequently globular or lobulated and while possessing a thin capsule are usually clearly invasive. The cut surface of the tumour is yellowish or variegated. Occasionally, areas of calcification are present at the periphery.

Cushing's syndrome *(Continued)*

Carcinoma *(Continued)*

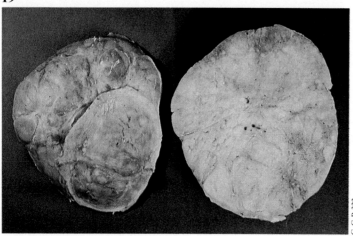

19 Cushing's syndrome due to carcinoma weighing 566g in a woman of 34. On the left the tumour can be seen arising from the adrenal. The cut surface is on the right.

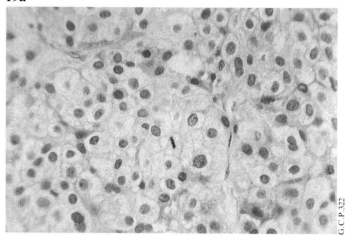

19a Same case. The carcinoma is well differentiated. The cells are fairly regular with moderately rich lipid content but there is some variation in nuclear size and one mitotic figure can be seen. *(H&E ×500)*

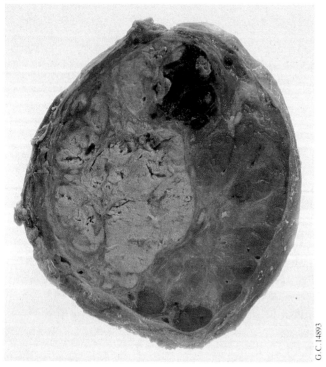

20 This tumour was discovered in a man of 48. Biopsy revealed that the tumour was adrenal carcinoma. Post-operatively he received radiotherapy and 12 weeks after the original laparotomy the tumour was removed.

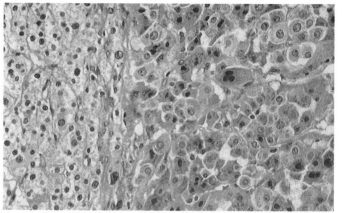

20a The tumour measured 22cm in maximum diameter and weighed 1020g. A large portion is pale and necrotic (left) but elsewhere it is brown and vascular. A micro-section of the tumour contrasts with the adjacent adrenal cortex on the left. The tumour is well differentiated. A number of cells are multinucleated and several show nuclear pyknosis – possibly a radiation effect. *(H&E ×250)*

21

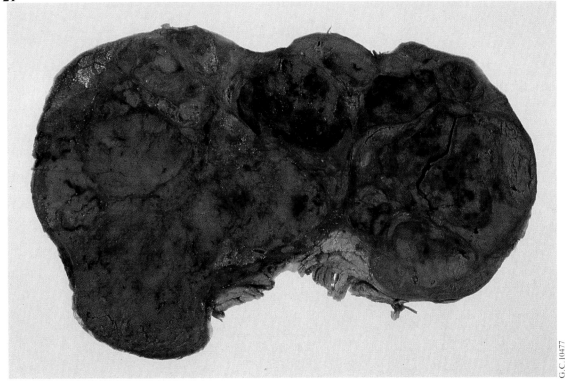

21 A man of 47 had experienced a few attacks of abdominal pain and sickness for nine months. He did not seek medical advice and it was only on routine medical examination that a large mass was discovered projecting beneath the left costal margin. The patient showed gynaecomastia and adiposity of female distribution which had gradually developed over three years. At operation the large lobulated tumour illustrated was discovered. It was ovoid measuring 20cm in greatest diameter and was composed of yellow tissue mottled by necrosis and haemorrhage, and irregularly sub-divided by fibrous septa. His sudden collapse and death 14 hours after operation was, at necropsy, attributed to adrenocortical insufficiency, the contralateral adrenal being atrophic.

21a

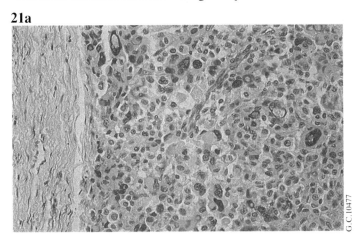

21a A subcapsular portion of the above tumour. The tumour is rather poorly differentiated with many bizarre nuclei and some lipid depletion. *(H&E ×250)*

Other hormonal effects

Most adrenocortical carcinomas have a hormonal effect. In addition to the tumours associated with Cushing's syndrome, there are some which result in virilisation in men and women, and in feminisation in men. Hyperaldosteronism may also result (p. 282).

Spread

Invasive carcinomas locally involve the posterior abdominal wall, the diaphragm, the kidney and on the right side the liver, lungs and lymph nodes. Adrenocortical tumours which are palpable are usually frankly malignant.

Aldosterone

Aldosterone release from the zona glomerulosa may be effected by three mechanisms:

1   By the release of ACTH in the large quantities following any trauma or haemorrhage.

2   By the renin, angiotensin II mechanism.

3   By a direct effect of an elevation of the serum potassium upon the zona glomerulosa itself.

22

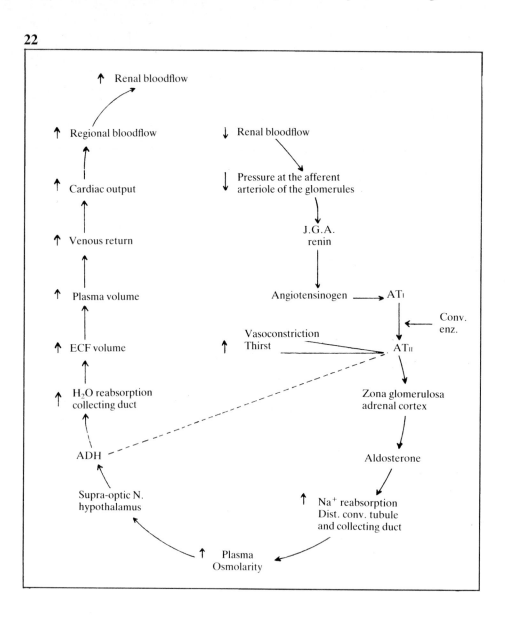

Causes of increased renin output

1   Decreased pressure at the afferent arteriole of the glomerulus.

2   Decreased [Na^+] at the macula densa segment and ascending limb of the loop of Henle.

3   S.N.S. stimulation via B receptors.

4   Decreased stimulation of atrial volume receptors.

Aldosterone causes reabsorption of sodium ions in exchange for either potassium or hydrogen ions in the distal convoluted tubule and collecting ducts of the kidney. It also causes sodium reabsorption in the salivary glands, gastric mucosa, terminal ileum, colon and sweat glands. Aldosterone is the principal mineralocorticoid secreted by the adrenal cortex; others which are less potent include corticosterone and deoxycorticosterone.

Long-term regulation of ECF volume and hence blood pressure is via the retention of sodium chloride and water. Sodium ions account for approximately half of the plasma osmolarity.

Plasma osmolarity = 282m Osmoles/L

Osmolarity due to Na^+ = 140m Osmoles/L

With changes in sodium ion concentration, go changes in ECF volume.

23

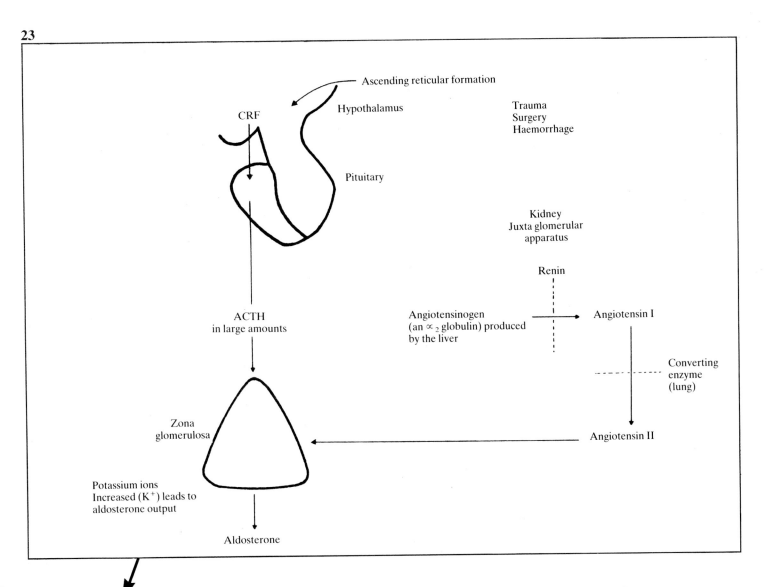

Possible mechanisms

1   A direct change in serum (K+)

2   Changes in intracellular (K+)

3   Change in flux of K^+ across the adrenocortical cell membrane.

Primary aldosteronism

(Conn's syndrome)

Primary aldosteronism is due to the presence of a hormone secreting tumour and is associated with a benign solitary or multiple adrenal cortical adenoma or less commonly a cortical carcinoma. It is approximately three times more common in women than in men. The majority of cases occur during the third and fourth decades but children with primary aldosteronism have been reported.

The tumour produces a continuous secretion of aldosterone which causes an increased exchange of sodium ions for potassium or hydrogen ions in the distal nephron. The sodium retention leads in turn to an increased extra-cellular fluid volume and an elevation in blood pressure.

The principal features are hypertension with excessive renal loss of potassium and resultant hypokalaemia. At an early stage in the disease the blood pressure may be only mildly elevated, the potassium may be marginally depressed and the patient may have no symptoms. In an established case, however, the hypertension is persistent though never severe and may show marked postural changes. Headaches are present. The total body potassium is reduced resulting in an extracellular alkalosis and an intracellular acidosis. The serum potassium level may fall below 3.5mm/L. In most cases the hypokalaemia is associated with a hypochloraemic alkalosis with an increase in plasma bicarbonate and arterial pH. The ECG shows changes compatible with hypokalaemia.

Diagnostic tests

Specific diagnostic manoeuvres are required to identify primary aldosteronism and to distinguish it from renin-angiotensin based hyperaldosteronism.

1 Estimation of plasma renin level. This is low in patients with primary aldosteronism.

2 Failure to increase a low level of plasma renin activity during volume depletion (sodium restriction).

3 Failure to suppress aldosterone secretion during volume expansion (sodium loading and deoxycorticosterone).

4 Increased urinary potassium loss during volume expansion.

5 In the presence of an aldosterone-producing adrenocortical adenoma the urinary excretion of 18-hydroxycortisol is increased 10 to 20 fold.

These tests should not be undertaken until base line levels of plasma and urinary aldosterone, plasma renin and plasma potassium have been obtained.

The majority of signs, symptoms and laboratory findings are related to the chronic potassium depletion.

1 Neuromuscular – muscle weakness and fatigue. Tetany may occasionally occur in association with the metabolic alkalosis.
2 Renal – polyuria, polydipsia, nocturia and a reversal of the usual clinical rhythm. On occasions the urine may be mildly alkaline. Failure to concentrate urine even with overnight dehydration (vasopressin resistant). As a secondary effect there is a reversible renal tubular vacuolation.

Mild azotaemia may occur but it is rare to have chronic renal failure. The sodium-potassium ratio in both sweat and saliva is reduced to less than one, an observation that may be used as a screening test in hypertensive patients. Serum sodium is usually within normal limits or slightly increased and there is an expansion of the extracellular fluid volume.

Patients with primary aldosteronism do not show significant oedema because of an escape phenomenon. If the plasma level of aldosterone is persistently elevated the effect of aldosterone on the kidney causing retention of sodium disappears and the rate of sodium excretion rises. The mechanism of this effect is not known for certain but it may be due to alteration in the Starling forces in the peritubular capillaries surrounding the proximal convoluted tubule as a result of increased plasma volume.

Although the effects of aldosterone on the kidney causing sodium retention are reduced, its effects on the increased secretion of potassium or hydrogen ions in the distal convoluted tubule and collecting duct are unchanged. Restriction of sodium on the other hand leads to renal conservation.

Normal values

Plasma aldosterone level	1– 5ng% resting
Aldosterone excretion (urine)	1– 5μg/24 hours
As di- and tetra-hydroaldosterone glucuronide	20–30μg/24 hours
Plasma renin level	1– 2.5ng/ml/hr

Differential diagnosis: (a) Hypertension from other causes, e.g. steroid treatment
(b) Potassium depletion – G.I. loss
– Renal loss
Renal tubular acidosis
(c) Familial periodic paralysis
(d) Secondary aldosteronism – CHF
– Starvation
– Cirrhosis
– Nephrosis

In view of the small size of the primary tumour the usual diagnostic investigations are of little benefit but venacaval and renal vein cannulation with angiography and sampling for aldosterone estimation is of value.

Primary aldosteronism *(Continued)*

Pathology

The tumours are usually single and small mostly measuring between 1 and 5cm in diameter. The round or ovoid tumours are usually composed of well demarcated yellow or orange-yellow or brownish tissue.

Most cases of primary aldosteronism are caused by a functioning adenoma of the adrenal cortex. About one third are associated with adrenocortical hyperplasia, sometimes bilateral. A few are due to the presence of a cortical carcinoma.

24

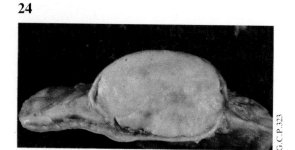

24 A woman of 59 who suffered from hypertension and hypokalaemia showed some response to spironolactone. Primary aldosteronism was diagnosed. The adenoma responsible measured 2cm in diameter. The colour is well shown.

The adenomas are composed of easily recognisable adrenocortical cells usually with a good lipid content. Their arrangement may be haphazard but when it is organised it more often resembles that of the z. fasciculata than the z. glomerulosa. Mitotic figures are rare but nuclear pleomorphism is not uncommon.

25

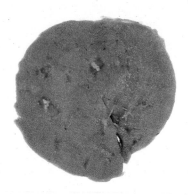

25 The patient presented with the characteristic symptoms and signs of Conn's syndrome. BP 215/100mm Hg. There was a partial and short lived response to potassium replacement and to the administration of sodium citrate. Urinary aldosterone was raised but fell with no treatment to 1.5μg per day.

At operation a 5cm adenoma of the left adrenal was identified and removed. The patient made an uneventful recovery and three months later the serum potassium was found to be normal. Unfortunately impaired renal function became evident and persisted.

26

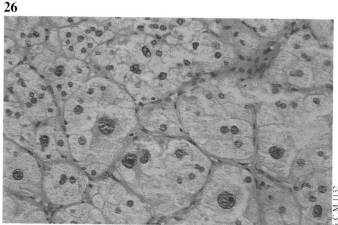

26 Histological appearance of part of the adenoma. The cells vary both in nuclear and cytoplasmic size and the large nuclei are hyperchromatic. In this field the arrangement resembles z. glomerulosa. *(H&E ×250)*

Androgens

Dehydroepiandrosterone is secreted by the z. reticularis in the male and female. The secretion of adrenal androgens is controlled by ACTH. The sex hormone activity of adrenal androgens is only 20% of the activity of testosterone and thus has only a minor effect on masculine characteristics when secreted in normal amounts. It causes, however, anabolism and growth. Secreted in abnormal amounts, as in adreno-cortical tumours or in enzyme deficiencies, it causes masculinisation.

Oestrogens

Oestradiol formed in the adrenals and secreted is usually in too low a concentration to have any apparent physiological effects.

Adrenal virilism

Results from an overproduction of C_{19} androgenic steroids and may occur in:
1 Congenital adrenal hyperplasia.
2 Benign or malignant cortical tumours.
3 Acquired post pubertal adrenal hypersecretion.

Congenital adrenal hyperplasia

The clinical presentation may be:

1 Simple virilism.
2 Virilism with renal sodium loss (21ß hydroxylase deficiency).
3 Virilism and hypertension (11ß hydroxylase deficiency).

In congenital adrenal virilism, the main factor is an enzymatic defect and may be of more than one type. Cortisol synthesis is diminished, and the depressed plasma levels stimulate ACTH production, which in turn stimulates the adrenal cortex to produce steroids. Steroid intermediates build up behind the enzymatic block and are converted via unblocked paths to androgens. The excessive production of androgens leads to masculinisation.

3ß dehydrogenase deficiency produces a pronounced glucocorticoid and mineralocorticoid deficiency which is usually fatal. 21ß hydroxylase deficiency is usually incomplete and enough glucocorticoids and mineralocorticoids are produced to sustain life. However, approximately 30% of patients with this enzyme deficiency show an increased loss of sodium and therefore have a reduced ECF volume. This is the salt losing form of the adrenogenital syndrome.

With 11ß hydroxylase deficiency there is excessive secretion of 11 deoxycortisol and deoxycorticosterone. These have mineralocorticoid properties and cause retention of sodium chloride and water resulting in an increased ECF volume and hypertension, the hypertensive form of the adrenogenital syndrome.

Virilism

Signs of congenital adrenal hyperplasia

Biochemical findings

1 Increased excretion of 17 ketosteroids in the urine.

2 In addition for 21ß hydroxylase deficiency (salt losing form of adreno genital syndrome).
Hyponatraemia and dehydration.
Periods of acute adrenal insufficiency.
Decreased cortisol and aldosterone secretion.
Increased blood levels of 17-OH Progesterone and increased urinary pregnanetriol.

3 For 11ß hydroxylase deficiency (hypertensive form of the adreno genital syndrome).
Increased production of 11-deoxycortisol and 11-deoxycorticosterone.
Increased blood levels of 11-deoxycortisol.
Increased amounts of tetra hydro 11-deoxycortisol in the urine.
Decreased metabolites of cortisol.

The condition may be arrested by the administration of glucocorticoids which repair the glucocorticoid deficit and inhibit ACTH secretion. This in turn prevents the secretion of abnormal amounts of androgens and other steroids.

Clinical features

In both sexes there is a rapid increase in growth and stature together with early osseous maturation. Bony epiphyses fuse prematurely with ultimate stunting of growth. Hirsutism and acne are early signs. Hyperpigmentation. Muscle hypertrophy – muscles are strong due to stimulus to protein anabolism by androgens. Change to a deep voice.

Boys Precocious secondary sexual development (Precocious Pseudopuberty) but testes are infantile. Androgens secreted in excess depress secretion of the gonadotrophins from the pituitary.

Adult males Accentuation of existing male characteristics.

Girls Clitoral hypertrophy. The development of a masculine body build and male distribution of pubic hair. They do not commence puberty, again because of gonadotrophin suppression.

Women Similar changes to prepubertal girls, but ovarian function is depressed leading to amenorrhoea and the mammary glands atrophy. Increase in libido. Feminism is rare although oestrogen secreting tumours of the adrenal cortex have been described.

Signs in newborn babies

Female The excessive androgen secretion leads to abnormality in the external genitalia. Clitoral hypertrophy, labial fusion and formation of a urogenital sinus may be present (27). In all cases of anomalous sex, cytogenetic and biochemical studies must be undertaken to determine the cause.
Male No abnormality in genitalia is obvious. In all cases the diagnosis should be suspected when signs of virilisation are present or where, as in the salt-losing form, there is excessive vomiting.

27

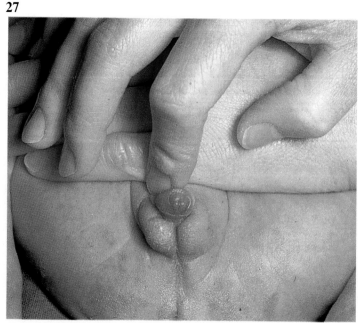

27 A female of one month showing virilism with hypertrophy of the clitoris and fusion of the labia with a small urogenital sinus opening at the base of the clitoris.

Benign or malignant adrenocortical tumours

The majority of tumours occur pre-pubertally (83% occur in females). They may be benign or malignant but assessment on the basis of histology may be difficult until invasion or distant spread has occurred.

With adrenal virilising tumours, there is a large increase in urinary 17 ketosteroids, especially with adrenal carcinomas. Plasma testosterone levels are elevated, but plasma cortisol levels are normal (no associated Cushing's syndrome). In the case of an adrenal tumour, the increased urinary excretion of 17 ketosteroids will not be reduced by dexamethasone suppression. Suppression will be seen in adrenal hyperplasia.

Virilism due to ovarian tumours

In the female virilism may also be caused by certain ovarian tumours. In these cases there is only a moderate increase in 17 ketosteroid output which is not suppressed by dexamethasone.

Other causes of virilism

Virilism in boys may result from androgen-secreting Leydig cell tumours of the testis. Tumours in or near the hypothalamus, particularly pineal tumours, may result in virilism (**28**). Rarely, other disorders of the hypothalamus, e.g. post-encephalitic, may also be responsible.

28

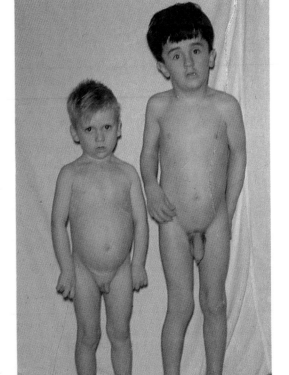

28 The appearance of a boy with hydrocephalus and virilism contrast with those of a normal boy of the same age.

Adrenocortical insufficiency

Acute

Acute adrenocortical insufficiency arising *de novo* almost invariably results from bilateral adrenal haemorrhage or apoplexy. This is classically associated with septicaemia, e.g. meningococcal, as in the Waterhouse–Friderichsen syndrome, but may arise in a number of other conditions. Stages in its development are shown below in the paired adrenal glands.

29

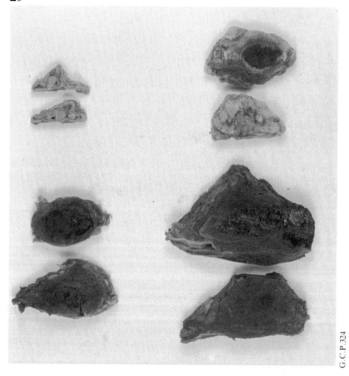

Small foci of necrosis and slight interstitial haemorrhage in both adrenals.

Necrosis and enclosed haemorrhage above. Cortical necrosis only below.

Bilateral haemorrhage mainly confined to adrenals.

Massive bilateral haemorrhage escaping into periadrenal tissue.

G.C.P.324

Acute adrenocortical insufficiency complicating corticosteroid therapy

Corticosteroid therapy suppresses the hypothalamic – pituitary – adrenal axis and if prolonged leads to atrophy of the adrenal cortex. In these circumstances sudden stress or abrupt withdrawal of the corticosteroids leads to acute adrenocortical insufficiency and may cause sudden death.

Chronic

This may result from any of the following.

1 Failure of the adrenal cortex because of damage by local disease. Mineralocorticoid and glucocorticoid insufficiency results. There is also defective negative feedback to the pituitary and hence hyperpigmentation of the skin.

2 Failure of pituitary ACTH production leading to atrophy of zonae fasciculata and reticularis. The z. glomerulosa, which is not under the direct influence of ACTH, is at first not affected so that only glucocorticoid production is deficient. Later the z. glomerulosa tends to undergo secondary atrophy.

Causal lesions

Auto-immune adrenocortical atrophy, tuberculosis, histoplasmosis, other granulomas, amyloid, carcinomatous metastasis, surgical removal.

Causal lesions

Anterior pituitary tumour. Anterior pituitary necrosis. (Sheehan's syndrome.)

In women the deficiency of adrenal androgen production results in loss of axillary and pubic hair.

Acute insufficiency may also arise in chronic forms of the disease either because of progression of the adrenal lesion or due to superadded stress.

Addison's disease

Bilateral destruction of the adrenal cortex leading to chronic adrenocortical deficiency was first recognised in 1855 by Addison and the disease is now generally known by his name. It may be caused in a variety of ways; in the past, tuberculosis was the main cause but other granulomatous conditions may also be responsible. Nowadays most cases appear to result from an autoimmune reaction with lymphocytic infiltration and destruction of cortical cells.

Addison's disease resulting from granulo-matous adrenalitis.

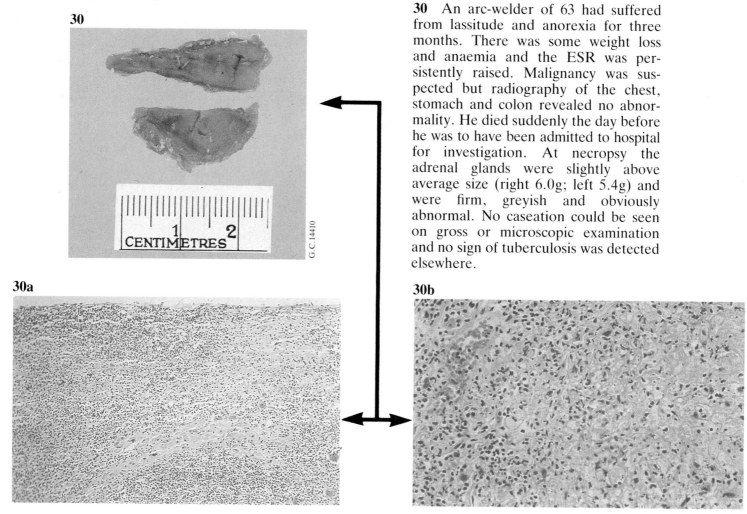

30 An arc-welder of 63 had suffered from lassitude and anorexia for three months. There was some weight loss and anaemia and the ESR was persistently raised. Malignancy was suspected but radiography of the chest, stomach and colon revealed no abnormality. He died suddenly the day before he was to have been admitted to hospital for investigation. At necropsy the adrenal glands were slightly above average size (right 6.0g; left 5.4g) and were firm, greyish and obviously abnormal. No caseation could be seen on gross or microscopic examination and no sign of tuberculosis was detected elsewhere.

30a Addison's disease. The cortex is extensively infiltrated by lymphocytes. Only a few pink-staining cortical cells survive. *(H&E ×50)*

30b Same case. Granulomatous adrenalitis resulted in necrosis, hyalinisation and ultimately fibrosis. *(H&E ×250)*

The pathogenesis of the disease in this case is not certain. A granulomatous reaction has occurred in the adrenals but no micro-organisms could be demonstrated. It is possible that auto-immunity was involved but the appearances of the thyroid and gastric mucosa lent no support to the hypothesis.

Tuberculosis

A classical cause of Addison's disease.

31

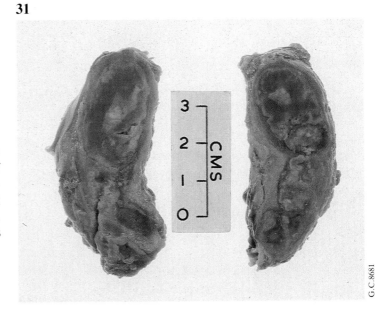

31 A man of 45 had suffered from progressive debility for two years. Three months before his death a patch of lupus appeared on his forehead and tuberculosis abscesses developed in the right cervical lymph nodes. At necropsy old tuberculosis was found at each lung apex. Both adrenals are enlarged and tuberculous caseous necrosis is widespread.

32

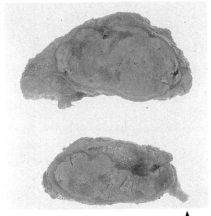

32 A male of 67 developed Addison's disease and was successfully treated by steroids for three years. He then developed obstruction due to a carcinoma of the pelvic colon which, at laparotomy, was found to have spread extensively in the peritoneal cavity. At necropsy both adrenals were seen to be virtually destroyed by tuberculous caseation. No tuberculosis was discovered elsewhere.

32a

32b

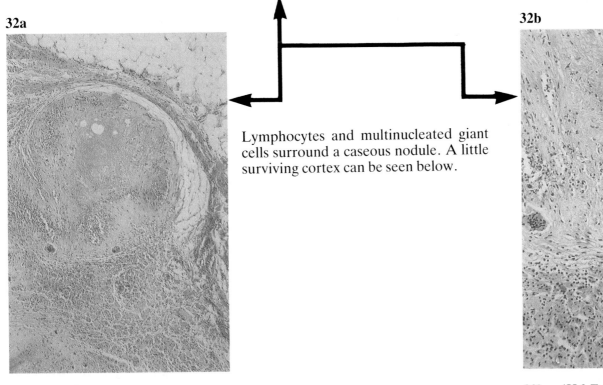

Lymphocytes and multinucleated giant cells surround a caseous nodule. A little surviving cortex can be seen below.

32a *(H&E ×50)*

32b *(H&E ×125)*

The adrenal medulla

The adrenal medulla is made up of interlacing cords of cells which lie in close relation to venous sinuses. These cells, of which two types can be distinguished, contain granules and are densely innervated. Adrenaline secreting cells have large, less dense granules. Noradrenaline secreting cells have small very dense granules. Adrenal medullary cells are APUD cell type, and secrete:

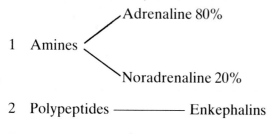

1 Amines
- Adrenaline 80%
- Noradrenaline 20%

2 Polypeptides ———— Enkephalins

Biosynthesis of the amines

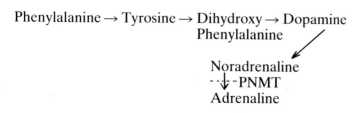

Phenylalanine → Tyrosine → Dihydroxy → Dopamine
Phenylalanine

Noradrenaline
--↓-PNMT
Adrenaline

The enzyme Phenyl enthanolamine N methyl transferase (PNMT) is present in all cells which produce adrenaline. The amines adrenaline and noradrenaline are stored in granules bound to ATP and a binding protein chromogranin.

On stimulation of the preganglionic neurones innervating these amine containing cells, acetylcholine is released, which initiates the release of either adrenaline or noradrenaline from these cells.

The adrenal medulla is part of the sympathoadrenal system, the other component being the sympathetic nervous system (SNS) itself. The SNS is widespread in its ramifications, but on stimulation of the adrenal medulla in states of 'fight or flight' adrenaline and noradrenaline are released into the blood stream and produce effects on cells not directly innervated by the SNS, i.e. the two components of the sympathoadrenal system are mutually supportive.

Effects of adrenaline and noradrenaline

In general these hormones have similar effects to SNS discharge. However, they have slightly different effects from each other which are dependent upon their differing abilities to stimulate the various types of adrenergic receptor.

Hormone	Receptor		
	α	β_1	β_2
Noradrenaline	++	++	0
Adrenaline	++	++	++

	Noradrenaline	Adrenaline
Heart rate	↑	↑
Cardiac contractility	↑	↑
Coronary vessels	Dilatation	Dilatation
Cardiac output	Up, then down due to reflex brachycardia	↑
Peripheral resistance	↑ Vasoconstriction, skin, splanchnic area, muscle.	↓ Vasodilatation of blood vessels in skeletal muscle.
Blood pressure elevation	Marked	Slight
Free fatty acid release	++	++
Stimulation of CNS	++	++
Increase blood sugar	+	++++

The normal plasma noradrenaline level is 300pg/ml and that for adrenaline is 30pg/ml. These values increase by 50–100% on standing. The main site of catabolism of these catecholamines is the liver. Circulating adrenaline and noradrenaline are 0- methylated by the enzyme Catechol 0 Methyl Transferase (COMT) and oxidised to Vanillyl Mandelic Acid (VMA). This product is then excreted in the urine.

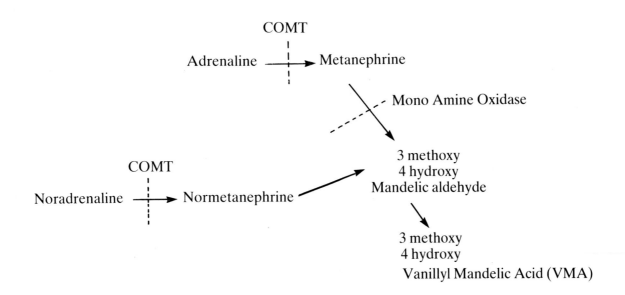

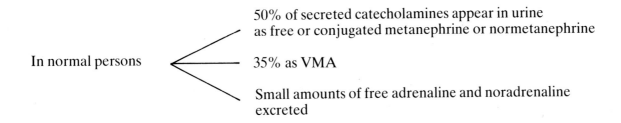

Approximately 700µg of VMA are excreted in the urine per day.

Medullary tumours

These tumours may arise from any or all of the medullary cell types and from any stage in their development. The primitive cell of the adrenal medullary tissue, the sympathogonia, is capable of differentiation both into the sympathoblast or neuroblast to form the adult ganglion cell, and into the phaeochromoblast to form the phaeochromocyte which has an affinity for chrome salts and an ability to produce adrenaline and noradrenaline. Medullary tumours may therefore be classified according to the preponderant cell type.

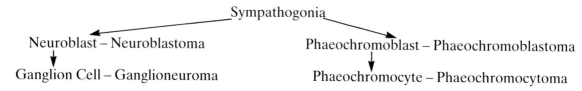

It should be remembered that although these terms refer to tumours with the majority of cells of one neoplastic type, mixed tumours are not infrequent. Tumours arising in the medullary part of the adrenal gland may also be divided into those with and those without hormonal activity. The majority of the non-hormonal tumours arise from the ganglion cell type or its precursor. They are tumours of nerve tissue and therefore may also arise in sympathetic ganglia.

Neuroblastoma

This tumour most frequently arises in childhood and may affect both adrenals. 50% of cases occur below the age of two years and congenital cases are recorded. The earlier the age of onset the less differentiated is the histological pattern of the tumour. When the tumour arises in later life the prognosis is better and fibril formation, with the presence of ganglion cells, shows a degree of transition to the ganglioneuroma described below. Both sexes are equally affected. The tumour is associated with a very high mortality but cases of spontaneous regression have been recorded.

33

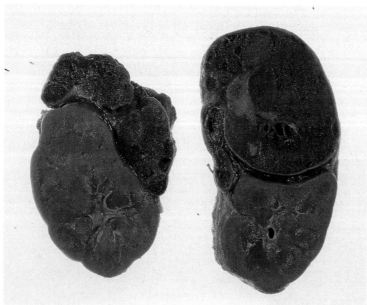

33 From the necropsy of an infant admitted to hospital at the age of seven weeks because of adrenal enlargement. The abdomen continued to enlarge and the infant died suddenly. The liver was greatly enlarged by metastases.

Neuroblastomas are present in both adrenals. It is not possible to be certain that the smaller tumour is not metastatic from the larger neuroblastoma which has caused renal distortion.

The tumour is invasive and destroys the cortical layer of the adrenals. On section it is soft, greyish, fleshy, with areas of haemorrhage and necrosis.

G.C. 660

Histology

Neuroblastomas are composed of cells resembling lymphocytes with darkly staining nuclei surrounded by a narrow rim of ill-defined cytoplasm. There is little supporting stroma. In the least differentiated tumours occurring in the youngest infants the cells are closely packed so that the tumour resembles a lymphosarcoma. In rather better differentiated neoplasms rosettes may develop. Rosettes are formed by rings of cells around a space occupied by neurofibrils which are demonstrable by silver impregnation or by electron microscopy. In still older tumours all stages of transition to ganglioneuromatous differentiation can be seen.

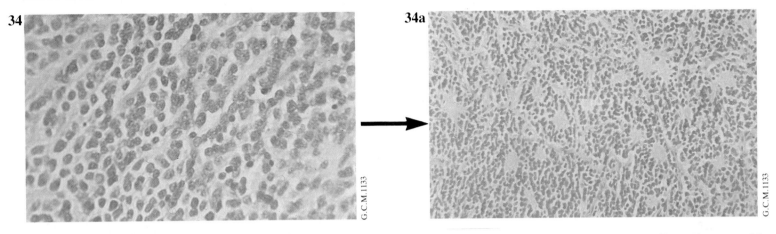

34 Adrenal neuroblastoma composed of sheets of neuroblasts resembling lymphocytes. *(H&E ×500)*

34a Adrenal neuroblastoma. The cells again resemble lymphocytes but are sometimes arranged around pale-staining amorphous-looking material to form rosettes. *(H&E ×125)*

Metastasis

40% of infants afflicted by a neuroblastoma usually come under medical care when metastases have developed. Fever, leucocytosis, abdominal upsets, diarrhoea, and wasting may call attention to the disease. Involvement of the liver and the bones is frequent.

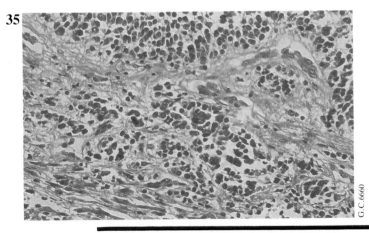

35 Neuroblastoma – metastasis in liver. The darkly staining cells of the neuroblastoma contrast with the paler liver cells. The spindle-shaped cells at bottom left are compressed hepatocytes. *(H&E ×200)*

Laboratory investigations

The urine in 75% of cases contains an increased amount of the end products of catecholamine metabolism. Hormonal effects are not clinically obvious but the investigation is useful in diagnosis and follow-up.

Prognosis

A highly malignant but radiosensitive tumour. If complete surgical excision is possible a high cure rate may be obtained with the aid of radiotherapy and chemotherapy. Spontaneous regression sometimes occurs.

Medullary tumours (Continued)

Adrenal neuroblastomas may spread widely in the retroperitoneum and in lymph nodes. Blood spread tends to affect liver and bones more markedly than lungs. Two presentations are mainly of historic interest, Pepper's syndrome and Hutchinson's syndrome.

36

Pepper's syndrome

Pepper's syndrome first described in 1901 is characterised by massive metastasis to the liver of a neuroblastoma particularly of the right adrenal gland. Abdominal swelling due to the enlarging liver is later increased by ascites.

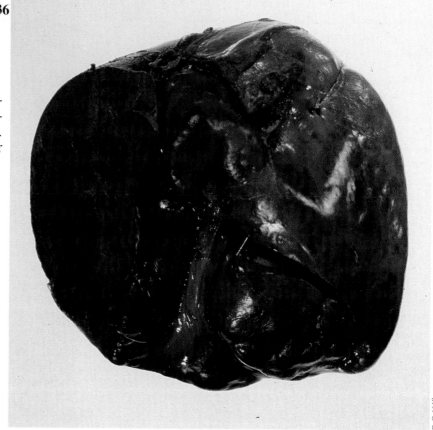

36 Hepatic metastases of the right adrenal neuroblastoma (**33**, **35**). Note how closely the primary tumour is applied to the liver.

G.C.6660

Hutchinson's syndrome

37

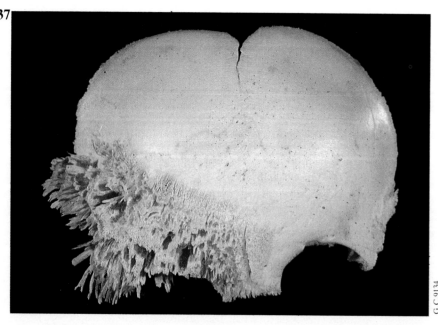

Hutchinson's syndrome was first described in 1907. The essential feature is the presence of a suprarenal tumour associated with cranial metastases, characterised by projecting spicules of bone from the surface of the skull and usually exophthalmos.

37 From a male aged one year, illustrating the features of Hutchinson's syndrome. There was a primary neuroblastoma of the adrenal with unilateral exophthalmos and cranial metastases.

G.C.9134

Ganglioneuroma

This is a rare tumour. Most frequently found in females during the second decade. The rate of growth is very slow and consequently asymptomatic. Cases have been described as an incidental finding at post mortem. Alternatively a palpable rounded tumour can be detected and there may be pressure on adjacent structures. Malignant change is rare. Generally after excision the prognosis is excellent.

Gross appearance

The tumour is firm, grey-white, well encapsulated and easily shelled out. The cut surface is usually homogeneous but areas of myxoid change may be apparent.

Ganglioneuromas, identical to those described also arise in sympathetic ganglia and from sympathetic nerves, especially in the abdomen and thorax.

38

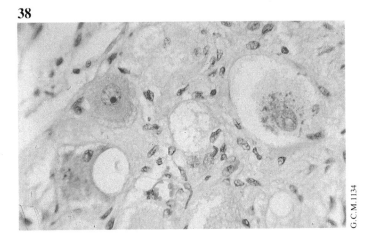

38 Ganglioneuroma showing the variation in ganglion cells and the presence of neurofibrillary material and Schwann cell nuclei. *(H&E ×375)*

Histology

Many neurofibrils, nerve bundles and Schwann cell nuclei may be present. Ganglion cells are characteristic, vary in size and shape, and tend to occur in small groups sometimes sparsely distributed. Occasionally neuroblasts may also be present. They tend to undergo maturation but rarely are the source of neuroblastomatous transformation.

Malignant change

39

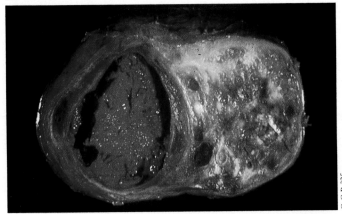

39 From a 55-year-old sailor. Asymptomatic swelling in the abdomen was found on examination. This was thought histologically to be an innocent ganglioneuroma. Ten years later he died from a metastasizing neuroblastoma.

The specimen shows degeneration in the tumour with cystic change resulting from necrosis and haemorrhage. Presumably this change destroyed the histological evidence of neuroblastomatous transformation.

This case illustrates the rare malignant change in ganglioneuroma and emphasizes the relationship of the two types of tumour.

Medullary tumours *(Continued)*

Phaeochromocytoma

40

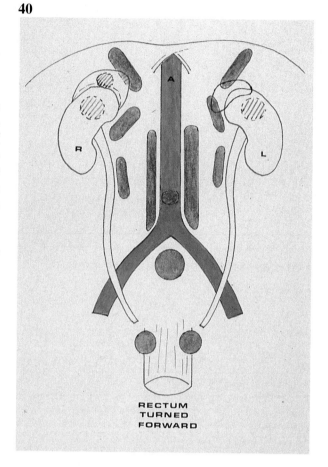

40 A hormonally active tumour arising from the phaeochromocyte of the adrenal medulla and characterised by an affinity for chrome salts and by an output of adrenaline and noradrenaline resulting in hypertension, often paroxysmal. 90% of phaeochromocytomas arise in the adrenal glands. The remainder develop in the organ of Zuckerkandl or in sympathetic ganglia (fully shaded areas).

The striped areas in the diagram indicate other subdiaphragmatic sites of phaeochromocytoma.

10% of these tumours are bilateral.

Incidence

Sex incidence – equal.
Age incidence – usually adults up to middle age.
   A familial incidence has been reported and an association with neurofibro-matosis is recognised.

Pregnancy

Hypertension in pregnancy has on occasion been found to be due to the presence of a phaeochromocytoma.

Familial phaeochromocytomas

About 6% of all cases.

In 50% both adrenals are affected.

About 25% also have a medullary carcinoma of the thyroid – multiple endocrine adenoma syndrome.

Pathology

The tumours vary in size. Some tumours which are small but hormonally active appear to have no capsule. Larger tumours are round or ovoid and develop a pseudocapsule formed by compressed cortical tissue and stroma. In well preserved tumours the cut surface is soft, grey and homogeneous. Many with a high catecholamine content turn brown on exposure to light and air and when left in fixative discolour the fluid. Chrome salts accelerate this colour change. In large tumours necrosis and haemorrhage may occur and may result in cyst formation.

41

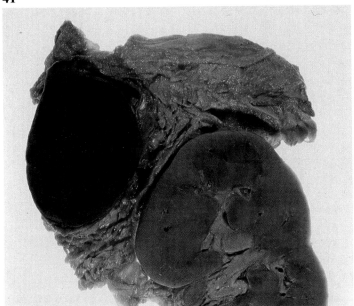

G.C.14691

41 From a middle-aged woman who had suffered from headaches and hypertension for nine years. The left adrenal phaeochromocytoma found at necropsy. Note the dark colour after exposure to light.

42

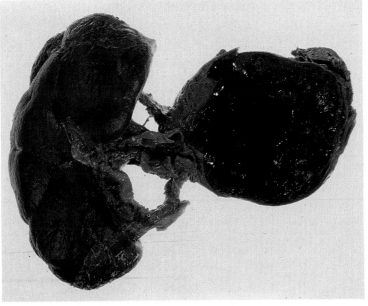

G.C.14779

42 An extra-adrenal phaeochromocytoma from a man who died of a massive myocardial infarct. The tumour was partly cystic as a result of old necrosis and haemorrhage.

Medullary tumours *(Continued)*

Phaeochromocytoma *(Continued)*

Histology

Phaeochromocytomas are usually well differentiated and thus exaggerate the appearances of normal adrenal medulla. They are composed of large cells varying considerably in size and shape and supported usually by delicate stroma containing many small thin walled blood vessels. The cytoplasm is ample and amphophilic and may contain brown granules particularly if chrome-containing fixatives have been used. The nuclei vary considerably in size and in chromatin content and more than one may be present. The pleomorphism merely reflects that of normal medullary cells and mitotic figures are few.

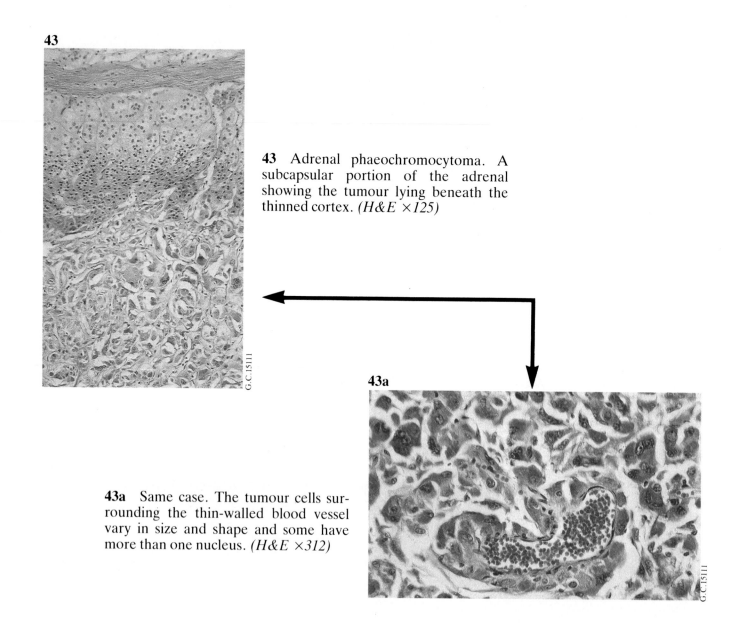

43 Adrenal phaeochromocytoma. A subcapsular portion of the adrenal showing the tumour lying beneath the thinned cortex. *(H&E ×125)*

43a Same case. The tumour cells surrounding the thin-walled blood vessel vary in size and shape and some have more than one nucleus. *(H&E ×312)*

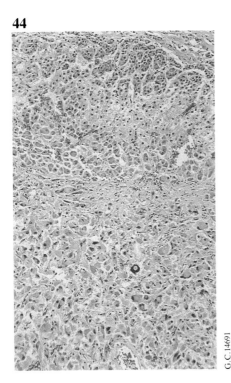

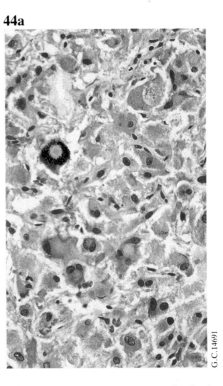

Microphotographs of the phaeochromocytoma shown in (**41**).

44 A pseudocapsule separates the phaeochromocytoma (below) from the compressed cortex (above). *(H&E ×100)*

44a The tumour is composed of pleomorphic cells often multinucleated. Note the brown granules in one of the cells. *(H&E ×312)*

Malignancy

Malignancy is rare (10%) and is difficult to assess on microscopic examination. The true proof is metastasis.

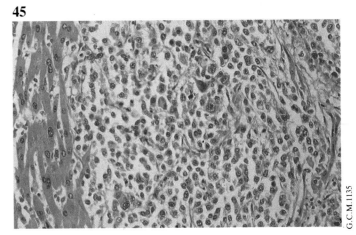

45 Hepatic metastasis from a malignant phaeochromocytoma. Mitotic activity is present and many cells are small and uniform but otherwise they differ little from non-metastasising tumours. *(H&E ×250)*

Diagnosis

If a phaeochromocytoma is suspected to be the cause of hypertension two initial tests must be undertaken:

24-hour excretion of VMA or metanephrines	Phentolamine Test
Total metanephrine increased in 85–100% of cases. VMA increased in 70–95%	Intravenous injection of 5mg of phentolamine, an ∝–receptor adrenergic blocker, causes a fall in B.P. in those cases with sustained hypertension

Drugs may interfere with both tests and must be omitted or taken into account when assessing the results.

Localisation of suspected phaeochromocytoma

Radioisotope imaging after intravenous administration of iodine-131-meta-iodo-benzylguanidine has been shown to be of value in locating the tumour in known or suspected cases of phaeochromocytoma.

James Fraser   M. O. Wright

301

The carotid body is the largest of the non-chromaffin paraganglia, the other important ones in this region being the aortic body and the glomus jugulare.

Anatomy

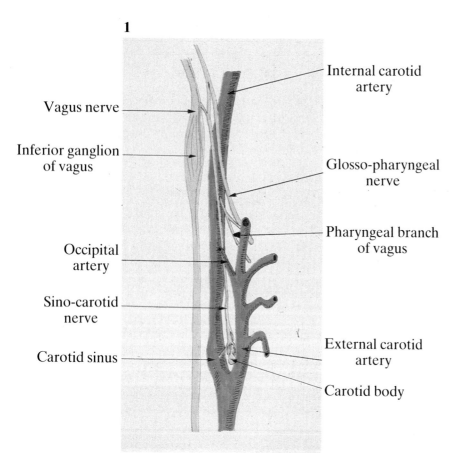

1 Diagram showing anatomy of the carotid bifurcation, carotid body and carotid sinus.

The carotid bodies develop from a condensation of the mesenchyme around the artery of the third pharyngeal arch. They are oval structures (usually one on each side) $6 \times 3mm$ in size and weighing 2mg and lie in close proximity to the bifurcation of the common carotid artery and the carotid sinus. They receive a large blood supply in relation to their size, approximately 0.04ml/minute (2,000mls/100G/min).

The sensory nerve supply is from the glossopharyngeal nerve (the nerve of the third arch) through a branch of the carotid sinus nerve, the information being passed to the respiratory centre within the medulla. There is also an innervation from a fine nerve plexus made up of the IX, X and sympathetic nerves.

Function

The carotid bodies, along with their companion structures, the aortic bodies, are arterial chemoreceptors. They are sensitive to the partial pressures of oxygen and carbon dioxide and to the hydrogen ion concentration within the perfusing blood.

A fall in the arterial pO_2, a rise in the arterial pCO_2 or a rise in the hydrogen ion concentration stimulates the afferent nerves to the medullary respiratory centres and causes an increase in the rate and depth of respiration.

2

Structure

The carotid body has a fibrous capsule from which extensions pass into the substance of the body to divide it into lobules. Within the lobules there are two types of cell, the Type I or glomus cell and the sustentacular or Type II cell. The Type I cells, the more numerous, are surrounded by Type II cells and are separated by them from the vascular sinusoids. The Type II cells may be glial cells. The Type I (glomus) cells are large with abundant cytoplasm, have dendritic processes extending from the cell body and contain vesicles with dense granules which are present throughout the cytoplasm and near the plasma membrane. They are members of the APUD cell series which synthesize and store dopamine, noradrenaline, and met- and leu-enkephalin.

Non-myelinated nerve fibres (the chemo-sensitive afferent fibres), make contact with the glomus cells by reciprocal synapses, as well as by the normal post synaptic relationship. As the axons emerge from the carotid body in a branch of the carotid sinus nerve they gain a myelin sheath and subsequently ascend to the medulla in the IX nerve. The cell bodies of these afferent fibres are in the sensory ganglia of the IX nerve. Adjacent Type I cells make contact with each other via reciprocal synapses thereby allowing them to influence each other's activities.

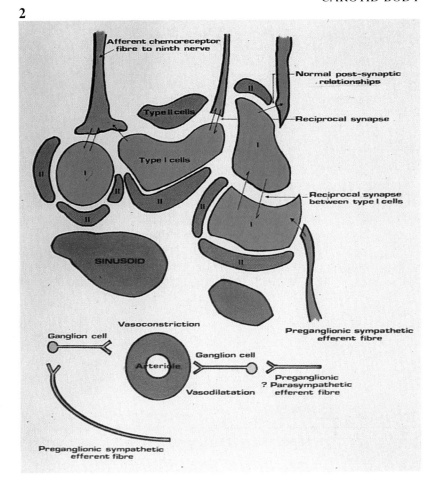

Sympathetic preganglionic fibres from the cervical sympathetic trunk also synapse with the Type I cells. Scattered throughout the carotid body are ganglion cells belonging to the sympathetic and parasympathetic systems, and these receive the appropriate preganglionic fibres. Postganglionic fibres pass to blood vessels within the carotid body, sympathetic fibres causing vasoconstriction and parasympathetic fibres vasodilatation.

The situation is complicated by the fact that vasoactive intestinal peptide (VIP) and substance P have been found in nerve fibres of uncertain type within the carotid body. The exact mechanism of chemical transduction in the carotid body is not yet known, but it is probable that the afferent nerve endings which make contact with the Type I cells and which pass into the glossopharyngeal nerve are the true chemoreceptors, sensitive to a fall in pO_2, a rise in pCO_2 or a rise in hydrogen ion concentration. The Type I cells modify the sensitivity of these chemoreceptor endings by way of a dopamine and noradrenaline release.

Carotid body tumour

(Chemodectoma: Potato tumour)

Tumours of the carotid body (chemodectoma) are rare and are found most often about puberty, though they may occur as late as the eighth decade. They form round or ovoid, slow-growing, rubbery swellings which lie beneath the sterno-mastoid at a lower level and deeper than branchial cysts. They are almost always benign, are mobile in the horizontal plane and are usually symptomless until they are large enough to press on the vagus and glosso-pharyngeal nerves and give rise to dysphagia or dysphonia. The tumour tends to grow around and between the carotid arteries widening the bifurcation but does not involve the tunica media and can usually be separated from the arterial wall in the sub-adventitial plane. Although it may become adherent to surrounding structures, or be surrounded by numerous tortuous vessels, the tumour is usually encapsulated. The cut surface is pink or greyish red and is divided by septa which grow in from the capsule. Their shape and lobulation and the colour of the cut surface have given rise to the term 'potato tumour'.

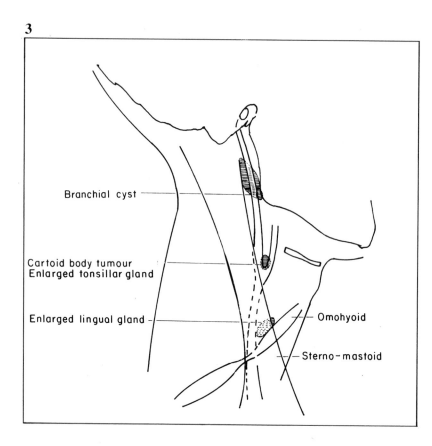

3 Relative position in the neck of branchial cyst, carotid body tumour and enlarged lymph glands.

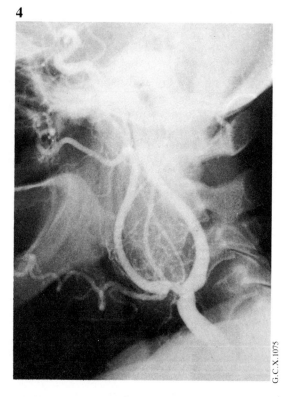

4 Female aged 64 years. Angiogram shows typical splaying of the internal and external carotid arteries due to a mass arising at the bifurcation.

Note the extensive blood supply of the tumour and the incidental atheromatous narrowing at the carotid bifurcation.

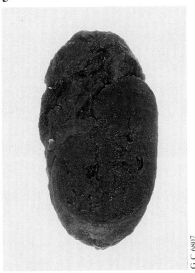

5 Male aged 16 years. Painless swelling right side of neck. A carotid body tumour which was bulging between internal and external carotid arteries was excised. Lobulated, brown and vascular with a homogeneous, rubbery consistence.

Histology

The histological appearance is variable, the most characteristic being of clumps of granular polyhedral cells arranged round very numerous sinusoidal-like blood vessels. Nerve fibres may be seen in the capsule and in the bundles. The same histological picture is seen in the glomus jugulare tumours which arise from the tympanic paraganglia and differ only in their tendency to local extension and recurrence after attempted removal. Metastases from either tumour are very rare.

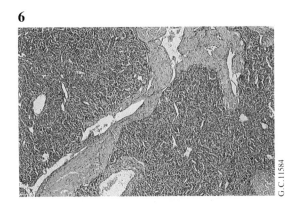

6 Carotid body tumour. Bands of dense fibrous tissue containing vascular channels subdivide the tumour. (*H&E ×50*)

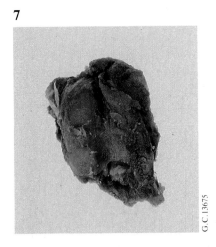

7 Carotid body tumour removed from a female aged 19 years. Note the groove in which the internal carotid artery lay.

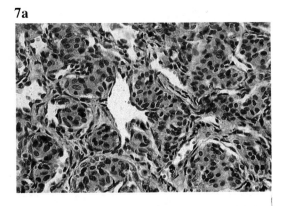

7a Carotid body tumour. A high power view shows the high vascularity of the tumour. Thin walled blood vessels run between tumour cells which characteristically are arranged in small, round or ovoid clumps. The closely packed cells have granular cytoplasm and ovoid nuclei. No mitoses are present. (*H&E ×250*)

A. I. S. Macpherson

It is recognised that a number of syndromes occur in which the endocrine disturbance is caused by lesions affecting more than one endocrine gland. In such instances the pathological basis lies in the presence of tumours or a combination of tumours and hyperplasia affecting different organs.

When more than one endocrine tumour is present the condition is referred to as multiple endocrine adenomatosis (MEA). It may be familial and in such cases those who develop one endocrine tumour may later be expected to show others. Two types of MEA have been described, Sipple's syndrome (type 2) and Wermer's syndrome (type 1).

Sipple's syndrome

The tumours arise from the parathyroid gland, the 'C' cells of the thyroid, and from the medullary cells of the adrenal. The clinical features depend upon the activities of its various components.

(a)   The parathyroid component either hyperplasia or an adenoma giving rise to hyperparathyroidism is a relatively infrequent part of the syndrome.

(b)   The calcitonin-producing 'C' cells of the thyroid give rise to a medullary carcinoma (*see* p. 242) which in addition to calcitonin sometimes secretes ACTH, prostaglandin or serotonin.

(c)   The phaeochromocytomas arising from the adrenal medullary cells are bilateral in about 70% of cases of Sipple's syndrome.

Sipple's syndrome may also be associated with a number of neuro-ectodermal abnormalities such as mucosal neuromas of the lips, tongue and conjunctivae; ganglioneuromatosis of the gastrointestinal tract causing constipation and sometimes dilatation of the colon; occasionally muscular weakness and features of Marfan's syndrome.

When Sipple's syndrome is familial it is inherited as a Mendelian dominant.

A case of Sipple's syndrome

The material in this case is from a middle-aged woman with a medullary carcinoma of the thyroid (*see* p. 242), bilateral phaeochromocytomas (p. 242), and lingual neuromas. The left adrenal tumour measured 5.5 cm in diameter and the right 2.5 cm.

1

1a

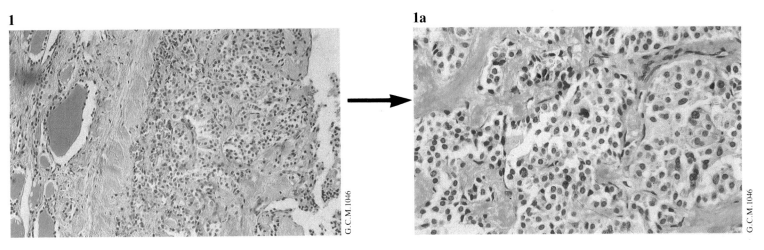

1 This section of a biopsy of the medullary carcinoma of the thyroid includes a portion of the capsule and the surrounding thyroid (left). Both the capsule and the tumour stroma show amyloid change. *(H&E ×162)*

1a No mitotic activity is obvious in this field of the thyroid tumour. There is some variation in nuclear size and a few cells are multinucleated. Stroma is abundant. *(Congo red ×312)*

2

2a

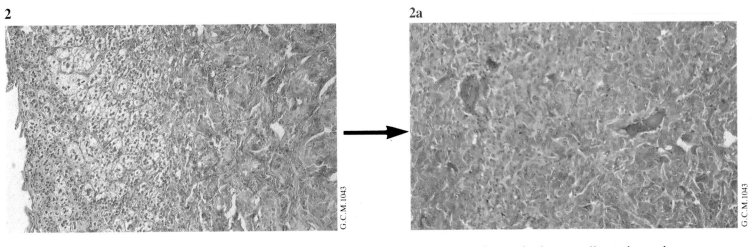

2 A small portion of the larger phaeochromocytoma lies beneath the adrenal cortex (left). *(H&E ×125)*

2a A section of the smaller phaeochromocytoma showing the vascularity. Both tumours are well differentiated. The cellular pleomorphism merely reflects that of the normal adrenal medulla. *(H&E ×125)*

Wermer's syndrome

In this condition the tumours arise from the parathyroid glands, pancreatic islets, and/or the anterior pituitary. The clinical effects may therefore be diverse.

(a)   The parathyroid adenoma or hyperplasia results in hyperparathyroidism.

(b)   The pancreatic islet tumours vary in the nature of their hormonal secretions and may change in character as the tumours develop. For example, the main effects of some of the tumours are:

Insulinoma   – hypoglycaemia

Gastrinoma   – Zollinger–Ellison syndrome

Vipoma   – watery diarrhoea

Glucagonoma – necrolytic migratory erythema and zinc deficiency with a tendency to venous thrombosis and pulmonary embolism.

(c)   The anterior pituitary adenoma, usually chromophobe or acidophil, may produce an excess of prolactin or growth hormone or both, and may cause pressure effects on the optic chiasma and hypothalamus.

Other forms of MEA

Recently other associations have been reported.

(a)   Duodenal carcinoid secreting somatostatin, with phaeochromocytoma and neurofibromatosis.

(b)   Pancreatic islet cell tumours, with phaeochromocytomas and Von Hippel–Lindau syndrome (vascular tumours of retina, cerebellum and liver, with cysts of pancreas, liver and kidneys, and adrenal adenomas).

The number of known associations shown below suggests that others may yet be described.

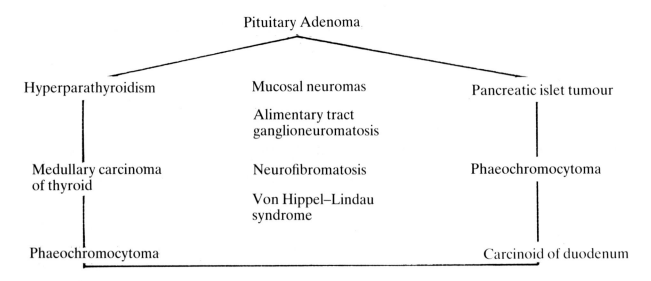

N. Maclean

Part III – Breast

The primitive milk streaks (mammary lines), from which the breasts develop, have been identified at the 6th week of foetal life and extend from the axilla to the inguinal region on both sides of the thoracic and abdominal walls.

In certain animals mammary gland formation is multiple and located at differing points along these lines. In the human, mammary development normally occurs in the pectoral region but additional nipple or breast formation is occasionally found (polythelia and polymastia).

The adult breast is a composite exocrine gland lying in the subcutaneous tissue of the chest wall. Its detailed structure is dependent upon age, menstruation and pregnancy. It comprises glandular, fibrous and adipose tissues, the adipose tissue giving the breast its shape.

The breast is made up of 15 to 25 lobes arranged radially about the nipple, but there is no distinct line of separation between adjacent lobes. Each lobe has a main milk duct plus its branches. The lobes are made up of ducts, blood vessels and lobules separated by fatty fibrous tissue. A lobule comprises a terminal duct (or ductule) and its dependent acini of which there may be 10 to 100. The latter are more evident during the menstrual phase but show their full functional potential during pregnancy.

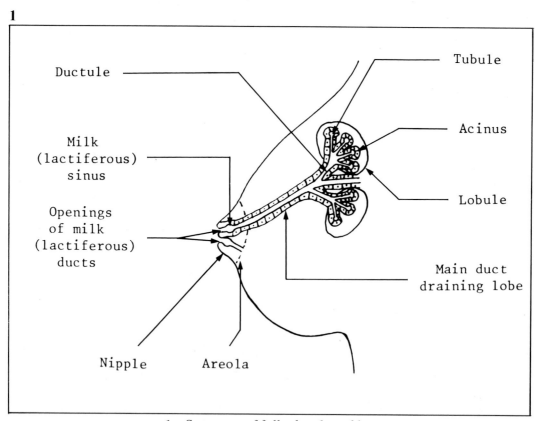

1 Structure of fully developed breast.

The acini are lined by a layer of cuboidal/columnar epithelial cells which are responsible for the manufacture and secretion of the components of milk.

Beneath the epithelial cells, and lying between them and the basement membrane of the acinus, are the myoepithelial cells. These cells have the ability to contract under the influence of the hormone oxytocin and play an important role in the movement of milk from the acinus into the larger ducts during the milk 'let down' mechanism at the commencement of each suckling process.

2

Acinus

Acinar cell

3 The acinar cells have the appearance typical of secretory cells. They have a prominent rough surfaced endoplasmic reticulum near the base of the cell, numerous mitochondria and a Golgi apparatus situated between the nucleus and the luminal surface of the cell. Within the cytoplasm of the cell there are vesicles containing protein and lactose (secretory granules) and also lipid droplets. The luminal surface of the cell is rich in microvilli.

3

Each main milk duct draining a lobe (15 to 25 milk ducts in total) converges on the areola, underneath which it forms a dilatation, the milk sinus (lactiferous sinus). Beyond this sinus the duct narrows once more and passes to the nipple to open on its surface. Each main milk duct opens separately on the nipple.

Within the nipple, each main milk duct is lined by squamous epithelium for a short distance, but before the milk sinus is reached the lining has changed to columnar type and this is continued right to the acini.

Histology

In the female the histological structure of the breast varies greatly with age, pregnancy, lactation, and after the menopause. The picture described already is for the fully developed lactating breast.

Development

Breasts of new-born baby

The breast at birth is represented by 15 to 25 epithelial tubules extending into the subcutaneous fat. The epithelial downgrowths begin as solid cords, but by the 6th month of foetal life they are canalised.

At term, the baby's breasts may enlarge and secrete a small amount of fluid (witch's milk) which comes from small acinar (alveolar) buds at the distal ends of the epithelial tubules. This secretion is caused by the elevated levels of maternal oestrogen and progesterone and foetal prolactin.

Following delivery, the child is removed from the source of oestrogen and progesterone (the placenta), foetal prolactin levels fall and the secretions cease. The tubular system of the breast regresses to the resting state (the buds disappear and only tubules remain). Further development is minimal until puberty. The main milk ducts and their larger branches are present but there are no lobules or intra lobular connective tissue.

4

5

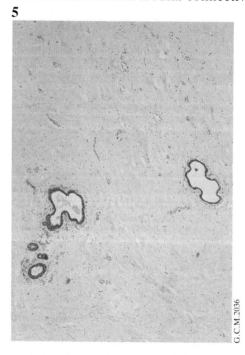

4 Breast, full term foetus. (*H&E × 40*)

5 Breast, infantile. (*H&E × 40*)

Puberty

At puberty in girls, largely under the influence of oestrogen derived from the ovarian follicles, the milk ducts lengthen and branch to form ductules and tubules with buds at their terminal ends (lobules formed). The bud formation may be influenced by progesterone. True acinar formation does not occur at this time. The new ducts, including their terminal ductules, are surrounded by the looser intralobular stroma (accommodative space). The duct epithelium often shows two layers of cells. The process of development is gradual and continues until the age of 20 years. The menstrual cycles become regular, and the breast tissues are regularly exposed to oestrogen and progesterone, leading to some further development of the ducts, acini and lobules. Glucocorticoids from the adrenal cortex may also be necessary for development at this time. There is deposition of fat in the breast leading to an increase in size (also under the influence of oestrogen).

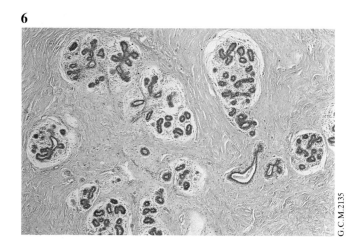

6 Breast, nullipara aet 21. (*H&E × 40*)

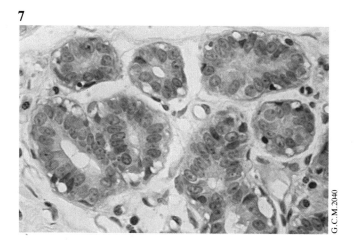

7 Breast – lobular epithelium. The inner layer is formed by columnar epithelial cells. Many of the outer myoepithelial cells are vacuolated. (*H&E×500*)

Menstrual cycle

During the luteal phase of the menstrual cycle in the days preceding the next menstrual period, there is swelling and tenderness of the breast. Some authorities believe that there are proliferative epithelial changes in the terminal ductules with new acinar formation. However, some oedema of the breast and increased blood flow certainly occur, with increased breast volume. Histamine and prolactin released by oestrogen stimulation may be responsible for these changes.

Pregnancy

From the commencement of pregnancy, changes occur in the breast in preparation for lactation, and these involve hypertrophy of the ductular – lobular – acinar system. Initially, the ductules elongate and repeatedly branch, and then later proliferation of the epithelium of the terminal ductules occurs with formation of true acini and obliteration of the accommodative space. Prominent lobules with acini grouped in clusters appear. There is a decrease in the amount of connective tissue stroma and the interstitial fat disappears. Vascularity of the breast increases.

The hormones required for this development include oestradiol, progesterone, glucocorticoids, insulin, human placental lactogen (HPL) and prolactin. Growth hormone does not appear to be necessary. Oestrogen stimulates growth of the ducts, and progesterone causes development of the lobular acinar system. By the end of the 4th month of pregnancy full development of the breast has taken place as described. The acinar cells contain secretory vesicles and fat droplets, but actual lactation does not occur until after parturition.

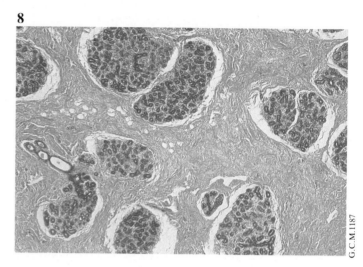

8 Breast showing increase in size and number of lobules (adenosis) of early pregnancy. (*H&E × 40*)

The role of prolactin in pregnancy and lactation.

Prolactin is a hormone produced by the acidophil cells of the anterior pituitary. It is similar in structure to growth hormone and human placental lactogen (a single chain polypeptide produced by the syncytio-trophoblast of the placenta). Its release is under the control of prolactin inhibitory hormone (dopamine) from the arcuate nucleus of the hypothalamus and perhaps a prolactin releasing hormone.

Factors causing the release of prolactin include:
    Oestrogen
    Mechanical stimulation of the nipple
    Suckling
    Thyroid releasing hormone

Oestrogen in the presence of prolactin causes development of the breast ducts as previously noted.

Progesterone plus prolactin cause the development of the lobulo-acinar system. During pregnancy, under the influence of oestrogen, progesterone, prolactin and human placental lactogen, the breast undergoes full lobulo-acinar development. From the first trimester until term there is a progressive increase in serum prolactin concentration from the non-pregnant level of 8ng/ml to 200ng/ml at term. This rise is paralleled by a rise in the level of human placental lactogen. Lactation does not occur during pregnancy despite the raised levels of prolactin, as the effects of prolactin on the breast to stimulate milk secretion are inhibited by oestrogen and progesterone. These steroids appear to exert their inhibition by acting directly on the acinar cells. Progesterone is known to inhibit lactalbumin synthesis.

Lactation

With the decline in oestrogen and progesterone following delivery of the foetus and placenta, prolactin can act to cause milk secretion (lactogenesis – the initiation of a plentiful flow of milk). Prolactin controls the volume of milk, the formation of the milk protein (lactalbumin and lacto-globulin) and the fatty acid and lactose content. The quantity and quality of milk are also dependent on the thyroid hormones, insulin, cortisol, and on the state of nutrition and fluid intake. The breasts begin to fill on the 3rd to 4th day after delivery.

The cells of the acini contain fat droplets and granules which are extruded into the lumen of the acini and ducts which become distended between sucklings.

In addition to the actively lactating elements, some additional lobules are found which are apparently inactive. These are regarded as reserve lobules, either to replace exhausted lactating cells, or to meet the increasing demands of the growing infant.

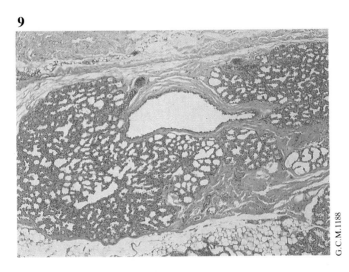

9 Breast – showing a large lactating lobule. (*H&E × 40*)

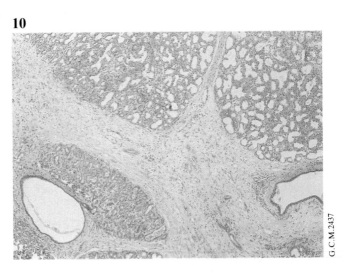

10 Breast – two large lactating lobules and a small reserve lobule. (*H&E × 40*)

During the first few days of lactation, colostrum is secreted. It differs from the mature milk in having greater concentrations of proteins and fat soluble vitamins and lower concentrations of fat, lactose and water soluble vitamins. It also contains immunoglobulins. Gradually, the composition changes to that of mature milk.

By a neuro-endocrine reflex suckling stimulates the release of oxytocin from the posterior pituitary and this causes the myoepithelial cells surrounding the acini to contract. The milk thus ejected into the ducts is removed from the breast by the act of suckling.

The long neuro-endocrine pathway accounts for the 30 second delay between the onset of suckling and milk release. Inhibition of oxytocin release, and thus milk ejection, occurs under conditions of stress, fear, or embarrassment.

Involution — Post-lactational

If the mother ceases to suckle her child or mechanically empty her breasts, lactation stops within two weeks, prolactin levels return to normal and the breast structure involutes. The process of involution is usually complete in four months after cessation of breast feeding, but shows much individual variation.

When breast feeding ends, the accumulating milk distends the acini and milk ducts causing increased intramammary pressure and flattening of the lining cells. Degenerative changes in the acinar cells become evident and desquamation occurs. Distension of the acini also compresses the blood supply to the glandular tissue, rendering it hypoxic. This will potentiate the degenerative changes occurring in the acinar cells. Some acini rupture, causing spaces (holes) in the glandular tissue. The milk products are gradually discharged or absorbed and the acini disappear. The removal of milk products and cell debris is associated with the appearance of phagocytic cells. There is a reduction in numbers of lobules and acini, but the ductular pattern remains. Vascularity decreases, and there is a progressive re-appearance of stroma and breast fat. The pattern is similar to that of the pre-pregnancy state, but the breasts tend to be larger, due to the presence of more fat.

11

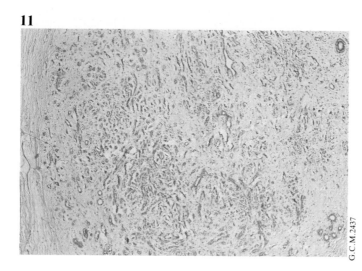

11 Breast — post-lactational involution. Here the epithelial atrophy is marked and the lobules are ill-defined. (*H&E × 40*)

Variations in the changes associated with involution are common.

1   The process of involution may be uneven or delayed.

2   The distension of the terminal ductules and acini may persist with the formation of multiple small cysts. The lining epithelium shows degenerative changes. In some instances the cytoplasm becomes markedly eosinophilic. The epithelium may disappear entirely and the cystic spaces then contain only a small quantity of clear fluid.

3   Localised adenosis persists.

4   Areas of increased fibrosis develop.

5   Limited areas of lymphocytic infiltration are seen which is possibly an inflammatory response to retained milk products. This infiltration is scanty and transient.

Post menopausal breast

The age at which the menopause (the last episode of menstrual bleeding) occurs is variable in women throughout the world, but normally occurs between the ages of 44 and 52 years.

It occurs because of ovarian failure: there is a reduction in the number of ovarian follicles, and an increased resistance of the remaining follicles to the actions of the gonadotrophin FSH and LH produced by the anterior pituitary. With ovarian failure, the plasma oestradiol concentration falls to low levels, and FSH and LH concentrations rise due to lack of negative feedback. The FSH and LH levels remain elevated for up to 15 years.

After the menopause the breast undergoes major involution and atrophy. The process is variable in time and degree, leading to a correspondingly variable histological picture. Ultimately there is a progressive atrophy of the ducts with eventual disappearance of the smaller terminal branches and obliteration of the accommodative space by fibrosis. Only the major ducts and their larger branches remain, embedded in dense fibrous tissue.

12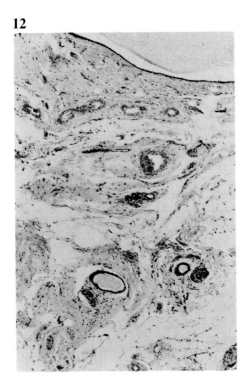

12a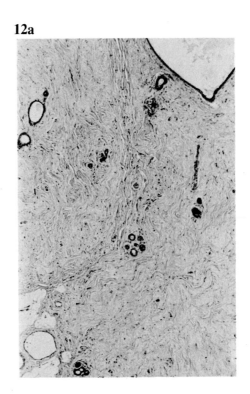

12 and **12a**   Post-menopausal breast. In each section a small portion of a main duct can be seen. Elsewhere epithelial atrophy is marked. On the left there is fibro-fatty replacement, whilst to the right the fibrous tissue is dense. ($\times 50$) G.C.M.1252

Senile breast

In advanced age, the breast is greatly shrunken with only residual main ducts being present traversing fibrous and fatty tissue.

M.O. Wright

Cystic hyperplasia

Benign, non-neoplastic disease, the commonest cause of a palpable lump in the breast, is a subject of complex, imprecise and often confusing terminology reflecting both the variable pathological features and the imperfect understanding of its aetiology and pathogenesis. The disease is commonest in the reproductive years and hormonal effects would thus seem to play some aetiological role. In support of this, two of the frequent components, epithelial hyperplasia and cyst formation, may be produced by oestrogenic activity. The other principal feature, fibrosis, may reflect an involutional change. Thus the variable stromal and epithelial responses to cyclical hormonal activity result in histological appearances which range from normality to an arbitrarily defined pathological lesion.

Terms that have been applied to the lesion include chronic mastitis, cystic hyperplasia, fibrocystic disease, cystic mastopathy, fibroadenosis, Schimmelbusch's disease and benign mammary dysplasia. The latter term, with an additional phrase to indicate which features predominate, is currently popular but is not entirely satisfactory in view of the connotation which the term dysplasia would hold in other contexts, e.g. as a potentially pre-malignant epithelial alteration. It is thus important that pathologist and clinician communicate in terms which are mutually understood and that the pathologist describes and evaluates those features of the condition which may have pre-malignant potential such as atypical epithelial hyperplasia.

Cyst formation is a frequent component. The cysts are often numerous and visible in a macroscopic specimen. The central clear fluid, visualised through an attenuated cyst wall, may give a bluish impression (blue domed cyst of Bloodgood).

13

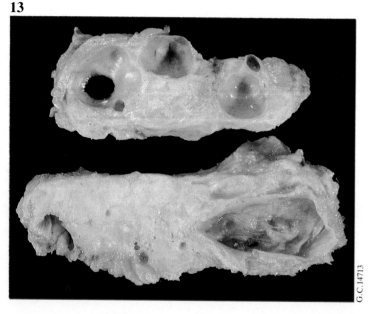

G.C.14713

13 Two sections of a breast showing gross cystic disease. Above, the cysts are mainly large and thin-walled.

Below there are several minute cysts and one large thicker-walled cystic cavity.

The microscopic appearance of the cysts is variable, the epithelial lining being at times attenuated or absent and the lumen containing inspissated secretory material, foamy macrophages and cholesterol debris. In other areas there may be varying degrees of epithelial hyperplasia or apocrine metaplasia. Cyst rupture may have elicited a chronic inflammatory reaction round the cyst with reactive fibrosis.

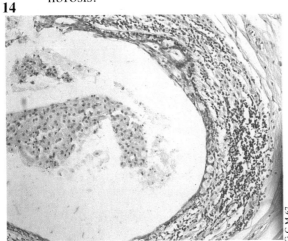

14 Breast cyst. The lumen contains desquamated epithelial cells and macrophages. In the inflamed cyst wall foamy macrophages and numerous lymphocytes can be seen. (*H&E × 125*)

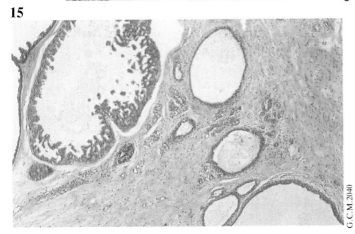

15 Breast – cystic hyperplasia. Several distended ducts and small cysts are shown. Most are lined by a single or double layer of epithelium. The others (top left) show papillary formation of apocrine epithelium. (*H&E × 40*)

Apocrine metaplasia may be found in either normal or dilated terminal ducts. The affected cells are eosinophilic and may show evidence of hyperplasia in the form of papillary infolding and nuclear variation. The surface of the cells exhibits apical blebbing; this decapitation secretion is typical of apocrine glands.

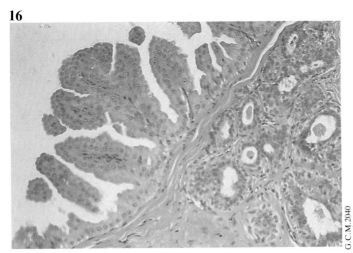

16 Breast – papillary ingrowth of apocrine epithelium from cyst wall. (*H&E × 160*)

Fibrosis

The degree of fibrosis is variable, usually occurring between lobules, surrounding ducts and sometimes constituting the major element of an excised specimen. When other features of benign cystic disease are present, fibrosis is accepted as an element in the pathology, perhaps hormonally related to involution or due to periductal inflammation resulting from previous cyst rupture. On occasion, however, the fibrosis constitutes the predominant feature. There is considerably less implication for any future malignancy in a pure stromal reaction of this nature.

17

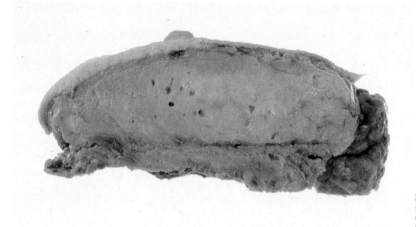

17 Breast – cysts and stromal hyperplasia. From a woman of 60 years with a diffusely nodular breast. Numerous small cysts are present in this breast showing stromal hyperplasia. Many of the features of cystic hyperplasia were seen on microscopic examination.

Adenosis

Adenosis, an increase in number of lobular and terminal duct units, is a variable feature.

18

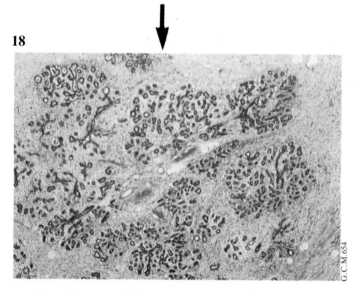

18 (*H&E × 40*)

19

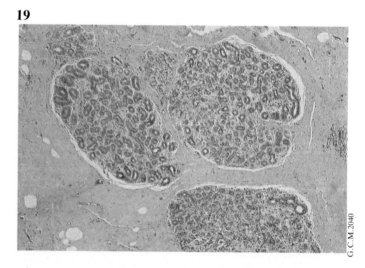

19 Breast – adenosis. Breast lobules are numerous and enlarged by increase in the number of their acini. (*H&E × 125*)

Epitheliosis

The proliferation of epithelial lining cells (epitheliosis) varies greatly between cases and between areas in one specimen but it is this feature which requires the most detailed pathological study and evaluation. The changes vary from multilayering of lining cells to papillary infolding, small intraduct papilloma formation − papillomatosis − to a more solid cellularity. It is the latter feature which may mimic the cribriform pattern which occurs in intraduct carcinoma. True cribriform pattern, atypical nuclei, mitoses and necrosis suggest intraduct malignancy. The distinction can be difficult. The term atypical ductal hyperplasia is used to indicate cellular atypia within the epithelium. It is this feature which has greatest significance in assessing the risk of the future development of carcinoma.

It is now appreciated that most of the epithelial proliferative changes and cyst formation of fibrocystic disease occur in the terminal ductule and its dependent lobule and this unit is the probable source of the majority of pathological changes in the breast.

20

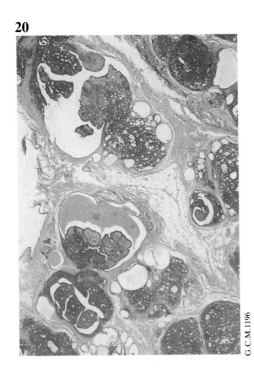

21

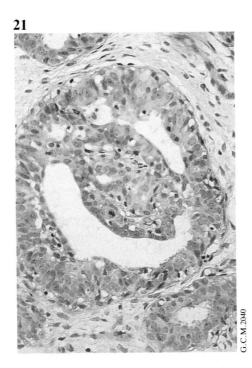

22

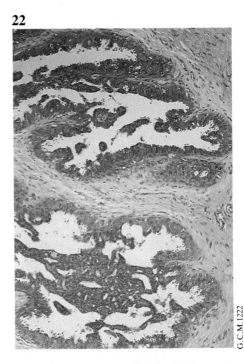

20 Breast − epitheliosis. Distended ducts show degrees of hyperplasia of the epithelium varying from simple heaping up to complete filling of the lumen by epithelial overgrowth. (*H&E × 12.5*)

21 Breast − epitheliosis. The epithelium is atypical and a cribriform pattern is developing. One mitotic figure is present. (*H&E × 250*)

22 Breast. Atypical ductal hyperplasia. Much of the epithelium is atypical with multilayering of cells, papillary pattern, nuclear pleomorphism and occasional mitoses. (*H&E × 100*)

Epitheliosis – malignant change

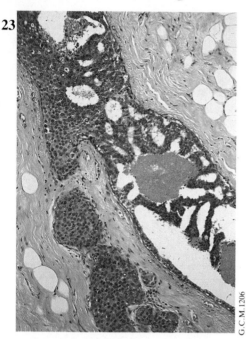

Assessment of the frequency with which benign breast disease may predispose to malignancy is complex but in some forms there does seem to be a risk of subsequent malignancy though the latter may be in the contralateral breast. Histological features of importance are the presence and degree of epithelial hyperplasia and, in particular, cellular atypia, i.e. variation in size and shape of cells and nuclei, mitoses, cell necrosis etc.

23 Breast – epitheliosis with malignant change. A cribriform pattern can be seen and there is focal necrosis.

Sclerosing adenosis

The changes which may occur in the lobule in benign breast disease are well illustrated in the condition sclerosing adenosis. This is a highly proliferative form of benign breast disease and is usually found in the context of the other changes previously described. It is, however, a rather discrete focus within the breast and may form a small, firm mass.

Microscopically it shows a retention of lobular architecture. It is, however, highly cellular, comprising proliferating terminal ducts and lobules distorted by associated proliferation of the lobular connective tissue. The retention of a double layer of epithelial elements, cytological regularity and absence of necrosis are additional features which aid in the diagnosis.

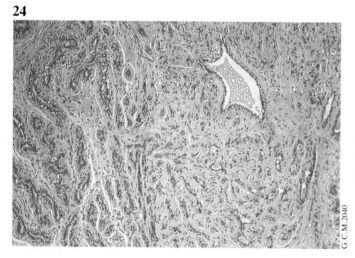

24 Breast – sclerosing adenosis. To the left the lobular pattern is clearly shown. Elsewhere fibrosis and epithelial distortion blur the histological picture. (*H&E × 100*)

Duct ectasia (periductal mastitis)

The confused terminology in this area reflects imperfect understanding of the disease. It may be termed plasma cell mastitis; since plasma cells are neither a specific nor necessary element, the term periductal mastitis is preferable. This condition, found most often in the 4th and 5th decades, is characterised histologically by dilatation of ducts with inspissation of luminal content; the latter may achieve a cheese-like consistency and may be squeezed from the ducts. There is thus an impression of duct stasis. Histologically the lining epithelium may be attenuated or lost, the lumen contains lipid-rich acellular material with foamy macrophages, the periductal tissues are the site of a variable chronic inflammatory infiltrate with fibrosis. The duct dilatation may amount to apparent cyst formation resembling that seen in fibrocystic disease but staining for elastic will demonstrate the presence of, albeit fragmented, elastic fibres in periductal mastitis. This supports the view that this condition is of basically inflammatory nature, related to duct dilatation and rupture as opposed to the initial epithelial hyperplasia and cyst formation of the terminal ductule-lobular unit in cystic hyperplasia. As one might predict, the duct dilatation with possible rupture and inflammation may lead to abscess formation and in the region of a chronic abscess the presence of periductal mastitis may point to such an aetiology for the abscess.

In the course of the disease, episodes of a more acute inflammatory nature may occur, suggesting a possible infective element in which anaerobic organisms have been implicated; infection as an initial cause is unproved.

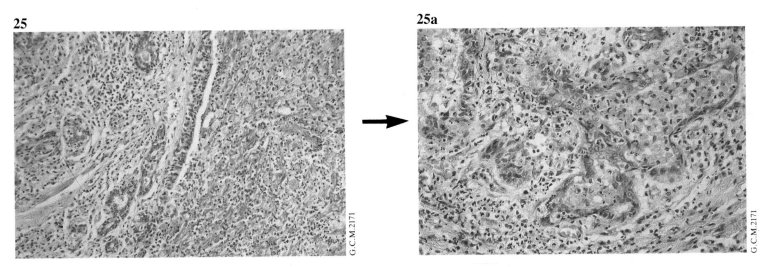

25 Duct ectasia (periductal mastitis) The duct (right) is distended by inspissated secretion infiltrated by inflammatory cells and lipophages. Lymphocytes and plasma cells infiltrate the periductal tissue. (*H&E × 160*)

25a Duct ectasia (periductal mastitis). A small duct is distended by foamy macrophages. In some places the duct contents have escaped through the wall, causing inflammation in the surrounding tissue. (*H&E × 250*)

Adenoma

Certain of the circumscribed solitary lesions occurring in young adults are characterised histologically by a predominant glandular element comprising numerous closely opposed small duct-like structures with epithelial and myoepithelial lining. Since the stroma is sparse the term adenoma is justified though these may be closely related to the fibroadenoma.

26

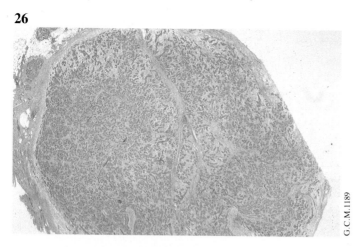

26 A small encapsulated adenoma from a female of 21. (*H&E × 12*)

26a

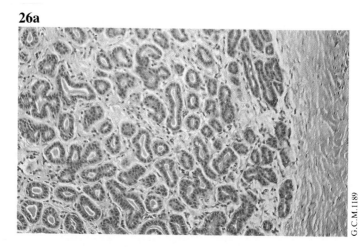

26a Breast adenoma. The degree of epithelial overgrowth contrasts with the relatively sparse increase on stromal elements. (*H&E × 50*)

Lactating adenoma

A lactating adenoma, found during pregnancy or in the puerperium, is a circumscribed area of florid lobular and ductular proliferation with secretory lining cells and luminal secretion.

28

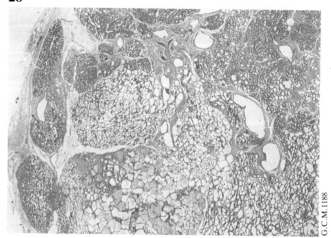

28 Breast – lactating adenoma showing acini distended by secretion. (*H&E × 10*)

Adenoma − nipple

The adenoma of the nipple found in a subareolar site may show a disturbing histological appearance with florid proliferation of duct elements embedded in a variably hyalinised stroma. The epithelial component consists of a two-cell layer with infrequent mitoses. The entrapment of small duct elements in a hyalinised stroma may mimic malignancy but these lesions are benign.

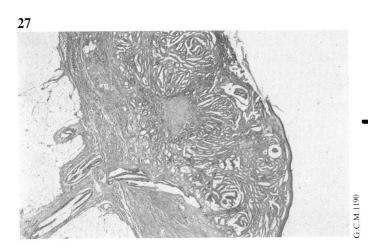

27 Adenoma of the nipple. Marked proliferation of well differentiated duct epithelium. Stromal hyalinisation can be seen (bottom) and in a central nodule. (*H&E × 10*)

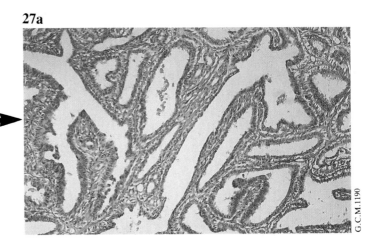

27a Same case. The inner layer of epithelium is darkly staining and cubical or columnar. The outer myo-epithelial layer tends to be vacuolated. (*H&E × 100*)

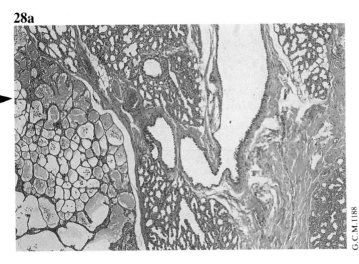

28a Same case. The acini are lined by a single layer of epithelium. (*H&E × 40*)

Fibroadenoma

This, the commonest benign breast tumour, is found most often in the 20–35 year age group and is multiple in about 20% of cases. The typical lesion is sharply demarcated, firm, pale with a whorled pattern on section.

29

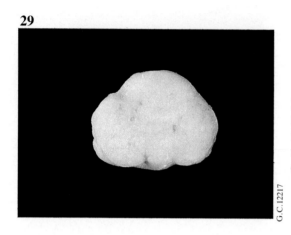

29 Breast – fibroadenoma. This painless mobile lump removed from the breast of a young woman is a typical fibroadenoma. It measures 3.5cm in maximum diameter and is composed of firm grey-white tissue with delicate septa and occasional minute cystic spaces.

30

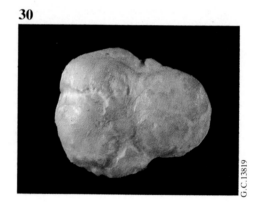

30 Fibroadenoma – calcification. This asymptomatic calcified fibroadenoma shelled out easily from the left breast of a woman aged 65 years. It measured 2cm in maximum diameter, was ovoid and slightly lobulated.

Histology

The histological appearances vary throughout one lesion due to the contribution of both epithelial and stromal connective tissue to the tumour. The tumours are termed pericanalicular when the proliferating small duct elements are surrounded by a commensurate increase in connective tissue and intracanalicular when the growth of the stroma invaginates the ducts, the resultant compressed lumina appearing as clefts and slit-like spaces. The epithelium of these lesions may show varying degrees of proliferative activity with multilayering of cells; apocrine metaplasia may also be present. The stroma may be fibroblastic and cellular or rich in acid mucopolysaccharides and may undergo hyalinisation, calcification or even osseous metaplasia. The epithelial proliferation is not thought significant in the growth potential of the lesion, the occurrence of carcinoma in fibroadenomas being exceptionally rare.

31

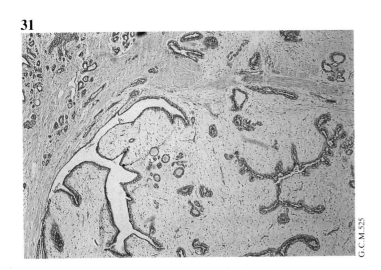

G.C.M.525

31 Breast – fibroadenoma. Part of a fibroadenoma occupies most of this field. The tumour is of mixed type. The overgrowth of fibrous tissue compresses the epithelium into slit-like channels. (*H&E × 40*)

31a

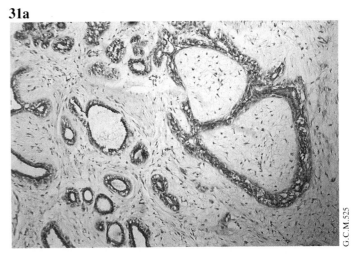

G.C.M.525

31a In this field the fibroadenoma shows both pericanalicular (left) and intracanalicular patterns (*H&E × 100*)

32

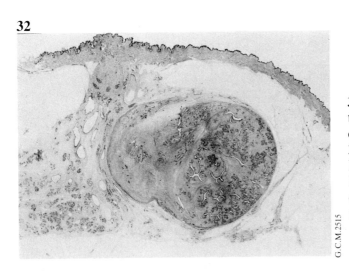

G.C.M.2515

32 Breast – Fibroadenoma. This section from a woman aged 41 shows an ovoid fibroadenoma which measured 3.5cm in maximum diameter. To the left, stromal overgrowth predominates. Elsewhere the combined stromal and epithelial proliferation has resulted in a mixed pattern.

Giant fibroadenoma and cystosarcoma phyllodes

A fibroadenoma may attain great size (giant fibroadenoma) and even ulcerate through the skin, but retain, histologically, its benign appearance. Rarely, the stromal element may exhibit malignant potential, the lesion then being termed cystosarcoma phyllodes or better, phyllodes tumour.

Phyllodes tumours are rare. They may arise de novo, without a pre-existing fibroadenoma. Most occur after the age of 40. There is no single definitive method of establishing the diagnosis, the features of importance being size, stromal cellularity and differentiation. The majority are larger than fibroadenomas though 50% may be less than 5cm in size. They are mobile in the breast. Larger tumours may ulcerate. They show a variable but often highly cellular stroma. The epithelial elements, distributed throughout in the manner of a fibroadenoma, may show varying degrees of proliferation, sometimes with cyst formation, but lack cytological criteria of malignancy. The stroma, however, shows varying cellular atypia with large pleomorphic fibroblastic cells, nucleomegaly and variable mitotic activity. The outlook may depend on size, cellularity and proliferative activity, but when the stromal element loses its relationship to the glands and exhibits histological criteria of a sarcoma then local recurrence and even metastatic disease may occur. The latter is more often blood-borne than lymphatic but does not usually occur in more than 10% of cases.

33

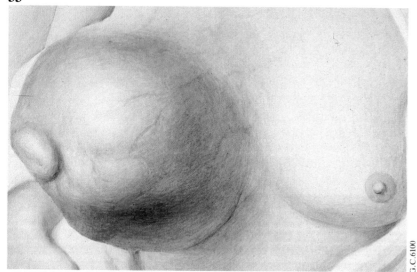

G.C.6100

33 Breast – giant fibroadenoma. A drawing of a rapidly growing breast tumour in a multipara aged 52. Numerous dilated veins are present in the skin covering the slightly nodular tumour. Microscopic examination revealed a cellular fibroadenomatous pattern. The patient was alive and well 13 years after simple mastectomy.

34

34 Breast – cystosarcoma phyllodes. A woman of 59 had noticed a breast lump for 9 months. Latterly it had grown rapidly.

The well circumscribed tumour measured 9cm in maximum diameter. Several cysts are obvious on the cut surface and masses of firm grey tissue project into some of them.

Histology showed a malignant stroma.

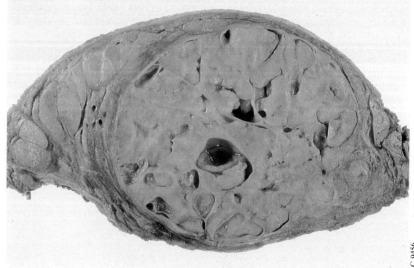

G.C.9456

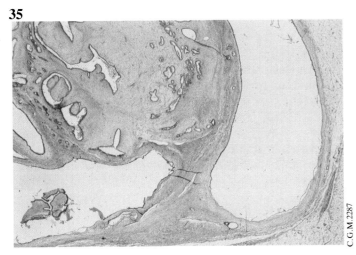

35 Breast – cystosarcoma phyllodes. Stromal overgrowth is well marked but quite large cystic spaces are also present. (*H&E×10*)

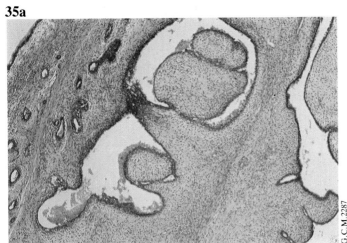

35a Same case. Proliferated stromal cells form small nodules projecting into cystic spaces. They are covered by epithelium but epithelial malignancy is not a feature. (*H&E×40*)

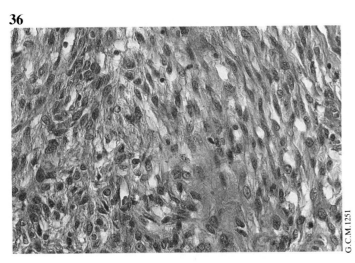

36 Cystosarcoma. The fibroblasts from a cellular part of the tumour are here arranged in interlacing bands. (*H&E×310*)

Intraduct papilloma

These usually small lesions may be difficult to identify after resection due to their soft and frond-like nature. They often lie in an area of duct dilatation and comprise a variably complex papillomatous growth, with a cytologically regular double-layered epithelium investing fibrovascular stromal cores. The appearances may be complex and may give rise to suspicion that malignant change has occurred. No single criterion is absolute but a cribriform growth pattern, absence of connective tissue stroma, or apparent invasion of the stroma of the tumour are features which suggest malignancy. However this is rare and local excision of intraduct papilloma is curative in the vast majority of individuals.

Papillomatosis, a type of epithelial hyperplasia, may form part of the proliferative elements of cystic hyperplasia (see p.321).

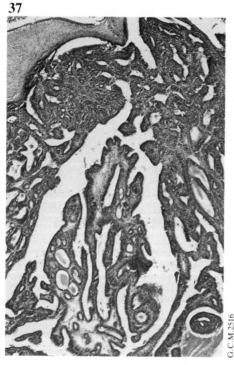

37 Duct papilloma. The epithelium is differentiated and the stroma well formed. (*H&E×40*)

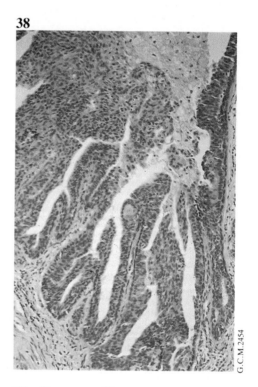

38 Duct papilloma – early malignant change. The epithelial cells have increased in size with multilayering. (*H&E×125*)

Whole sections demonstrating the distribution of papillomatous lesions in the breast.
From the E.K. Dawson collection.

39

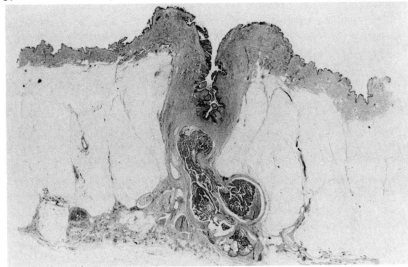

G.C.M.260

39 Breast – papillomatosis. A section of breast showing benign papillomatosis of the main ducts with marked indrawing of the nipple.

40

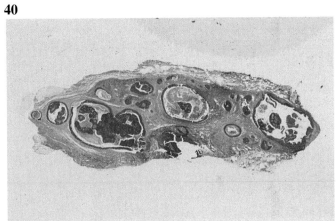

G.C.M.1243

40 Breast – duct papillomatosis. Many small ducts are distended by papillary ingrowths of epithelium. (×5)

41

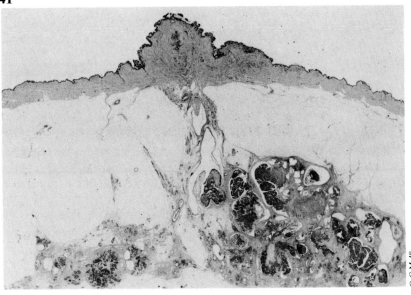

G.C.M.48

41 Breast – papillomatosis with malignant change.

A section showing florid papillomatosis of a large portion of the breast. Histological examination revealed that carcinomatous infiltration of the stroma of the tumours had occurred in several places.

Carcinoma

Epidemiology

There is a large variation in the incidence of breast cancer in different regions of the world. In general the incidence is highest in North America and northern European countries, intermediate in southern Europe and South American countries, and lowest in Asia and Africa. The reason for these differences is not known but studies of migrating populations suggest environmental factors are important.

In the United Kingdom 24 000 new cases are diagnosed annually, and it is estimated that 1 in 16 women will get breast cancer in her lifetime. This incidence is ten times greater than that in the East or in Africa.

42

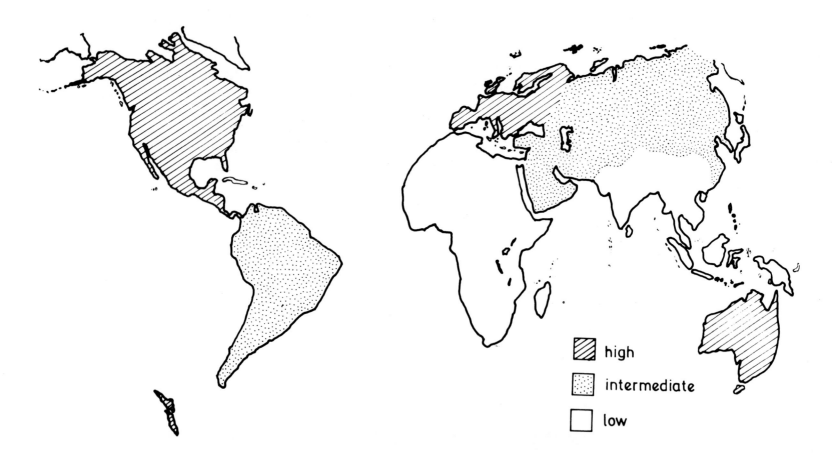

Risk factors

At the present time the cause or causes of breast cancer are unknown, but several factors have been described which are related to the risk of developing disease. These are summarised in the table.

Factor	High risk	Low risk
Age	over 45 years	under 30
Parity	nulliparous	parous
Age at 1st full term pregnancy	30 years	20 years
Family history	first degree relative	—
Previous benign breast disease	fibrocystic disease with atypical hyperplasia	—
Mammographic pattern (Wolfe's types)	dense prominent ducts ($DY+P_2$)	lucent ($N+P_2$)
Age at artificial menopause (oophorectomy)	—	early

Carcinoma

Pathology

The pathological classification of breast carcinoma may be based on:

(a) Its character, *in situ* or invasive.
(b) Its pattern, e.g. tubular or medullary.
(c) Its presumed site of origin, e.g. ductal or lobular.

The classification and terminology may thus be confusing. The various classifications and attempts at histological grading have not in general provided precise information as to growth potential, prognosis, response to treatment etc, and have largely been ineffective in elucidating aetiology. In any one case the pattern may be variable throughout the tumour and this often renders precise classification impracticable. Therefore observer variation in classification and grading on separate occasions of pathological study contributes to the difficulties in this area. The criteria should be as precise and reproducible as possible. Only by such means may the aetiology, innate growth potential and response to treatment be assessed.

43

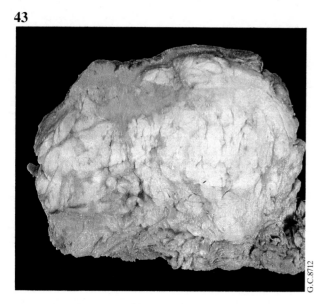

44

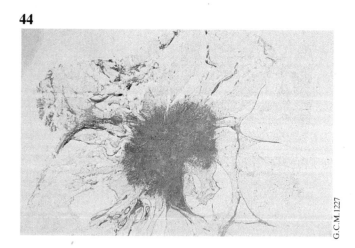

44 Breast − carcinoma. This section shows the characteristic appearance of a small, invasive carcinoma situated deep in an atrophic breast. (*H&E×3*)

43 Breast − carcinoma. In this large fatty breast the tumour has infiltrated the areola and has expanded beneath it.

Intraduct carcinoma

Intraduct carcinoma by definition is preinvasive and macroscopically may show gross duct distension, mimicking simple duct ectasia. Microscopically the problems of evaluation of epithelial proliferative states (see benign breast disease) obtain. There is often a haphazard cellular proliferation with cytoplasmic and nuclear pleomorphism, mitotic activity, and a cribriform growth pattern without supporting stroma; central necrosis and calcification may occur. Ducts may become distended by partly necrotic tumour − comedo carcinoma. On other occasions the epithelium may be attenuated and show only a micropapillary growth of cells or an elongated strand of malignant epithelium may traverse the duct without an apparent supporting stroma. The assessment of malignancy requires detailed study, as does the assessment of any invasive element.

Since lesions diagnosed as intraduct may (in one series, 18%) show axillary lymph node metastases, invasion may be missed. Moreover, the trabecular, solid growth pattern of invasive lesions may mimic duct formation giving a false impression of the occupation of a pre-existing duct. This may be confirmed or refuted by the use of elastic stains.

45

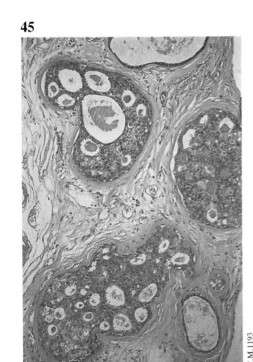

45 Breast − intraduct carcinoma. The duct lumen is filled with atypical epithelial cells showing nuclear pleomorphism, mitoses and loss of normal maturation. (*H&E×100*)

46

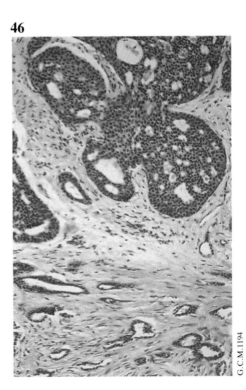

46 Breast − carcinoma. In this example, the neoplastic cells adopt a cribriform pattern. Invasive carcinoma is also present (bottom). (*H&E×125*)

47

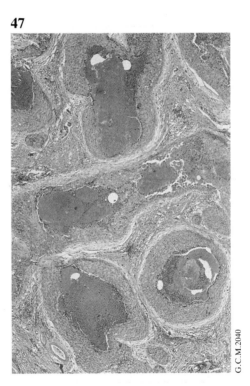

47 Breast − comedo carcinoma. Ducts are distended by carcinoma showing central necrosis. (*H&E×40*)

335

Invasive ductal carcinoma

Invasive ductal carcinoma is the commonest type encountered. It has the typical macroscopic appearance of a stellate, puckered area with a gritty resistance to the scalpel blade and radiating trabeculae of firm fibrous strands.

48

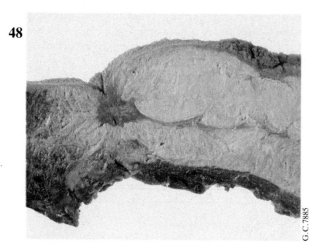

48 Breast – scirrhous carcinoma. A woman of 43 noticed a puckering of the breast skin near the axilla overlying a small hard lump. The tumour which has the typical appearance of a scirrhous carcinoma lies about 4cm lateral to the nipple.

The term scirrhous carcinoma reflecting this hardness should be reserved only for such macroscopic evaluation but is reflected at histological level by diffuse stromal invasion and resultant fibroblastic tissue response.

Microscopically there is great variation in cellular differentiation, the carcinoma infiltrating as small ducts, acinar structures or individual cords of cells. While the cells may show great nuclear variation and moderate mitotic activity they are frequently of moderate size and relatively monomorphic appearance. The production of abundant elastic tissue around intraduct and invasive tumour and in the walls of associated vessels within the breast, termed elastosis, is a frequent occurrence in invasive malignancy. It may, however, be found in non-malignant lesions, e.g. sclerosing adenosis. The origin of the mesenchymal fibres is unresolved, but is in part a response of stromal cells to tumour invasion. Around such an area of invasive carcinoma there may be evidence of *in situ* ductal malignancy, a presumed earlier stage of the disease.

49

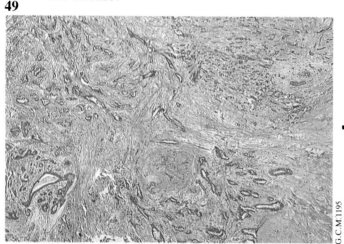

49a

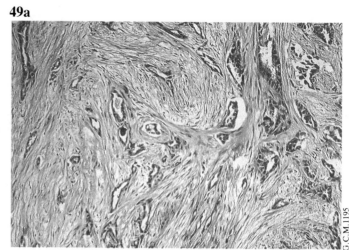

49 This invasive carcinoma is associated with a marked stromal reaction. The stroma varies in cellularity, some being hyaline and relatively acellular. (*H&E×40*)

49a Same case. Here the carcinoma has a ductular pattern and the spindle-cell stroma is cellular. (*H&E×125*)

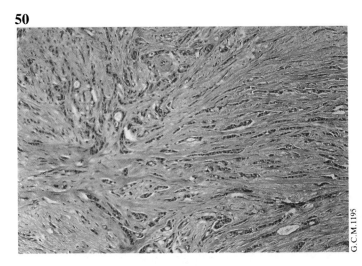

50 This pattern of radiating cords of tumour cells and associated fibrous reaction, producing the hard, 'scirrhous' feel, is typical of invasive carcinoma of breast. (*H&E×125*)

Elastosis

The production of elastin fibres may be found in several forms of breast disease but is most often associated with invasive carcinoma. The origin of these fibres has not yet been determined; local production by stromal cells in response to the tumour seems probable but a contribution of fibre from the tumour cells has been suggested. Elastosis is a very variable finding in any one case and indeed in different areas of the same lesion. There is a relationship between elastosis and the presence of oestrogen receptors in a tumour, and both have been suggested as favourable prognostic factors.

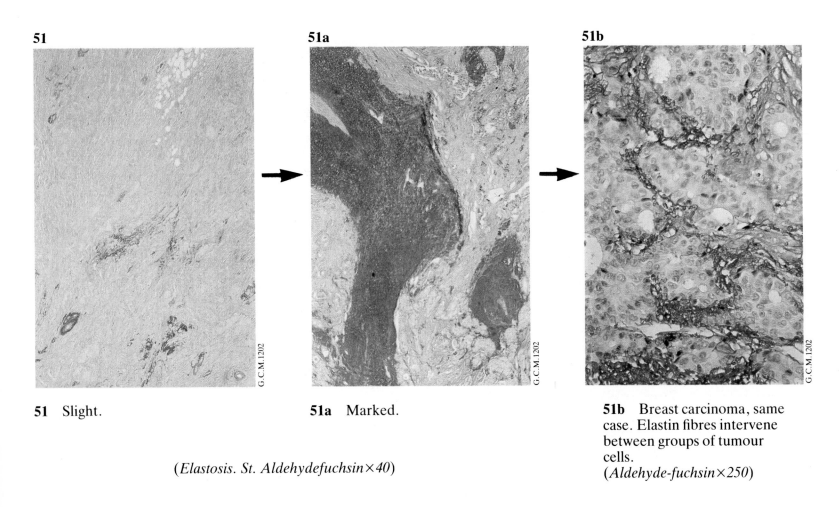

51 Slight.

51a Marked.

51b Breast carcinoma, same case. Elastin fibres intervene between groups of tumour cells. (*Aldehyde-fuchsin×250*)

(*Elastosis. St. Aldehydefuchsin×40*)

Paget's disease

This is the manifestation of intraepidermal invasion by subjacent ductal carcinoma. The excoriated eczematous lesions of nipple may be difficult to biopsy.

52

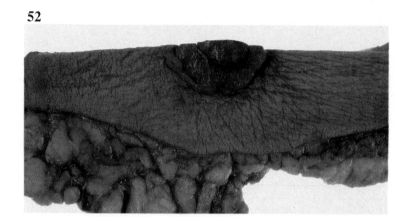

52a

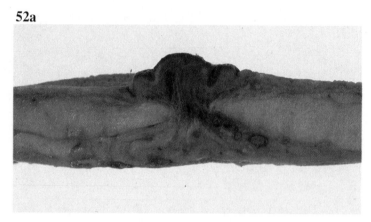

52 and **52a**   From a female aged 68 who had had a discharge of watery, and occasionally blood-stained, fluid from the right nipple, for over a year. Examination revealed a red granular area involving the nipple and whole areola. The skin in the affected area was a little thickened, but no induration was palpable in the breast. The axillary lymph nodes were not palpable.

In the specimen of half of the right breast the nipple and the areola are raised a little above the level of the surrounding skin, are reddish and granular, and on section are seen to be thickened.

The breast is small and atrophic. To one side the ducts are distended by largely necrotic intraduct carcinoma. No invasive tumour can be seen.

G.C.10084

52b

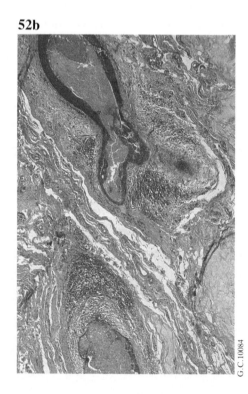

52b   The dilated breast ducts of the above specimen are mainly occupied by eosinophilic necrotic tumour and there is considerable inflammatory reaction around them. The intraduct carcinoma is only clearly seen in the uppermost duct where the necrotic material is surrounded by darkly staining malignant epithelium. (*H&E×40*)

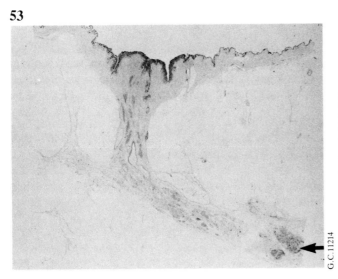

53 Paget's disease of the nipple. Histologically the characteristic appearances of Paget's disease are present in the nipple of this section. The epithelium of the ducts from the peripheral focus of intraduct carcinoma (arrow) upwards to the nipple shows almost continuous malignant change.

From the E.K. Dawson collection.

The typical histology shows a haphazard invasion of all layers of epidermis by large, pale cells of breast duct origin. They may contain mucin and, rarely, cytoplasmic melanin by cytocrine transfer from adjacent melanocytes. The subjacent carcinoma is usually found in major ducts and may be apparently *in situ* or show widespread stromal invasion.

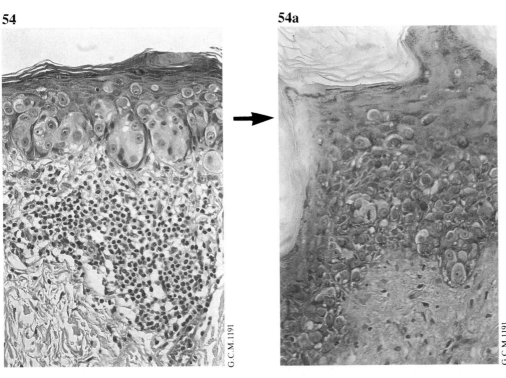

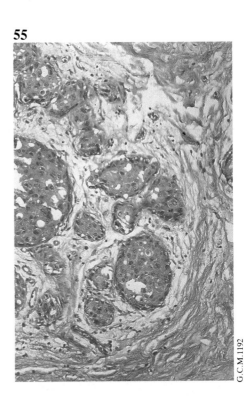

54 Nipple. Paget's disease. The epidermis is infiltrated by large pale carcinoma cells with prominent nucleoli. Lymphocytes infiltrate the underlying stroma. (*H&E×250*)

54a Same case. The carcinoma cells are numerous. Their mucinous content is, in this case, demonstrated by PAS staining, but mucin is not invariably present. (*×250*)

55 Case of Paget's disease of the nipple with foci of ductal carcinoma 2cm deep to the nipple. (*H&E×125*)

Lobular carcinoma

Lobular carcinoma occurs in *in situ* and infiltrative forms. It may account for up to 10% of breast carcinomas. It would seem that lobular carcinoma more often than other types may give rise to bilateral malignancy. The overall prognosis seems better than that of classical ductal carcinoma.

The *in situ* form, if small, may be found incidentally since it lacks the stromal response which would produce clinical palpability. Microscopically the enlarged lobules and terminal ducts produce a curious appearance being distended with bland, pale, monomorphic cells whose round or oval nuclei show little variation in size and shape.

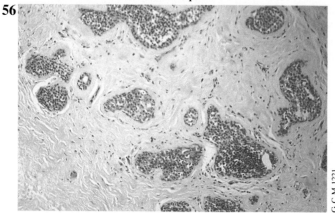

56 Atypical lobular hyperplasia reflects abnormal proliferation within the lobule and may be a potentially premalignant stage. (*H&E×100*)

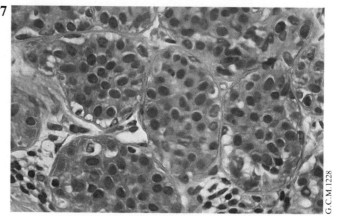

57 Breast − lobular carcinoma. In the *in situ* stage, the lobules are distended with rather monomorphic small epithelial cells. The cells may contain intracytoplasmic lumina with secretion. (*H&E×400*)

When invasive, the pattern is variable but classically shows a targetoid pattern of infiltration around ducts and lobules in a concentric manner. Elastosis is variable.

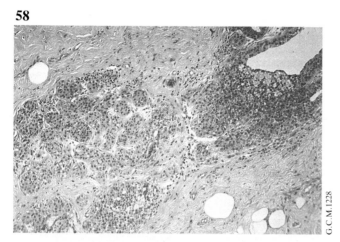

58 Breast − lobular carcinoma. To the left the tumour is entirely *in situ*. On the right early periductal invasion has occurred. (*H&E×100*)

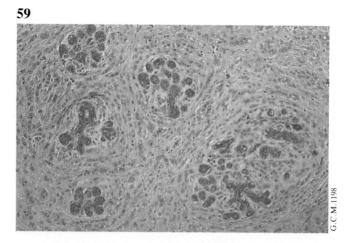

59 Breast − invasive lobular carcinoma. Pale carcinoma cells infiltrate the lobules and surround them in concentric fashion. (*H&E×100*)

The 'Indian-file' pattern of infiltrating single cells is typical and the cells frequently possess an intracytoplasmic lumen containing a small amount of mucin. These may be identified by mucin staining and by electron microscopy.

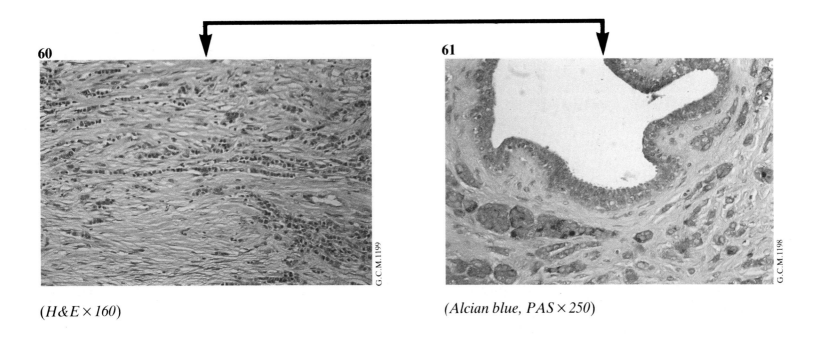

60

(H&E × 160)

61

(Alcian blue, PAS × 250)

Tubular carcinoma

This unusual variant shows a well differentiated tubular growth pattern, small single-layered epithelial-lined ductules lying in a haphazard distribution in a fibrous stroma. The pattern may mimic that of sclerosing adenosis but subjacent myoepithelial cells and a delineating basement membrane are usually absent in the tubular carcinoma. The lesion is often multicentric and may be bilateral (though the contralateral lesion may not be tubular); these features, reminiscent of lobular carcinoma, may imply a relationship between the two. The prognosis in tubular carcinoma is better than in the classical ductal type despite nodal involvement in approximately one third of cases at presentation.

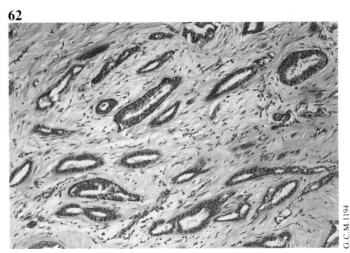

62

62 Breast, tubular carcinoma.
(H&E × 125)

Mucinous (mucoid, colloid) carcinoma

This term should be restricted to those lesions which show abundant mucin formation. The small eosinophilic tumour cells, often differentiating to microglandular structures, lie within pools of mucin. The prognosis may be better than that of classic ductal though recurrence is common.

63

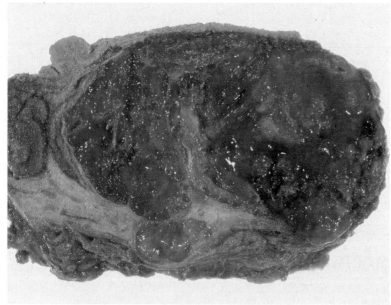

63 Breast − mucoid carcinoma. Lying mainly to one side of the nipple a tumour which measured 10cm in maximum diameter extends from skin to deep fascia. It is formed mainly by glistening mucin and at its margins is quite well defined.

64

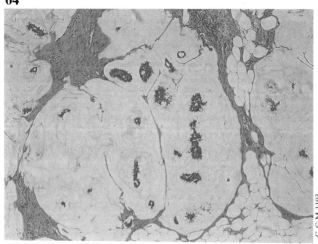

64 Breast − a highly mucoid carcinoma supported by stroma containing fat cells. Small groups of tumour cells in papillary formation lie in abundant mucin. (*H&E × 50*)

Medullary carcinoma

This lesion is often bulky, circumscribed, soft, and homogeneous.

65

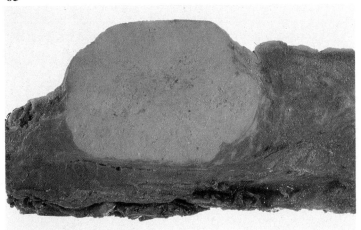

G.C.7486

65 A woman of 53 had noticed a painless breast lump for 10 months.

The tumour is ovoid measuring 10cm in maximum diameter. Its borders are clearly defined but it extends from skin to deep fascia.

66

G.C.11252

66 Medullary carcinoma from a 45 year old woman who was alive and well 9 years after radical mastectomy. The lobulated circumscribed appearance is well shown in this whole section of breast.

The histological appearance is of solid sheets of large pleomorphic cells with large nuclei, prominent eosinophilic nucleoli and a high mitotic index. There is little in the way of glandular formation and intraduct elements are not normally regarded as part of the lesion. At the delineated border of the tumour there is a prominent lymphocytic infiltrate.

67

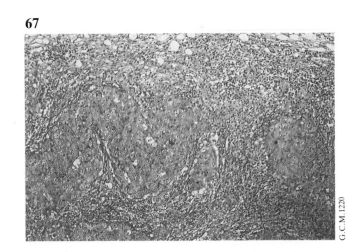

G.C.M.1220

67 Breast – medullary carcinoma. (*H&E×100*).

Despite the alarming cytological features the long term prognosis seems genuinely better in these cases. Similar cellular appearances and focal lymphocytic infiltrate may occur in other carcinomas, e.g. ductal, and only if the pattern constitutes 75% of the tumour should it be designated medullary.

Breast carcinoma during pregnancy

The aggressive growth pattern and metastatic potential of breast carcinoma developing during, or accelerated by, pregnancy may reflect the oestrogen and progesterone sensitivity of the malignant cells in the hormonal environment of pregnancy.

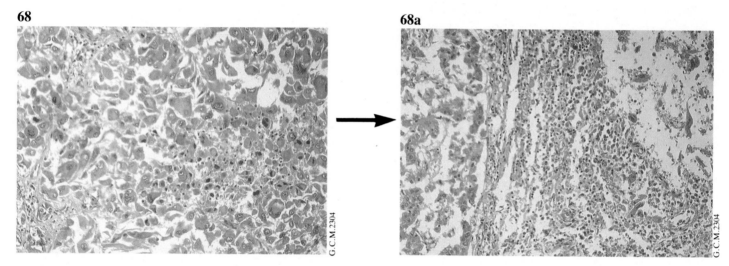

68 Breast carcinoma in pregnancy. The tumour is composed of large pleomorphic cells showing mitotic activity. Multinucleated tumour cells are also present. To right of centre there is a focus of necrosis where nuclear pyknosis and cytoplasmic disintegration are obvious. (*H&E×125*)

68a Same case. Here a considerably larger area of necrosis has provoked an inflammatory reaction. The preserved tumour on the left is separated from the disintegrated tumour by a broad band of inflammatory cells. (*H&E×125*)

'Inflammatory' carcinoma

This, a clinical pattern rather than a specific pathological type, is not synonymous with breast carcinoma during pregnancy. The lesion is characterised, usually, by widespread lymphatic invasion and dermal metastases and the production of an erythematous, oedematous breast. It is often of a large cell, poorly-differentiated type.

69

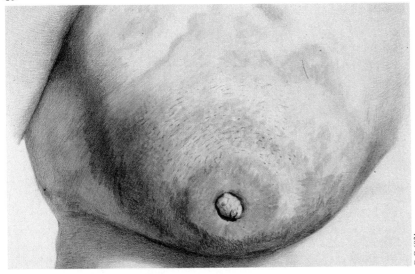

69 Breast — drawing of an 'inflammatory carcinoma'. The breast is swollen, firm and oedematous. Involvement of the skin has produced an erythematous thickening, limited by a fairly definite margin beyond which several irregular, smaller, erythematous areas appear. The nipple is retracted, the areola swollen and the erythematous portion of the breast shows discrete dimpling at the attachment of the suspensory ligaments.

69a

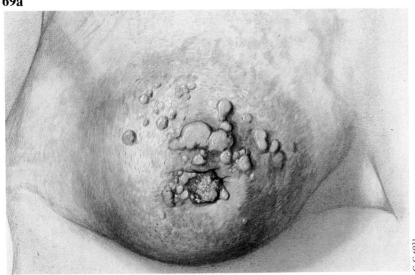

69a   5 weeks later. Erythema extends to the axilla and neighbouring chest wall. Around the apex of the swollen breast, especially superiorly, are numerous cutaneous nodules. The nipple is retracted and the areola is not distinguishable.

Carcinoma − male breast

Carcinoma of the breast accounts for only 0.15% of deaths from cancer in men. Its incidence is less than 1% of that in women and it tends to occur in a slightly older age group. In cases of Klinefelter's syndrome the incidence is increased at least ten-fold.

The histology resembles that of carcinoma of the breast in females although fibrosis is often less marked and there are differences in incidence of the less common histological patterns, e.g. lobular carcinoma is rare in male breast tumours. Men with carcinoma of the breast tend to present late so that infiltration of the skin and axillary node metastases are usual.

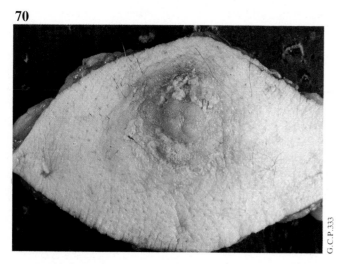

70 Male breast carcinoma. Tumour lying beneath the nipple has infiltrated skin causing excoriation and crust formation.

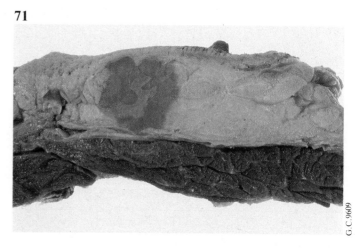

71 Male breast carcinoma. A man of 65 had noticed a painless lump in his left breast for 5 weeks. A grey-white tumour 2cm in diameter lay lateral to the nipple and extended almost from skin to deep fascia. There was some central necrosis.

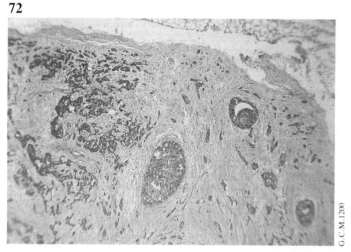

72 Male breast carcinoma. All histological types may be found but the most frequent will be an invasive ductal type, here showing the typical stromal response to infiltrating tumour cells. (*H&E × 40*)

Prognosis

Because of late presentation men fare worse than women. When, however, allowance is made both for stage of the disease and the age of the patient the behaviour is similar in both sexes.

Gynaecomastia

Gynaecomastia (enlargement) of the male breast is idiopathic in most cases. It may occur as a result of hormonal disturbances in the neonatal period, at puberty or in old age, or in association with testicular atrophy. Gynaecomastia in the presence of chronic liver disease may reflect abnormal metabolism of steroid hormones. Oestrogens given for control of prostatic cancer and drugs such as digitalis, cimetidine, spironolactone, antimitotic agents etc may also be implicated. Neoplastic change in gynaecomastia occurs only rarely.

The characteristic histological features are the epithelial proliferation of ducts and the connective tissue oedema and fibroplasia in periductal sites. Since elastic tissue is not a prominent feature, it may be that the terminal ductules are predominantly involved but lobule formation is excessively rare. The latter may be found, however, in cases of Klinefelter's syndrome, where the presence of an additional X-chromosome in the body cells (47 XXY) is associated with testicular atrophy.

73

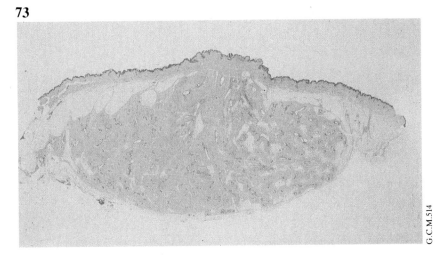

73 Gynaecomastia. This florid example developed in a boy 9 years of age. A substantial enlargement of the breast has resulted from increase in ducts and stroma. (*H&E × 1.5*)

73a

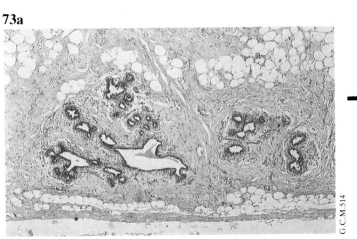

73a Gynaecomastia, same case, showing the development of a lobule – a rare occurrence. (*H&E × 50*)

73b

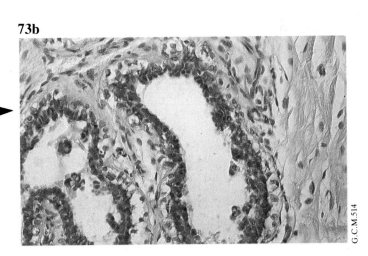

73b Same case. Ducts composed of darkly staining hyperplastic epithelial cells and pale myoepithelial cells are set in cellular stroma. (*H&E × 250*)

Carcinoma – spread

Carcinoma of the breast is often associated with extensive spread. The character of the spread determines the surgical treatment.

Intramammary spread

From the initial lesion, spread within the breast may occur by extension within the mammary ducts or by lymphatics within the breast. The spread may be localised resulting in but few evident metastases or may be extensive. In the latter instance the interpretation of the picture is difficult and doubt will remain whether the picture is that of widespread metastasis or of multifocal primary malignancy.

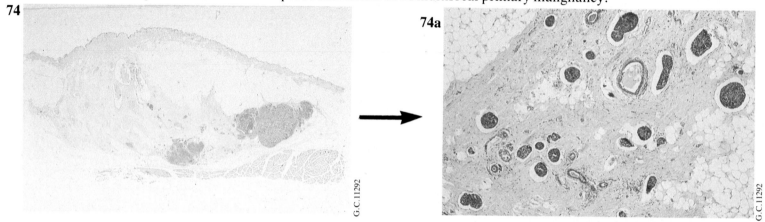

74 Breast carcinoma. Several nodules of tumour are present in this breast. (*H&E × 0.5*)

74a Same case. Many lymphatics are invaded by tumour. (*H&E × 40*)

Local spread

The breast is surrounded by fatty tissue. Superficially a layer of fat separates the breast from the skin. In this layer are numerous fibrous strands which bind the breast to the skin (Cooper's ligaments). Where carcinoma spreads along these ligaments it reaches and invades the skin which becomes hardened, thickened and roughened. To this state the term peau d'orange is applied. At a later stage ulceration occurs.

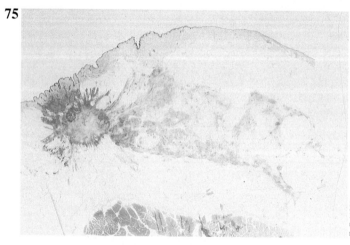

75 Breast – scirrhous carcinoma from a woman of 43 years. This whole section of the breast shows spread of tumour along Cooper's ligaments. The skin is involved and there is some spread into the retromammary adipose tissue. (*H&E × 0.5*)

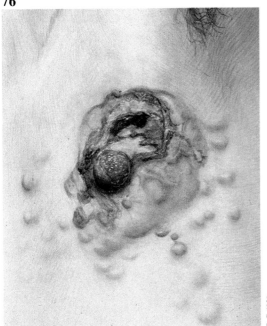

76 Spread along the ducts upwards to the nipple leads to retraction of the nipple and later ulceration. The drawing illustrates advanced local spread.

The tumour may spread deeply invading the retromammary space in which there are numerous lymphatics. Subsequent spread involves the pectoralis major muscle leading to fixation of the breast.

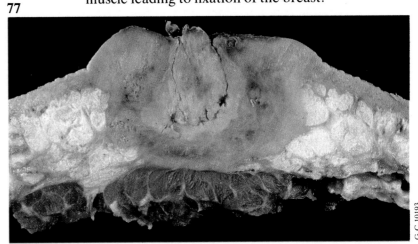

77 Breast carcinoma. The tumour has ulcerated through the skin and shows considerable central necrosis. On its deeper aspect it has penetrated the pectoral fascia and is beginning to invade muscle. The axillary lymph nodes were widely infiltrated by carcinoma and 4 months later spinal metastases were obvious on X-ray.

Lymphatic spread

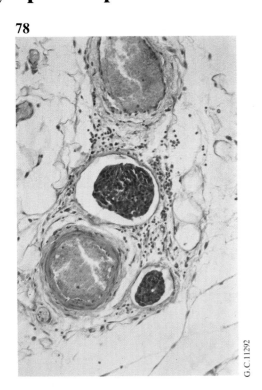

78 Carcinomatous invasion of lymphatics. (*H&E × 60*)

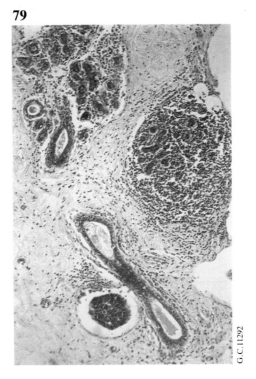

79 Tumour in periductal lymphatic. (*H&E × 100*)

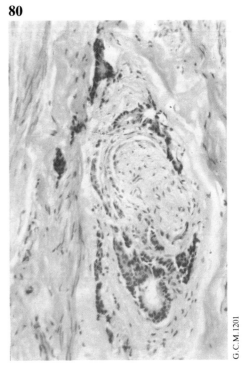

80 Perineural invasion. (*H&E × 160*)

Extramammary lymphatic spread

The lymphatic drainage of the breast is free and extensive. When carcinoma arises in the breast the direction of spread is determined in some measure by the site of the initial lesion. The majority of tumours of the breast arise in the upper and outer quadrant. Lymphatics from this part run upwards and outwards towards the axilla along the line of the lateral thoracic artery and thereafter reach the nodes lying in relation to the axillary artery with subsequent spread upwards into the root of the neck around the subclavian artery. The initial involvement may consist of relatively discrete secondary nodules but ultimately these tend to become fused together to form a fixed solid mass. The involvement of the axillary nodes will cause a degree of lymphatic obstruction to the arm with consequent swelling.

81

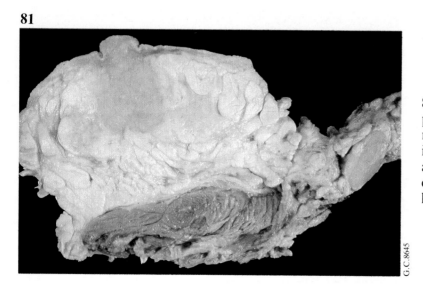

81 Breast carcinoma with axillary metastasis. The patient, a woman of 48 years, first noticed a swelling a month before mastectomy. A firm grey tumour measuring in cross-section 35 × 30mm lay beneath the nipple and had infiltrated it. Spread had occurred along the deeper breast trabeculae and the enlarged axillary lymph node shown was replaced by carcinoma.

Occasionally tumours in the medial quadrants of the breast appear to have a lymph drainage which communicates with the lymphatics of the opposite breast and this may be an explanation of some cases where malignancy develops in the second breast.

Posterior spread of the disease may affect the lymphatics which lie along the internal mammary artery. Spread backwards through the internal mammary chain may involve lymphatics running in association with the intercostal vessels and extend along these vessels to reach the paravertebral lymph nodes. Vertebral involvement may result particularly in TV 3, 4 and 5.

Haematogenous spread

Metastases arise in many sites. At death the organs most commonly affected are lungs (60%), liver (50%), bones (50%) and brain (20%).

Haematogenous metastasis in the past was regarded as occurring relatively late and in general developing during the period of five years after operative treatment. However, the modern view is that the escape of malignant cells into the blood stream or lymphatics occurs early and may even result from small, localised breast cancers which have been excised early. Further it is appreciated that malignant cells which escape into and settle out of the blood stream (micrometastases) may be widely disseminated and may not give rise to detectable secondary lesions for many years after the development of the original cancer.

Why a micrometastatic deposit remains latent and then assumes activity and develops into a macroscopic focus of disease is unknown. Alterations in body immunity or hormonal status due to ageing and other factors may be involved. The metastases may be single or multiple and while a majority become obvious within a period of five years of the development of the original mammary tumour, others may lie quiescent for 20 or more years.

Spread within the body cavities, the pleura, peritoneum and by the cerebrospinal fluid represent secondary spread from metastatic deposits in these regions.

Hormone receptors and carcinoma of the breast

The cells of some breast carcinomas have receptors with a high affinity for binding oestrogens such as oestradiol. These oestrogen receptors, which are protein in nature (oestrophilin), can be assayed using a variety of techniques, and are situated in the cytoplasm of the cell. Oestrogen passes through the cell membrane and binds to the receptor; the oestrogen-receptor complex then enters the nucleus, where it causes the transcription of DNA with the formation of mRNA which in turn leads to the formation of proteins in the ribosomes of the rough surfaced endoplasmic reticulum. Later, DNA synthesis, cell division and tissue growth occur.

Oestrogen receptors can be detected in 45% of breast tumours from pre-menopausal patients and in 65% of tumours from post-menopausal patients. The lower levels of detectable receptors in tumours from pre-menopausal women might in part be due to the fact that blood oestrogen levels are higher in these women, leading to an increased uptake of this hormone on to oestrogen receptors in the tumour. This binding of oestrogen to the receptors prevents the receptor from being detected by the radioactive oestrogen method of determination.

Besides oestrogen receptors some tumours have receptors for progesterone, glucocorticoids, androgens and prolactin. Receptors for these hormones usually occur in tumours which also have oestrogen receptors.

In the management of breast carcinoma, the response to hormone-ablation, i.e. removal of potential sources of hormones which may promote tumour growth, is an important factor. The assessment of oestrogen receptors on tumour cells may give some indication as to subsequent response and such studies are currently being evaluated. The majority of tumours without demonstrable oestrogen receptors fail to respond to endocrine manipulation. Approximately 50% of tumours with oestrogen receptors show some regression in response to endocrine therapy or ablation. The presence of a progestogen receptor may have similar predictive value. In addition the possession of such receptors may confer, or be associated with, a more favourable prognosis even without endocrine therapy. It is of interest that infiltrating lobular carcinoma, with its apparent longer survival, shows expression of oestrogen receptors more often than the invasive ductal variety.

The elastosis already described as a frequent but variable feature of invasive (ductal or lobular) carcinoma has been suggested as another histological feature which may reflect prognosis and may correlate with oestrogen receptor activity. Survival rates have been positively correlated with the amount of elastosis present.

Carcinoma

Statistical studies

Many clinical trials compare survival duration among cancer patients randomly allocated to different treatments. Outcome expressed in terms of 5 and 10 year survival rates can be misleading, as long-term studies show continued loss of life attributable to cancer for up to 30 years after treatment. Life table graphs and logrank P-values are more accurate and sensitive and these methods are more appropriate for expressing the results of clinical trials.

The life table

This is a graph or table giving an estimate of the proportion of a group of patients that will still be alive at different times after randomisation, calculated with due allowance for incomplete follow-up.

The logrank test and significance levels

The 'P-value' expresses the probability that the difference found in the two treatment groups is a chance occurrence and not due to a real difference in the efficiency of treatment A and treatment B.

Thus 'P < 0.05' means that there is a less than 1 in 20 chance that the differences found between treatment A and treatment B are due to a chance finding.

The logrank test involves counting the number of deaths observed in each group and comparing it with the extent of exposure to risk of death in that group.

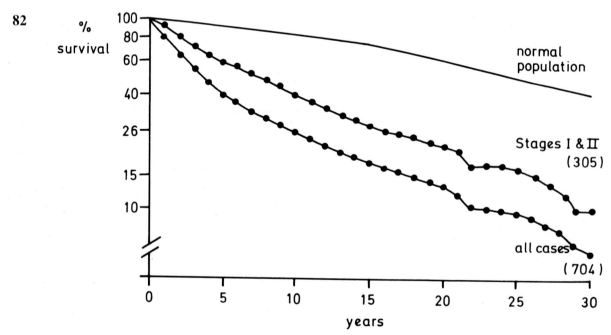

82 Fate of 704 women with breast cancer treated in East Anglia between 1947 and 1950. (From Brinkley & Haybittle 1980)

Prognosis

The outcome for breast cancer depends largely on the stage of the disease.

The 'TNM' system is now widely used for clinical staging. 'T' describes the size of tumour and whether the tumour has spread outside the breast parenchyma to involve the skin and chest wall. 'N' describes the clinical node status of the ipsilateral axilla and supraclavicular fossa. 'M' describes whether or not metastases are present. The accuracy of clinical staging is limited by the relative insensitivity of clinical assessment of the axilla and of presently available methods for detecting metastatic disease.

Clinical staging

T – Primary tumour

Tis *In situ* carcinoma

T0 No demonstrable tumour in breast (mammographic lesion).

T1 Tumour of 2 cm or less in its greatest dimension
  T1a With no fixation to underlying pectoral fascia and/or muscle.
  T1b With fixation to underlying pectoral fascia and/or muscle.

T2 Tumour more than 2 cm but not more than 5 cm in its greatest dimension
  T2a With no fixation to underlying pectoral fascia and/or muscle.
  T2b With fixation to underlying pectoral fascia and/or muscle.

T3 Tumour more than 5 cm in its greatest dimension
  T3a With no fixation to underlying pectoral fascia and/or muscle.
  T3b With fixation to underlying pectoral fascia and/or muscle.

T4 Tumour of any size with direct extension to chest wall or skin
  T4a With fixation to chest wall.
  T4b With oedema, infiltration or ulceration of skin of breast (including peau d'orange) or satellite skin nodules confined to the same breast.
  T4c With fixation to chest wall and skin oedema or ulceration or satellite nodules (T4a + T4b).

N – Regional lymph nodes

N0 No palpable ipsilateral axillary nodes.

N1 Palpable ipsilateral axillary nodes.
  N1a Nodes not considered to contain metastasis.
  N1b Nodes considered to contain metastasis.

N2 Ipsilateral axillary nodes fixed to one another or to other structures.

N3 Ipsilateral supraclavicular or infraclavicular nodes or oedema of the arm.

M – Distant metastases

M0 No evidence of distant metastases.

M1 Distant metastases present including skin involvement beyond the breast area.

Carcinoma (*Continued*)

Pathological staging

Axillary node status

The pathological staging of the axilla gives valuable prognostic information. Patients with axillary node metastasis have a worse prognosis than those without nodal involvement and the extent of nodal involvement adds further information.

83

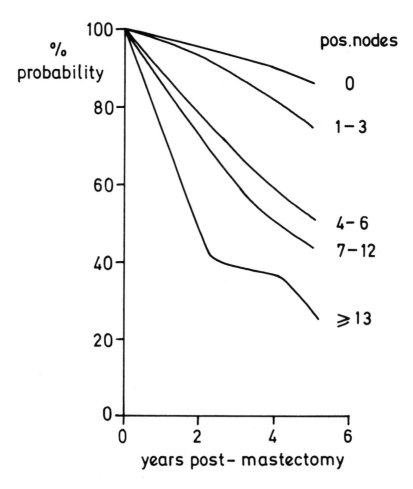

83 (After B Fisher et al)

Other prognostic indicators

Several other factors related to the outcome in patients with breast cancer, have been described and are summarised in the table. The effects of these factors are less than that of stage and axillary node status, and also, several are inter-dependent. For example, oestrogen and progesterone receptor content of breast cancer exhibit a strong correlation with the degree of tumour differentiation.

	Prognostic factor	Favourable	Less favourable
(a)	Oestrogen receptor content of tumour	High	Low
(b)	Progesterone-receptor content of tumour	High	Low
(c)	Histological type	Mucoid Medullary Tubular Lobular	Undifferentiated 'no special type' (usually ductal)
(d)	Histological grade (Bloom & Richardson)	Grade 1	Grade 11 Grade 111
(e)	Elastosis	Present	Absent
(f)	Regional lymph node sinus histiocytosis	Present	Absent

Histological grading (Bloom and Richardson)

Three grades of malignancy are suggested in this classification:

Low (Grade I); Intermediate (Grade II); High (Grade III)

These depend upon the degree of tubule formation (reflecting better differentiation), nuclear pleomorphism, hyperchromatic nuclei and mitoses (reflecting a worse grade).

Diagnostic imaging of the breast

Film/screen mammography

This is a soft tissue radiograph of the breast employing specially developed films and intensifying screens. The signs of a carcinoma include:

(a) An irregular opacity.
(b) An area of altered architecture
(c) Fine clustered microcalcification.
(d) Skin oedema.
(e) Increased vasculature.

The oblique mammogram shown, illustrates the appearance of a normal breast on the left side and a carcinoma on the right.

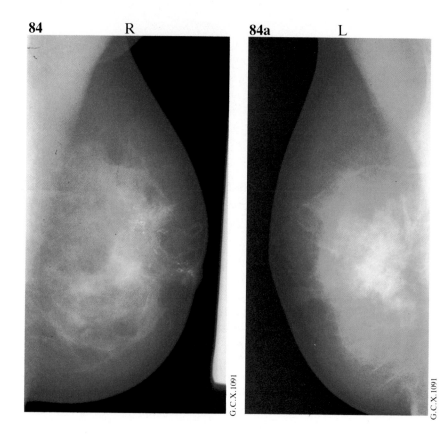

Mammography with moving grid

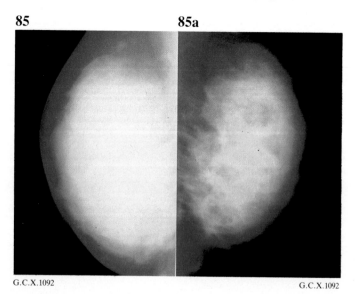

85 and **85a** Some women have breasts which are radiologically very dense and tend to scatter a large proportion of the X-rays which produce the image, giving an appearance similar to the film on the left.

The film on the right, a picture of the same breast, is produced with a moving grid attachment between the breast and the film cassette. Greater detail of the breast structure can be seen.

Xeromammography

This is also a soft tissue radiograph of the breast but uses a radioelectric process. The advantages of the xeroradiographic method are the enhancement of the margins of lesions, the highlighting of micro-calcification and the ability to penetrate dense dysplastic breasts.

Though the radiation dose is low, it is higher than that of film/screen mammograms and, therefore, less suitable for screening purposes.

86

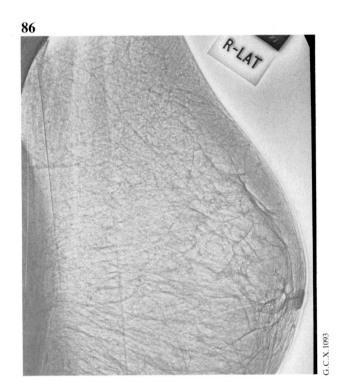

86a

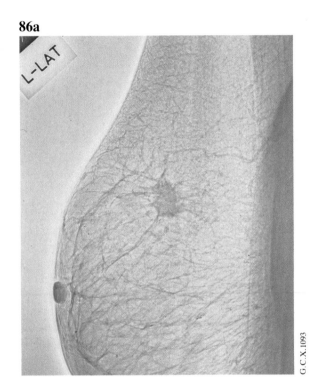

86 and **86a**   The xeromammograph of the left breast shows a spiculated opacity typical of a carcinoma.

The section on diagnostic imaging of the breast has been contributed by Dr A.E. Kirkpatrick.

Sonar scanning

The breast can be scanned, either by an automated system which scans the breast in up to 200 sequential images with the breast immersed in a water bath, or by contact real-time scanning using a high frequency (5–7.5 Mhz) hand held probe.

The technique is of particular value for confirming the nature of opacities seen on mammography when no palpable lesion is present. A high proportion of such opacities turn out to be cystic and can be aspirated under ultrasound control. The pre-aspiration scan shows a 15 mm cyst which was aspirated, and the post-aspiration scan shows the disappearance of the cyst.

88   Pre-aspiration

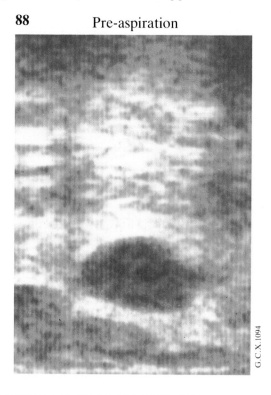

88a   Post-aspiration

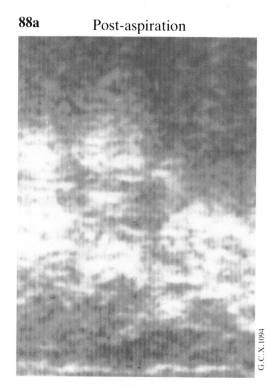

Ductography

90

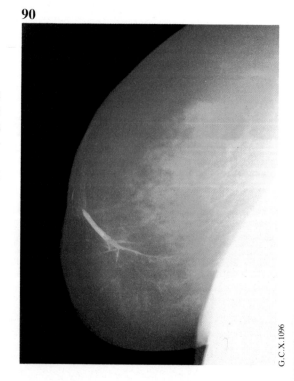

90 This technique is used to investigate nipple discharge, particularly when blood-stained. The discharging duct is dilated, a fine plastic catheter is introduced, and X-ray contrast is injected.

This example shows a dilated duct system containing a ductal polyp.

Magnetic resonance imaging (MRI)

MRI, otherwise known as nuclear magnetic resonance, is a new imaging technique which uses the combination of magnetism and radio-frequency radiation to produce changes in the behaviour of atomic nuclei. These are short-lived and generate signals which can be detected and converted into an image. This technique has the potential of generating information, not only from alterations in an anatomical structure, but also biochemical changes.

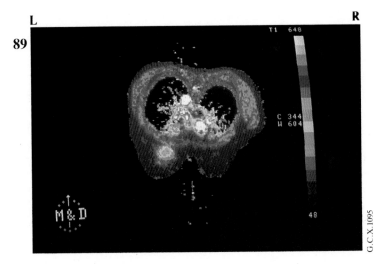

89 The example shows a normal breast on the right side, and a carcinoma on the left.

Aspiration cytology

Fine needle aspiration of breast lumps, with expert evaluation of the cytological appearances of the aspirated cells, has proved a sensitive and accurate method of pre-operative diagnosis. The cytological assessment includes details of nuclear size, shape and variation, chromatin pattern, nucleolar prominence, cytoplasmic outlines and staining and intercellular relationships.

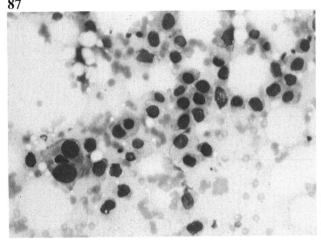

87 Aspirate from an invasive ductal breast carcinoma. Note the variation in cell size and shape, in nuclear size and outline and in chromatin staining.

359

Stewart–Treves syndrome

Oedema of the arm is a common sequel of the treatment of carcinoma of the breast whether by radical mastectomy with surgical clearance of axillary nodes or simple mastectomy and radiotherapy. The development of a lymphangiosarcoma in the grossly oedematous arm was first reported in 1948 by Stewart and Treves.

91

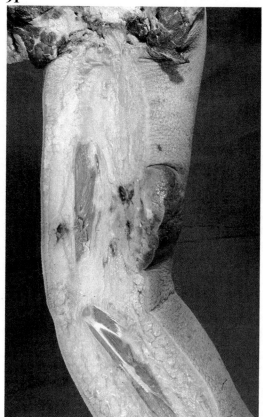

91 The patient, a housewife aged 55, was treated for an invasive ductal carcinoma of the left breast by a 'sub-radical mastectomy' and post-operative radiotherapy. Several axillary lymph nodes contained metastatic tumour. Severe lymphoedema developed 5 months after operation and persisted. 10 years later an angiomatous lesion developed in the left antecubital fossa. It grew rapidly and 6 months later formed an ulcerated haemorrhagic tumour measuring 14 × 9 cm surrounded by several purple-red nodules in the surrounding skin. After an unsuccessful search for metastases a forequarter amputation was performed. She died at home a year later with a pleural effusion and radiological evidence of solitary metastatic nodules in the skull and right lung.

Specimen. The illustration of part of the amputated arm shows the vascular tumour of the antecubital area.

GC 13475

Incidence and course of disease

The condition is rare and the tumour has been reported as developing at any time between 1 and 20 years after operation. It then grows rapidly and usually proves fatal within 2 years. It presents as a purple-red swelling generally on the medial aspect of the upper arm. The overlying skin is discoloured by ecchymosis resembling superficial bruising and tends to bleed easily.

Pathology

A highly vascular tumour with a uniform angiomatous pattern. There are numerous clefts lined with plump cuboidal endothelium and usually devoid of red blood cells. The superficial parts of the tumour are frequently less malignant in appearance than those more deeply sited. A meshwork of reticulin fibres is present. The tumour infiltrates diffusely and is multicentric in origin. Distal metastases are common in the lungs, pleura and abdominal viscera.

The tumour occurs only in oedematous limbs. Radiotherapy is significant probably only in that it may increase the incidence and severity of the post-operative oedema. The tumour may be simulated by metastasis of the breast carcinoma in an oedematous arm showing lymphatic distension and endothelial hyperplasia.

A tumour of similar character has been described in chronically oedematous lower limbs.

Histology

The histological illustrations are from another case, a woman who developed lymphoedema of the arm following mastectomy at the age of 57. Nine years later a tumour 11 cm in diameter had developed.

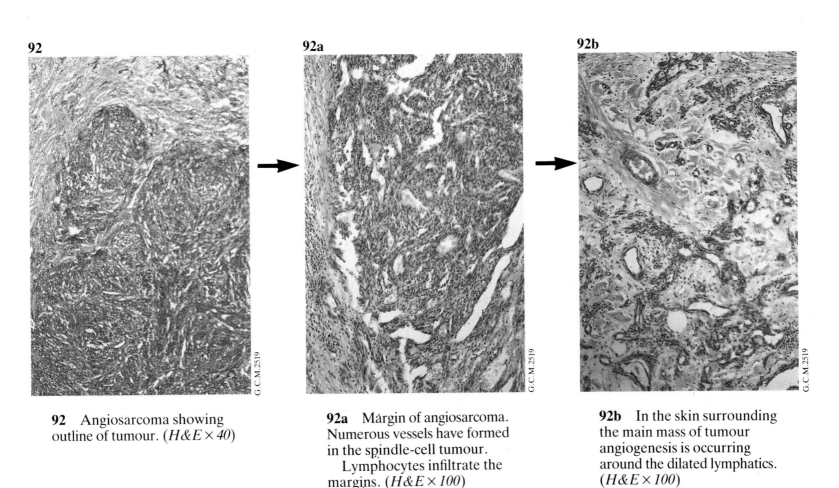

92 Angiosarcoma showing outline of tumour. (*H&E × 40*)

92a Margin of angiosarcoma. Numerous vessels have formed in the spindle-cell tumour.
Lymphocytes infiltrate the margins. (*H&E × 100*)

92b In the skin surrounding the main mass of tumour angiogenesis is occurring around the dilated lymphatics. (*H&E × 100*)

Other breast tumours

Both benign and malignant forms occur. All are rare.

Many types of skin appendage tumours may arise in the skin overlying the breast (see p. 396). The connective tissue of the breast, as elsewhere, may give rise to a number of simple tumours such as fibroma, lipoma and leiomyoma. In addition the breast is one of the sites of the rare Abrikossof tumour (granular cell myoblastoma) which also occurs in tongue (see p. 114), skin and vulva.

93

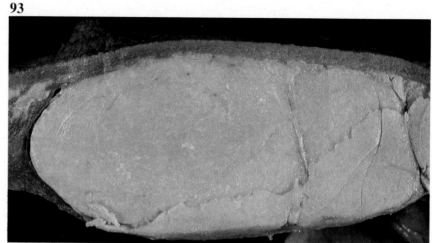

Lipoma

93 The ovoid lipoma present in this breast is composed of mature adipose tissue subdivided by fine fibrous septa. Two equally large lobulated lipomas (not shown) extended from it into the axilla.

Sarcoma

Osteoid and chondroid metaplasia may occur rarely in the stroma of breast carcinoma. There are, however, some breast malignancies which arise primarily from connective tissue. When both epithelial and mesenchymal elements are malignant, the term carcinosarcoma is used.

Carcinosarcoma

Well documented examples of these lesions are rare. The diagnosis implies malignancy in both stroma and epithelium. The stromal component may show differentiation to striated muscle, bone or cartilage. Some may arise in pre-existing fibroadenomas.

94

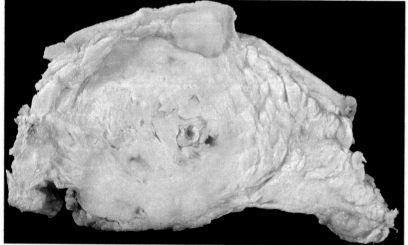

G.C.13678

94 Carcinosarcoma arising in a fibroadenoma.

Following an injury, a woman of 62 years had experienced some breast discomfort for 1 year before mastectomy. She was aware of a breast swelling for only 2–3 weeks.

The tumour measured 10cm in diameter. The cut surface is composed of firm grey tissue extending from skin to deep fascia. There are some small translucent areas. Larger yellow areas of necrosis are also present and some cavitation. There is a satellite nodule beneath the nipple.

Microscopically a spindle-cell sarcomatous component with foci of chondroid formation predominated. In one area trabeculae of unequivocal carcinoma cells were also present.

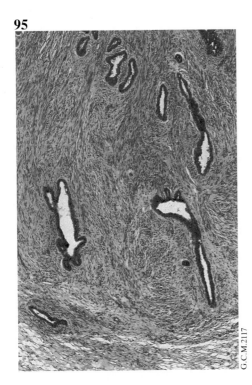

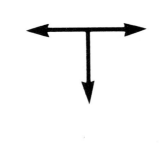

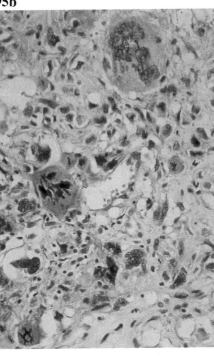

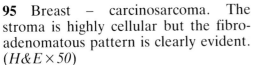

95 Breast – carcinosarcoma. The stroma is highly cellular but the fibro-adenomatous pattern is clearly evident. *(H&E × 50)*

95a Same case. Here both stromal and epithelial components have undergone malignant change. *(H&E × 100)*

95b Same case. In a further area the tumour is completely anaplastic. Numerous polyploid nuclei with abnormal mitoses are present. *(H&E × 250)*

Lesions which may be mistaken for true carcinosarcoma include:

1   The phyllodes tumour in which the epithelial element is not considered to be malignant.
2   A spindle-cell carcinoma in which recognisable epithelial differentiation may be scanty and spindle-shaped epithelial cells predominate. In such a case immunohistochemistry may help to demonstrate epithelial markers such as cytokeratin in the spindle cell epithelial components; and electron microscopy may demonstrate intercellular junctions and secretory features in the spindle epithelial cells and exclude any true mesenchymal differentiation.

Rarely chondrosarcomas, osteosarcomas, liposarcomas and angiosarcomas may arise as primary breast tumours. They metastasise by the blood stream, and angiosarcomas have a particularly bad prognosis.

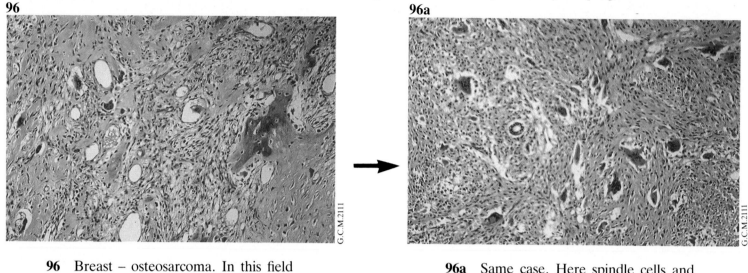

96 Breast – osteosarcoma. In this field osteoid and fibrous elements predominate. Focal calcification has occurred (right). (*H&E × 100*)

96a Same case. Here spindle cells and osteoclast-like cells are present. (*H&E × 100*)

Lymphoma of breast

While the breast may be involved by dissemination of malignant lymphoma, a primary presentation within breast parenchyma may rarely occur. Such lesions should be designated according to standard lymphoma classification. Thus the pattern, whether nodular (follicular) or diffuse, and the cell type (cell size, lymphocyte differentiation) must be evaluated. Most are of diffuse, follicle centre cell (centrocytic/centroblastic) B cell type.

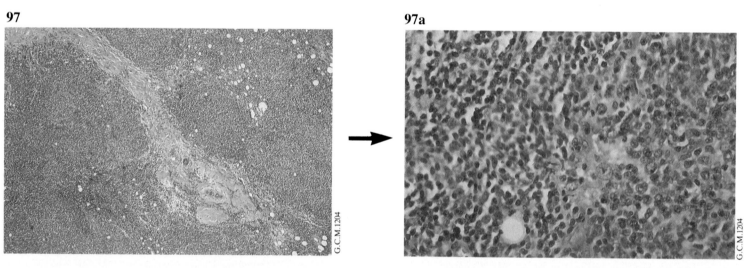

97 Breast – malignant lymphoma. The breast is widely invaded by a lymphoma that still shows some suggestion of a follicular pattern. (*H&E × 40*)

97a There is an admixture of small centrocytes and larger centroblasts. (*H&E × 400*)

Inflammatory lesions

Fat necrosis

This inflammatory reaction to degradation products of adipose tissue within the breast may give rise to a firm palpable lesion which may reach a large size, e.g. 6 cm. Up to one-third of patients may give a history of trauma. In other cases rupture of dilated ducts may be a contributory factor.

Microscopically fat necrosis is reflected by the presence of finely divided lipid within macrophages and sometimes by cholesterol crystals either extracellular or within the cytoplasm of giant cells, and by an admixture of chronic inflammatory cells and resultant fibrosis. With time, the digestion of the lipid may leave small cystic spaces surrounded by reactive macrophages, giant cells and fibrous tissue resulting in encysted fat necrosis.

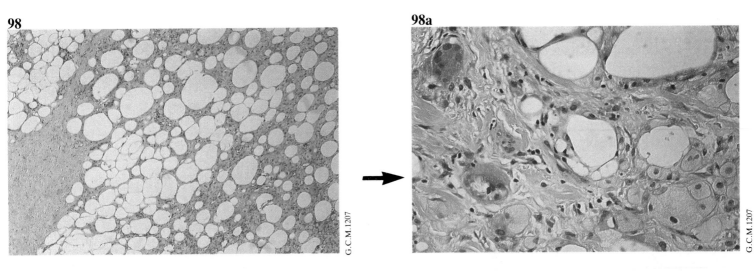

98 Breast – fat necrosis. Many of the fat cells have ruptured giving rise to microcysts. The stroma is thickened by chronic inflammation and fibrosis. (*H&E × 50*)

98a Breast – fat necrosis. Same case. Lipid-laden macrophages (foam cells) are present in the fibrous stroma, and foreign-body giant cells can also be seen. (*H&E × 250*)

Inflammatory lesions (*Continued*)

Galactocoele

Dilatation of a breast duct during lactation results from some relative obstruction; an aggravating factor may be the secretory content of the lactating duct. The resulting galactocoele may be large with a thin flattened epithelial lining and, depending on the presence and degree of escape of content, a periductal inflammatory and fibrotic reaction.

Pyogenic infection

Pyogenic infection of the breast occurs mainly in the puerperium and is related to nipple trauma and duct infection during suckling. The dilated, secretion-filled ducts are a favourable environment for multiplication of micro-organisms.

Streptococci and staphylococci are the main infecting agents and in the latter the infection is apt to result in abscess formation, often multiple. The abscesses tend to spread within the breast breaking down the interlobar septa in so doing.

The non-pregnant breast may also be the site of abscess formation which may follow the excoriation of an eczematous nipple.

In some cases an abscess develops beneath the areola and eventually discharges on the surface. The tract, lined by granulation tissue, may communicate with one of the lactiferous ducts giving rise to a *duct fistula*.

99

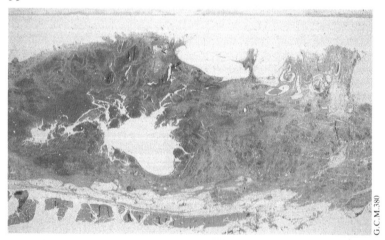

99a

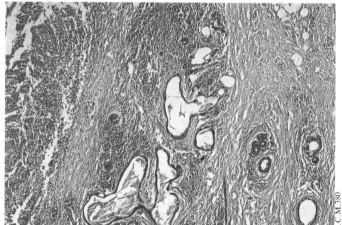

99 Breast abscess. A whole section of breast showing a breast abscess involving more than one lobe. There is a dense inflammatory infiltrate around it. (*H&E × 1*)

99a Breast abscess. A small part of the abscess (left) contains pus and necrotic debris. Outside its fibrous wall, chronic inflammatory cells infiltrate the breast tissue. (*H&E × 50*)

100

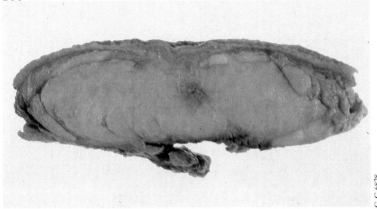

100 Breast – chronic abscess. Centrally in the breast there is a small chronic abscess surrounded by a thick wall of granulation and fibrous tissue. The nipple is retracted and there were two small sinuses, one on the areola and one just external to it. Microscopic examination showed non-specific inflammation.

Tuberculosis

Tuberculosis of the breast, always an uncommon lesion, is now rare in communities where tuberculosis in general has been brought under control. When it does occur it may be secondary to localised tuberculosis of underlying rib or pleura or may be part of more widespread disease. A tuberculous lesion of the breast presents as a firm mass which later caseates and breaks down into a tuberculous abscess leading to the formation of one or more sinuses. The microscopic features are similar to those of tuberculosis elsewhere.

101

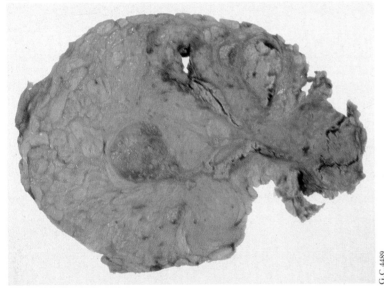

101 Breast – tuberculosis. There is considerable periductal fibrosis throughout. Deep in the breast there are substantial areas of caseation, a tuberculous breast abscess, and areas of fibrosis with tuberculous granulomas.

Other granulomas of the breast

Other granulomas of the breast may occur:

1 Sarcoidosis (rare).

2 A granulomatous mastitis may develop in which no causative organism is identified. It is presumably a response to secretory material from ruptured ducts and lobular units.

3 A rare cause of inflammation and necrosis in the breast is the ischaemic necrosis which follows arteritic occlusion. When the arteritis is of Wegener's type, the affected vessels exhibit a granulomatous inflammatory reaction in their wall.

U. Chetty

K.M. McLaren

Part IV – Skin

Burns and scalds are a form of trauma of importance because of the risk to life and the disfigurement which may follow. The subject is of special significance in that so often the victims are children. Burns and scalds must be considered from two aspects:

1 The local injury raises the problem of the physical damage to the tissues especially the skin and the resulting scarring, deformity and disfigurement.

2 The systemic effects of a burn vary according to the extent of the lesion and may cause death.

Heat damages tissues in proportion to the temperature and length of time of contact. Similar damage can be caused by corrosive chemicals or severe cold.

In the United Kingdom approximately 14000 cases of burns and scalds are admitted to hospital annually. The majority of admissions from home accidents are children under 4 years of age. Of the adults a large proportion have predisposing factors, e.g. alcohol, cerebrovascular insufficiency and epilepsy.

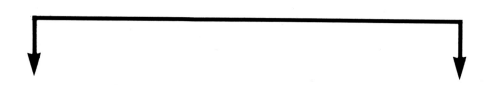

Analysis of burns cases by location of accident

Location of accident	Number	Percentage
Home	6790	48.9
Road	180	1.3
Other and Unspecified	6910	49.8
Total	13880	100.0

Analysis of burns in the home by age

Age (Years)	Total	Percentage
0–4	3510	52
5–14	880	13
15–24	360	5
25–44	660	9
45–64	590	9
65+	800	12
Total	6800	100

Source: Hospital In-patient Enquiry 1975

Local lesion

A burn damages or destroys the outer layers of cells, coagulating and disrupting them. Deeper tissues that are not completely destroyed are likewise damaged. In particular, capillary walls become permeable to protein molecules resulting in the loss of protein rich fluid from the circulation into the extracellular spaces. This gives rise to:

Oedema
Loss of circulating fluid volume

Relatively superficial burns disrupt the adhesion between epidermal cells allowing exudate to accumulate and split the epidermis just superficial to the basal layer thus forming blisters. These usually rupture.

Depth of burn

The depth of tissue damage determines how the burn will heal. Healing will occur from any epithelial cells of the basal layer which survive. Epithelial appendages (hair follicles, sebaceous glands, sweat ducts and glands) pass down into the dermis from the epidermis and may take part in the regenerative process of the epithelium.

1

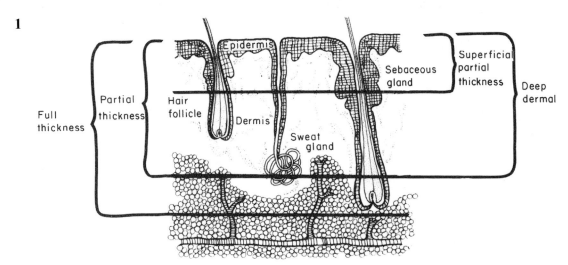

1 Burns may be *partial thickness* – where some dermis survives or *full thickness* where none survives. *Partial thickness* burns can be subdivided into *superficial* or *deep dermal* (deep partial thickness). They will heal from surviving epithelial elements.

Superficial burns

2

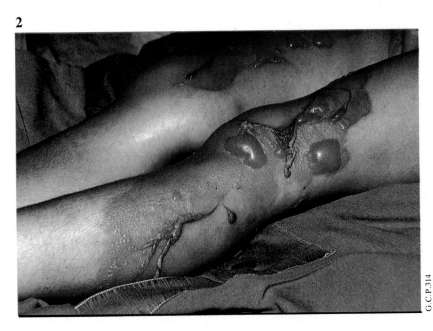

2 Superficial burn of leg. From a child aged 4 years scalded by boiling water.

Note the blisters, many of which are broken revealing a red raw weeping surface. This is very painful. It will heal without scarring in less than three weeks.

Deep dermal burns

Although some epithelial cells survive in the deepest layers of dermis, they are few and healing takes more than three weeks. Because only a little dermis survives, the quality of the healed skin is poor and hypertrophic scarring occurs.

3

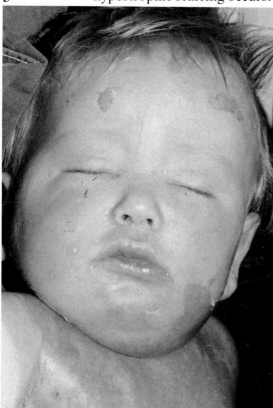

3a

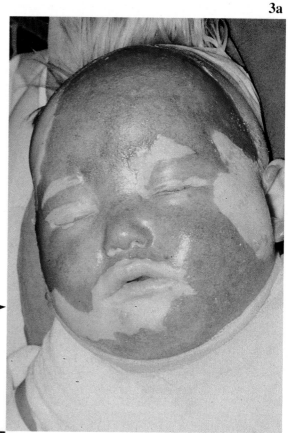

An 18-month-old boy with a scald of the face and chest caused by hot tea. The face is superficial and the chest deep dermal.

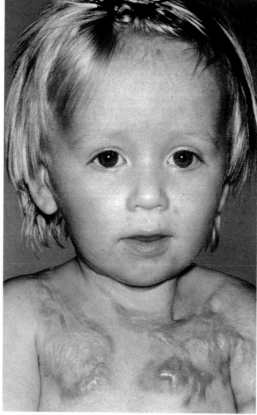

3   On admission – note early blistering of the face and mottled and pale areas on the chest.

3a   Face treated by exposure, crust formed. Note severe oedema. Chest dressed.

3b   Healed. No scarring on face. Note grafts on chest and hypertrophic scars where grafts failed.

G.C.P.315

Full thickness burns

Destruction of the whole depth of the skin results in a defect which can only heal from the edges by epithelialisation and contraction of the base. This results in unacceptable scarring and split skin grafting is required unless the burn is small.

4

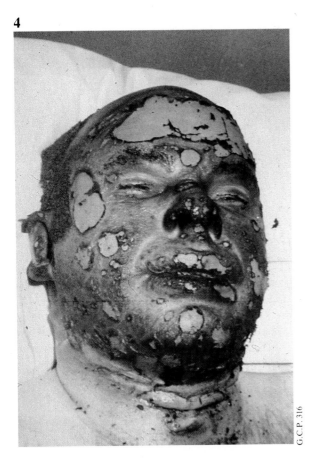

G.C.P. 316

4 Full thickness flame burns of head and face sustained in a house fire.

4a

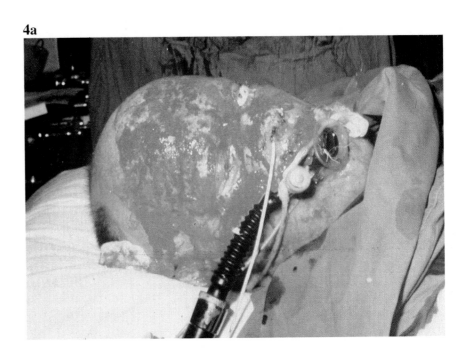

4a Same patient three weeks later after separation of eschar showing underlying granulations.

Grafting

Only autogenous grafts survive and require a vascular recipient bed to do so. Homografts and heterografts are ultimately rejected but during their period of survival can be useful as temporary biological dressings. The immune response is depressed after a big burn and rejection is therefore delayed.

Thin split skin grafts 'take' well on poor surfaces but are unstable and tend to shrink. Thick split skin grafts are stronger and shrink less but require a better recipient area. Medium thickness grafts are the most appropriate for covering burns.

Systemic effects

An immediate result of the injury is loss of protein rich fluid from the damaged capillaries causing oedema. There is also a copious loss from the raw surface. This dual loss leads to a fall in the blood volume which can be fatal. If the burn is large it will lead to the clinical manifestations of shock. The critical size is about 15% of the body surface area in adults but children will become shocked with burns of 10% or even less.

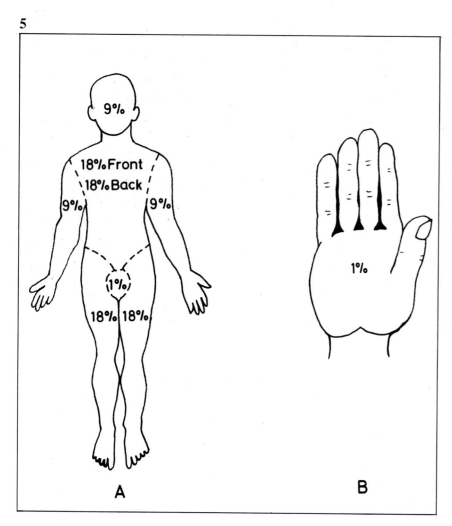

5

5 When a patient is admitted to hospital an assessment must be made both of the outlook and the corresponding appropriate treatment. The area of the involved skin must be assessed as a percentage and recorded. For an approximate calculation of the percentage of surface burned the 'rule of 9's' introduced by A. B. Wallace can be useful in the adult.

The volar surface of the patient's hand with fingers closed is approximately 1%.

A more detailed chart is used in children and for a more accurate assessment in adults (*see* page opposite).

The loss of plasma-like fluid from the circulation is greatest immediately after the burn and decreases as the damaged capillaries recover.

The oligaemia which is a major factor in the production of shock is associated with haemoconcentration and a raised haematocrit – often over 50%. This results in an increased blood vicosity and poor perfusion of the tissues.

6

NAME .... WARD .... UNIT NUMBER .... DATE ....

AGE ....

░░░	Superficial
▨	Deep

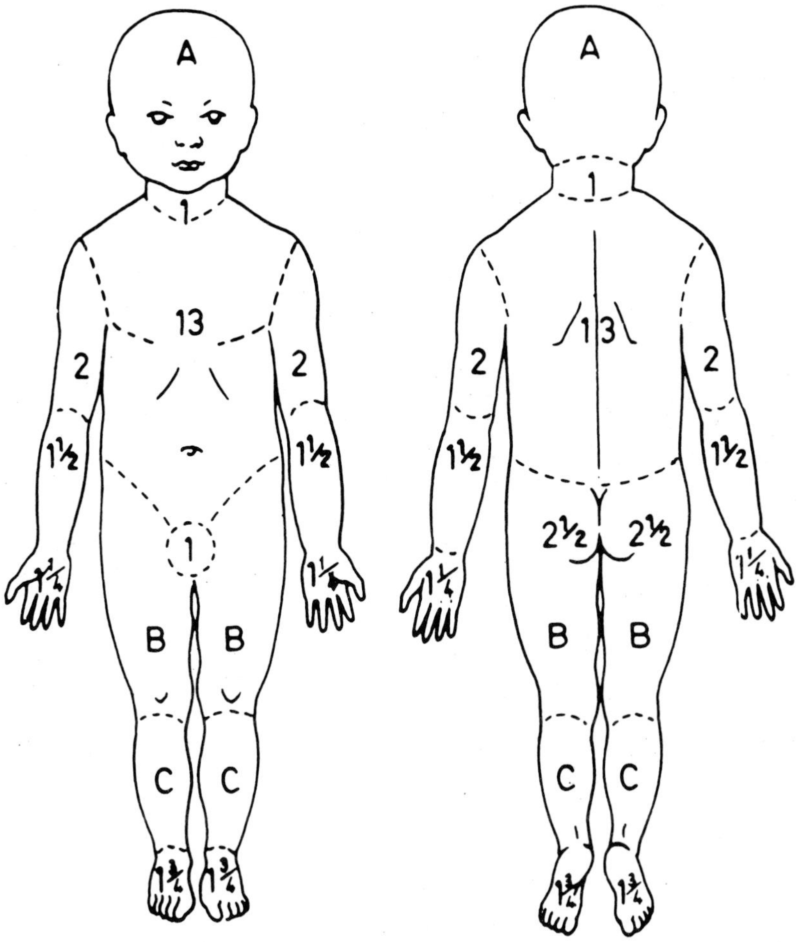

REGION	%
HEAD	
NECK	
ANT. TRUNK	
POST TRUNK	
RIGHT ARM	
LEFT ARM	
BUTTOCKS	
GENITALIA	
RIGHT LEG	
LEFT LEG	
TOTAL BURN	

RELATIVE PERCENTAGES AFFECTED BY GROWTH

AREA	AGE 0	1	5	10	15	ADULT
A = ½ OF HEAD	9½	8½	6½	5½	4½	3½
B = ½ OF ONE THIGH	2¾	3¼	4	4½	4½	4¾
C = ½ OF ONE LEG	2½	2½	2¾	3	3¼	3½

6   After Lund and Browder.

Systemic effects *(Continued)*

Oedema

In small injuries the oedema is restricted to the area of injury; in large burns it is found also outwith the burned area. The oedema may persist after the period of maximal loss because:

1 There is a mild increase in capillary permeability for 2–3 weeks and therefore continuing loss from the intravascular compartment.
2 The leaked plasma proteins from the intravascular to the extravascular space exert an osmotic effect binding the oedema.
3 The protein coagulum in the extravascular space can block lymphatic channels.

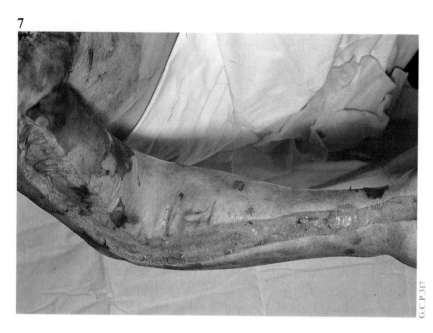

7

7 Oedema deep to a constricting circumferential deep burn can lead to compression of limb blood vessels and ischaemia or restriction of respiratory movements. This illustration shows a release incision in such a burn of the arm. Note how widely the incision is gaping.

Blood changes

Full thickness burns destroy many red cells which leads to haemoglobinaemia and anaemia.

1 RBCs have reduced life span as well as immediate destruction from heat. This can be as much as 30% of normal and is considered to be due to circulating plasma factors. Experimentally:

   RBCs from burn → injected into unburned → normal lifespan
   RBCs from unburned → injected into burned → reduced lifespan

2 Increased viscosity.

3 Early thrombocytopaenia followed by slow rise sometimes to above normal levels.

4 Fall in fibrinogen with increase in fibrin split products.

Cardiac function

There is an immediate drop in cardiac output which precedes any measured decrease in functional blood volume and has returned to normal long before functional blood volume is restored.

This also is thought to be caused by 'circulating plasma factors' but they are probably only significant in more extensive injury.

These features have been demonstrated experimentally in animals.

Renal function

The three most important factors requiring urgent treatment are as follows.

1   Diminished renal plasma flow.

2   Depressed glomerular filtration. Release of renin and angiotensin into circulation. This leads to oliguria (sometimes high output failure).
Note: early increase in antidiuretic hormone ensures urinary output stays low even if resuscitation is adequate.

3   The free haemoglobin pigment excreted in the urine following a large full thickness burn may obstruct the renal tubules.

8

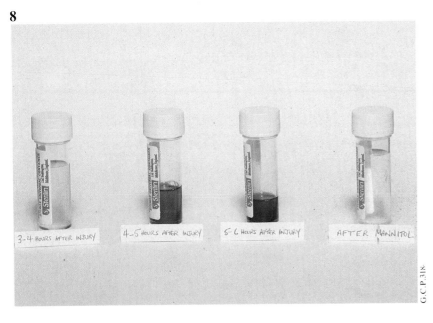

8   Four specimens of urine from a patient with extensive deep burns illustrating increasing haemoglobinuria which is associated with decreasing urine volume. The last specimen is after the administration of 20% mannitol which causes a diuresis and has cleared the urine.

Acute renal failure

These factors can produce acute renal failure characterised by a falling urine output in spite of restoration of circulating fluid volume, and a rising blood urea. This is a common cause of death when resuscitation of a burned patient is delayed.

Systemic effects *(Continued)*

Liver function

There is elevation of aspartate transaminase, alanine transaminase and alkaline phosphatase within 2–3 days of injury, but they remain high for several weeks in the major injury. The aetiology is thought to be inadequate perfusion in the early post burn phase.

Lung function

In the absence of inhalational injury there is little change in lung function apart from some increase in oxygen intake.

Metabolic changes

Nitrogen balance

In a major injury there is a period of prolonged negative nitrogen balance even in the face of increased protein intake. The nitrogen lost in the exudate from the burn wound makes a considerable contribution to overall loss. This loss will increase with infection of the surface.

There is a rapid and persistent drop in plasma proteins to about 40g/L, the drop being due to low albumin levels with a reversed albumin/globulin ratio and often persists until the wound is closed.

Potassium balance

Potassium balance follows the nitrogen balance closely. Again the surface loss is of importance.

Sodium balance

Initially the balance will be strongly positive due to the large volumes of sodium containing fluid required for resuscitation. This large load is only slowly released over the first 7–10 days following injury. Because of the changes in the intravascular and extravascular compartments this sodium retention is not reflected in the serum sodium level which is often lower than normal during this adjustment phase. Later because of the large surface losses the balance may become negative if intake is inadequate to correct the loss.

Water

Initially there is water retention, a diuresis usually being seen around the 4–5th post burn day.

There is an early loss of water in the plasma exudate which will be reduced as a surface coagulum forms. In the partial thickness burn the loss will be controlled in this way. In the full thickness injury the losses will be small initially but as the eschar develops there is a marked increase. Some reduction may follow as the eschar softens and separates, followed by a rise as granulation tissue develops. The losses can be in the order of 6–8 litres/day. Vapour pressure measurements confirm these losses, the pressure in the full thickness injury being about 32mm Hg compared to 2–3mm Hg in normal skin.

Metabolism – body weight

The metabolic rate increases as the extent of the injury increases until in the major injury the level may be 100% above normal or more. The cause for this is not completely understood and is not apparently related to increase in thyroid function. It may be related to increased catecholamine release from the sympathetic system and adrenal medulla. In addition there may be a change in central temperature regulation, burn patients showing temperature elevation not necessarily related to infection. The increased water loss from the surface may result in surface cooling and then stimulate heat production to maintain body temperature. The skin itself is a major thermal regulating organ which can no longer assume this role in the major injury. These subjects cannot vasoconstrict, insulate or regulate heat transfer from body core to surface.

It is considered that evaporative loss is not the main factor in the increased metabolic rate but that increased energy production is related to changes in metabolic activity at higher body temperature. Whatever the cause the caloric demand to meet the need is very high. 5,000 to 7,000K calories being recommended in patients with extensive injury.

Within the first week following injury and resuscitation there is an increase in weight due to oedema. Rapid loss follows of between 10–20% of preburn weight despite high levels of intake, levelling off at the end of the negative nitrogen balance phase (the catabolic phase) and slowly rising as skin cover is achieved (the anabolic phase).

Infection

The large unhealed raw area of a burn wound very readily becomes infected with all the attendant dangers both local and systemic. Burned skin is sterilised by the heat but bacteria may invade the dead tissue from the patient's surrounding skin, bowel, upper respiratory tract or by contamination from external sources.

Effects of infection on the burn wound

Delay in epithelialisation.
Tissue destruction, increasing the depth of injury.

Systemic effects if the burn is large

Suppression of bone marrow function.
Bacteraemia leading to metastatic infection – lungs, kidneys etc.
Septicaemia.
Many of the complications may be fatal.

Prevention of infection is one of the greatest priorities in treating the burn wound.

Scar formation

Disfigurement and deformity represent the late result of burns and scalds. Disfigurement may result from the nature of the epithelial healing when the scarred area is covered by a thin skin with varied colour and texture. The cause of deformity is excessive subepithelial fibrosis which progressively contracts over a period of weeks or months and is particularly important around the face and mouth. The degree of subepithelial scar formation is enhanced where there has been prolonged infection.

Occasionally a very late complication of burn is the development of squamous epithelioma in the scar. This is not infrequently seen in northern India as the result of a kangri burn (*see* p. 390).

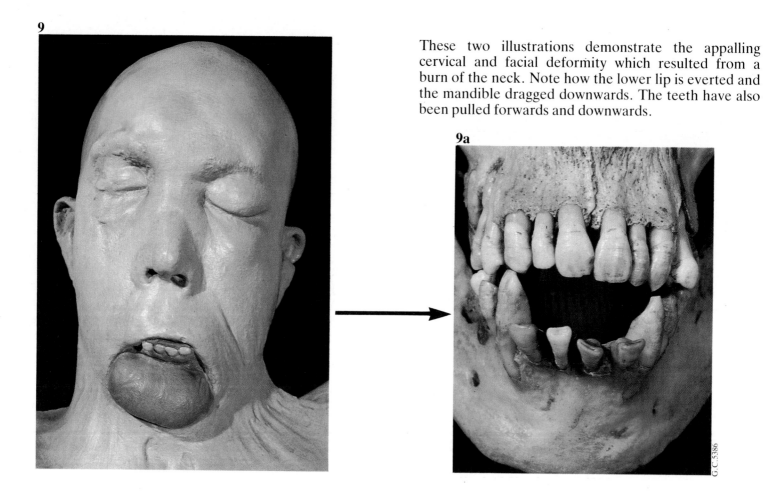

9

These two illustrations demonstrate the appalling cervical and facial deformity which resulted from a burn of the neck. Note how the lower lip is everted and the mandible dragged downwards. The teeth have also been pulled forwards and downwards.

9a

There is an interesting historical note regarding this case. The specimens were obtained from a man who died during the cholera epidemic in Edinburgh in 1834. The accident from which the deformity arose had occurred in childhood long before the age of plastic surgery. He was associated with the nefarious trade of providing corpses for the old anatomy schools which flourished at the beginning of the 19th century in Edinburgh.

Contracture of the limbs results especially where the flexor aspect is the site of scarring. This is most frequently seen in relation to the elbow and knee. It is also serious functionally where it involves the hands and fingers.

10

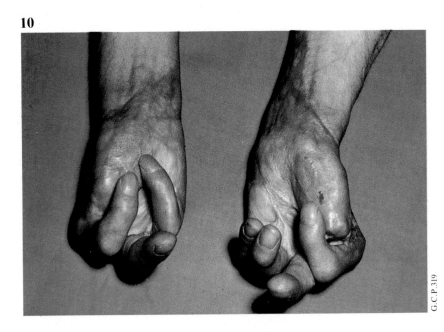

G.C.P.319

10 A case demonstrating the crippling deformities caused by severe burns to the hands.

Mortality

11

11 Burns and scalds are attended by a significant mortality which varies according to the age of the patient and the size of the burn as is illustrated in the chart. Accordingly, while more children are admitted to hospital for burns their mortality is much lower than that which occurs in the aged and senile patient. (From Muir and Barclay.)

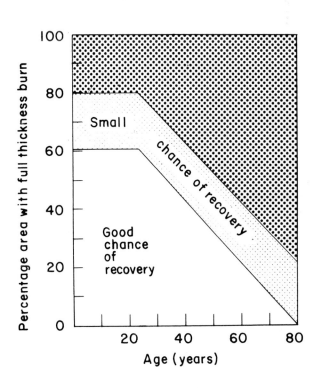

Anne B. Sutherland

A. C. H. Watson

Epidermal tumours

Viral wart

Common warts or verrucae are of viral aetiology. Though often found in childhood, they may occur at any age. These papillomatous, hyperkeratotic lesions are often multiple. Variants include the flat-topped plane wart, the often deeply invaginated plantar wart and the exuberant, papillomatous warts of the vulva, penis and peri-anal regions, the condylomata acuminata.

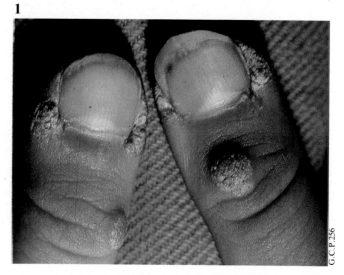

1 Multiple viral warts on fingers.

Histology

The viral wart comprises fronds of squamous epithelium growing in a papillomatous pattern with pronounced surface hyperkeratosis. Cells of the stratum granulosum and upper spinosum are vacuolated, a reflection of cellular damage induced by the human papilloma virus (HPV) which is intranuclear in site. Techniques of DNA analysis have revealed the existence of several subgroups of the virus, some of which, e.g. HPV-2 are more often associated with the common wart of skin. The viral wart is a benign lesion without malignant potential. Exceptionally, viral warts of the condyloma variety may show local invasion when the patient is subject to immune suppression.

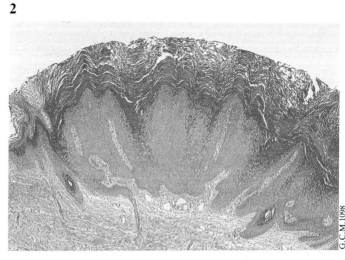

2 Viral wart (verruca vulgaris) showing papillomatous fronds of epidermis with marked hyperkeratosis. *(H&E ×40)*

3

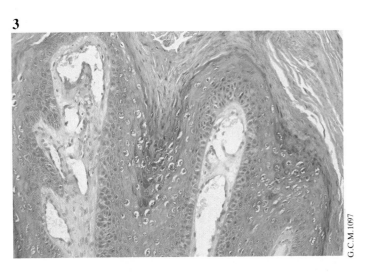

G.C.M.1097

3 Cell vacuolation in the granular layer reflects viral damage. Note the prominent vascular channels in the dermis. *(H&E ×125)*

4

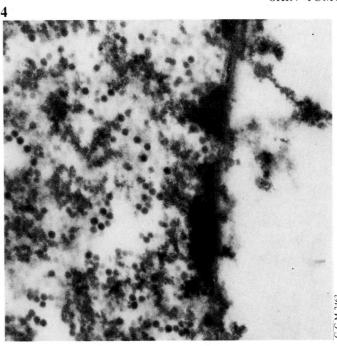

G.C.M.2463

4 Electron micrograph of human papilloma virus within the nucleus of the infected cells of a viral wart. Lead citrate and uranyl acetate × 37 500.

Squamous papilloma

Simple squamous papillomas occur which lack proof of a viral aetiology. Some may be hamartomatous in nature, e.g. epidermal naevi. The hyperkeratosis in basal cell papillomas may be very great and mimic squamous papillomas clinically.

5

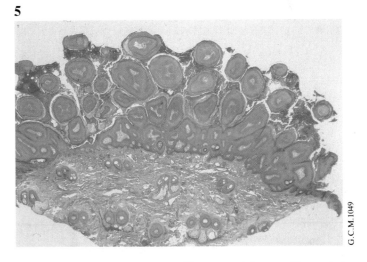

G.C.M.1049

5 Simple squamous papilloma with papillomatous fronds of squamous epithelium. In this case evidence of a viral aetiology is lacking. *(H&E ×15)*

Epidermal tumours (Continued)

Seborrhoeic keratosis

This common lesion comprises a focal benign proliferation of basal epidermal cells. Other names applied to this lesion include:

    basal cell papilloma
    seborrhoeic wart
    verruca senilis.

Typically a basal cell papilloma appears as an elevated waxy, hyperkeratotic and often papilliferous, fissured lesion and is variably pigmented. With the help of a lens, discrete milky dots (horn cysts) may be seen on or just under the surface. Although normally rough they may be smooth in areas subjected to friction (e.g. skin folds). Multiple lesions are often found on the back and chest and are common in older people. The lesions vary in colour from brown to black depending on the melanin content and changes in the surface keratin. Their dark colour and occasional traumatic inflammation and ulceration may mimic malignant melanoma, excision biopsy being required for diagnosis.

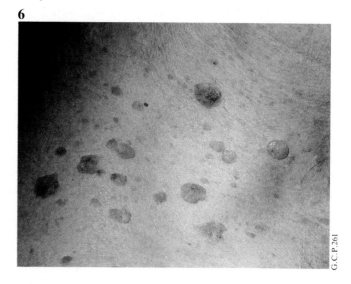

6   Multiple basal cell papilloma. Note the surface fissuring and pigmentation.

Histology

The histological picture shows a 'stuck on' appearance, the lesion being elevated above the surrounding epidermis, and comprising proliferating basal cells with associated keratin formation, often in the form of horn cysts. The constituent cells contain variable amounts of melanin. These tumours are benign without malignant potential.

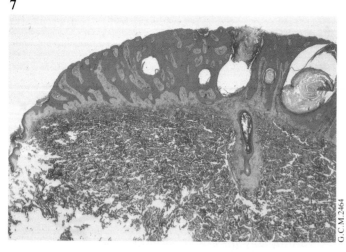

7   Basal cell papilloma. Note the elevated, 'stuck-on' appearance. The lesion lies above the general level of the surrounding epidermis and comprises proliferating basal cells showing abrupt keratin formation in horn cysts. (H&E ×20)

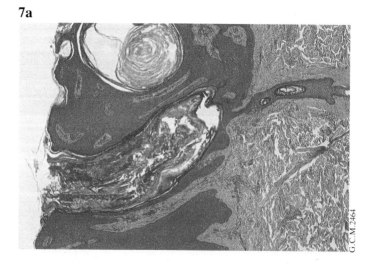

7a   Basal cell papilloma showing horn cysts enclosed by proliferating basal cells of uniform appearance. (H&E ×40)

Keratoacanthoma

This interesting lesion occurs most often on exposed areas and appears as a nodular dome-shaped tumour which grows rapidly to reach a maximum size in 6–8 weeks and thereafter regresses spontaneously in a variable time. The aetiology of these lesions is unknown but animal experiments would indicate that their usual origin is from the hair follicle.

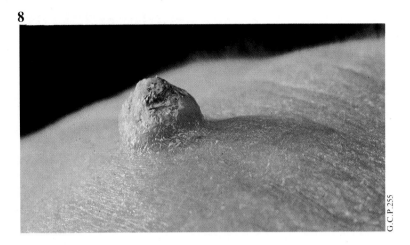

8 Keratoacanthoma with its epidermal shoulders and central plug of keratin.

Histology

The lesion is typically symmetrical and comprises proliferating fronds of epidermis which may penetrate to the level of the sweat glands and which exhibit mitotic activity but retain a well differentiated squamous appearance with much glassy keratin production. The centre of the cup-shaped mass is filled with keratin and at its margins it is delineated by a thinned shoulder of adjacent normal epidermis. Despite the deep penetration of islands of cells showing variable mitotic activity, regression is predictable and involves an associated and possibly destructive acute and chronic inflammatory cell infiltration of the lesion. It has many clinical and pathological features suggestive of malignancy but usually follows a benign course. Histological distinction from a squamous cell carcinoma is not possible unless the pathologist can assess the complete architecture of the tumour. Excision biopsy is therefore required for accurate diagnosis.

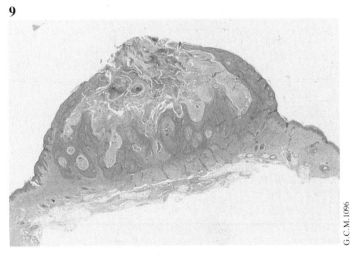

9 The symmetry of a keratoacanthoma is obvious. Elevated shoulders of epidermis delineate the central crater of keratin. *(H&E ×2.5)*

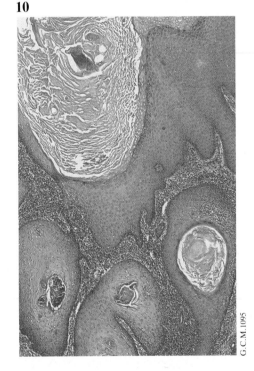

10 The proliferating squamous epithelium of the keratoacanthoma may penetrate to deep dermis. An associated inflammatory infiltrate is common. *(H&E ×40)*

385

Epidermal tumours *(Continued)*

Bowen's disease

This lesion, an intraepidermal squamous carcinoma, has a longer natural history than has a squamous carcinoma developing in a senile keratosis. Thus it remains as an *in situ* carcinoma for a long period.

The same aetiological factors as are cited for squamous carcinoma also operate here though the more frequent development on the trunk or limbs may indicate that ultra-violet light exposure is less important. The development of multiple foci of intraepidermal carcinomas may reflect the presence of visceral malignancy, often gastro-intestinal.

11

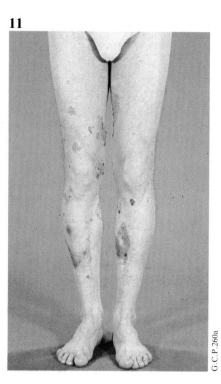

11 Bowen's disease. Multiple scaly patches are present on the legs.

Clinically, the lesion is often found on lower limbs or trunk and appears as an erythematous well-circumscribed scaly patch, which may mimic discoid eczema or psoriasis.

11a

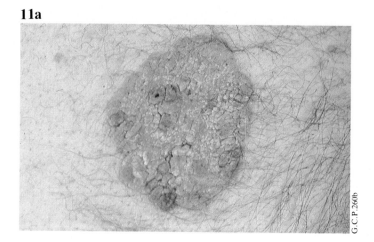

11a A patch of Bowen's disease is elevated, scaly and variably pigmented.

Senile or actinic keratosis

The common mixed hyperplastic and atrophic lesion found on the skin of elderly Caucasians, senile keratosis, is histologically and probably pathogenetically similar to the actinic or solar keratosis induced by chronic sun exposure. Its importance lies in its possible transition to invasive squamous carcinoma.

Clinically the lesions are pink, discrete, irregularly shaped with a warty surface. They may be felt more easily than seen and vary from 0.5 to 2cm in diameter. They occur most commonly on exposed areas especially on the backs of the hands (**16**) and on the bald scalp.

The histology of senile or actinic keratosis is variable but essentially exhibits alternating zones of hyper- and parakeratosis overlying an epidermis which may show both acanthosis and atrophy. An increase in basal melanin pigment is common. There is often a chronic inflammatory infiltrate at the dermal-epidermal junction and the dermal collagen may be degenerate and eosinophilic in staining (senile or solar elastosis). The epidermis may show variable aberration with occasional pleomorphic cells and a loss of the normal maturation pattern. These changes may be minor but on occasion the degree of dysplasia is sufficient to warrant the term 'intraepidermal carcinoma'. At this stage the lesion has the capacity for dermal invasion. Thus squamous cell carcinoma may arise in a senile keratosis.

Histology

The picture is that of an acanthotic and dysplastic epidermis showing lack of normal cell maturation, variable basal budding and surface hyperkeratosis. Individual cells are often large and pleomorphic exhibiting abnormal mitoses and frequently showing single cell keratinisation or dyskeratosis. A chronic inflammatory infiltrate is often seen at the dermo-epidermal junction, which is preserved.

12

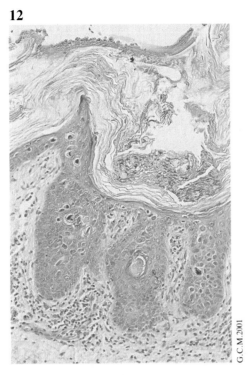

13

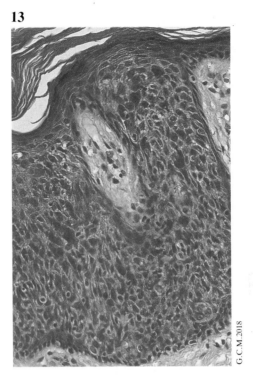

12 Bowen's disease showing acanthosis and hyper-keratosis with cellular atypia. A subjacent chronic inflammatory infiltrate is present. *(H&E ×40)*

13 At higher magnification the cellular pleomorphism and loss of normal maturation is seen. The appearances reflect intraepidermal carcinoma. *(H&E ×250)*

14 In this example the epidermis exhibits dysplasia with budding of the basal layer and nuclear pleomorphism. Such features reflect the biological potential for development of squamous carcinoma and are of practical importance in the management of such patients since early removal should prevent the development of malignancy. Note the marked elastosis – a fragmentation and homogenization of collagen fibres – in the dermis and the chronic inflammatory infiltrate. *(×64)*

14

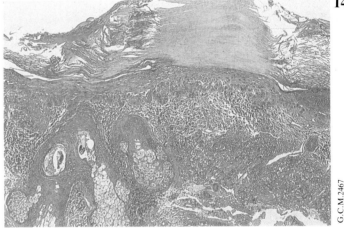

Epidermal tumours (Continued)

Squamous cell carcinoma

Aetiology

Certain rare genetic disorders involving impairment of DNA repair mechanisms, such as xeroderma pigmentosum, illustrate the importance of DNA alteration in the pathogenesis of malignancy. These concepts have been expanded by recent work concerning the integration of viral DNA within epidermal cells by the human papilloma virus (HPV). The common skin lesion caused by this agent, the viral wart or verruca, is not regarded as a pre-malignant lesion. However, under certain modifying circumstances (e.g. immunosuppression and in rare skin disorders such as epidermo-dysplasia verruciformis), specific subgroups of the HPV may play a part in the development of some squamous carcinomas. The search for viral DNA sequences in many malignancies including those of skin may show that the virus is a pathogenetic agent where, up to now, conventional signs of viral presence and infectivity have been lacking. It is possible that the synergistic operation of two or more factors is needed, e.g. viral infectivity, ultra-violet light exposure and immuno-suppression. The concept of two factors acting as initiator and promoter is also well illustrated in the chronic trauma with concomitant carcinogenic exposure that predisposes the pipe smoker to squamous carcinoma of the lip.

This malignant tumour most commonly arises in a pre-existing senile keratosis, usually in elderly individuals. Thus the assessment of cellular aberrance or dysplasia in a senile keratosis is an important predictor of malignant potential. When the lesion arises as Bowen's disease it remains *in situ* for a long period of time but many eventually infiltrate and metastasise.

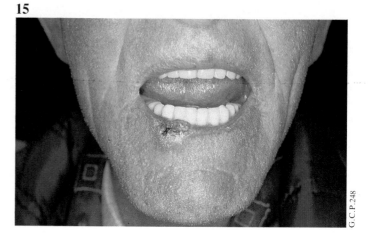

15 The classic clinical appearance is of an ulcerated hyperkeratotic nodule with an indurated base.

It is clear that cultural, social and occupational factors may determine the relative importance of specific aetiological factors but, as our knowledge of carcinogenic mechanisms increases, so hopefully the incidence of exposure to such risk factors will decrease.

Many of the best described factors are nowadays of greater historical than practical interest. A number of these are illustrated on the following pages.

Carcinogenic hydrocarbons

16

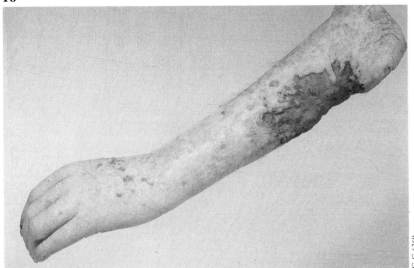

16 An ulcerated squamous carcinoma on the arm of a worker in the bituminous shale industry. Note the presence of multiple keratoses.

17

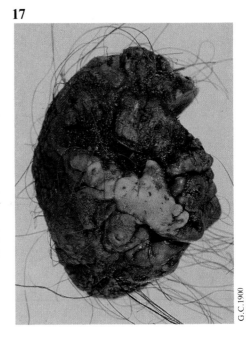

The development of carcinoma of scrotal skin in chimney sweeps following close and constant soot exposure with inadequate hygiene, described by Pott in the eighteenth century, remains a classic early description of carcinogenic action.

17 Squamous carcinoma, pale and hyperkeratotic in contrast to the skin on the scrotum of a chimney sweep.

Irradiation

18

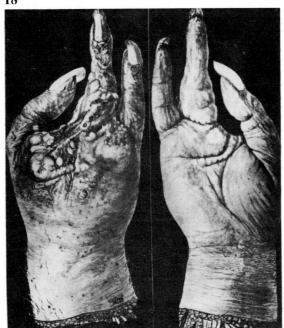

18 Multiple areas of squamous cell carcinoma in the skin of a radiologist's hand following repeated incidental exposure to x-irradiation before the risks involved and the requirement for protection were appreciated.

Epidermal tumours *(Continued)*

Thermal injury

19

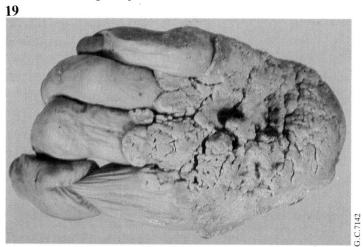

19 Squamous carcinoma developing after extensive burns to the hand.

20

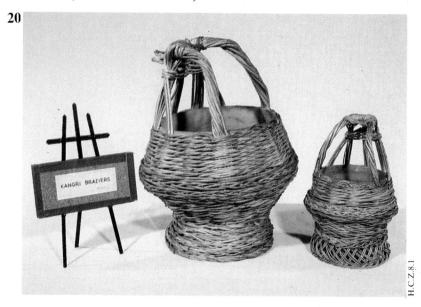

20 Thermal injury operates in the development of squamous carcinoma of the abdominal wall in northern Indians who practise warming of the body by the wearing of kangri baskets containing hot charcoal next to the skin.

Persistent ulceration

21

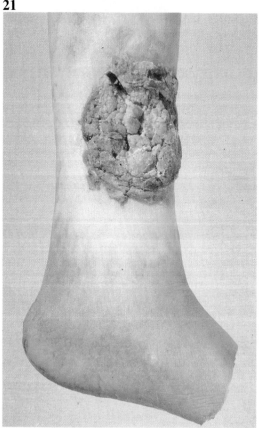

Chronic ulceration has phases of tissue destruction and of healing. This latter phase is associated with proliferation of the epithelium and in prolonged ulceration neoplastic change may occur.

22

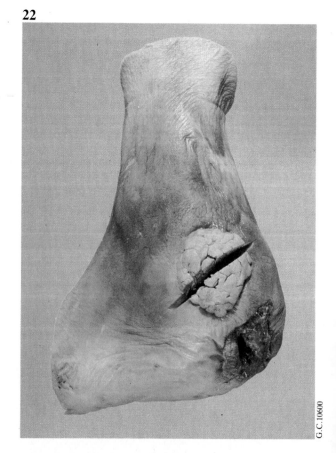

21 A large, ulcerating squamous carcinoma at the site of chronic varicose ulceration.

22 The hyperkeratotic and invasive squamous carcinoma complicated persistent osteomyelitis of the oscalcis which followed a shark bite.

23

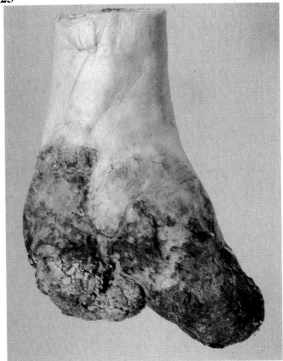

The early lesions present as a persistent ulceration but for diagnosis biopsy is necessary. In the photographs of the classical and more advanced lesions already illustrated the persistent large ulcer with protruding edges and exposure of the underlying tissues may be seen. These are the essential features of a malignant ulceration.

23 An extensive squamous carcinoma has developed at the site of long-standing tuberculosis of the foot.

Histology

The histological appearances vary greatly but when arising in a senile keratosis, show irregular strands of infiltrating squamous carcinoma of variable differentiation usually retaining the capacity for keratin production. The granular layer in the infiltrating areas is often lost. The invasive process usually results in an associated inflammatory cell reaction. The tumour cells may lack cohesion and this cell separation may result in clefts occurring in the infiltrating strands.

24

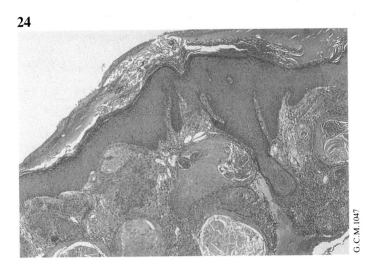

25

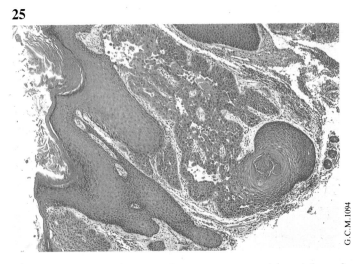

24 A moderately well-differentiated squamous carcinoma undermines a variably thickened epidermis. (*H&E ×40*)

25 Infiltrating strands of squamous carcinoma invade the dermis. (*H&E ×50*)

Spread

These tumours if neglected spread both locally and to lymphatics.

Epidermal tumours (Continued)

Basal cell carcinoma

This is the commonest malignant neoplasm of skin, and is rare under the age of 40. It is most often located on the head and neck. The clinical appearance generally reflects the different histopathological growth patterns. It usually presents as a slowly expanding ulcer with a pearly edge ('Rodent Ulcer'). Nodulo-ulcerative, cystic, cicatricial (morphoeic), superficial (multicentric) and pigmented types are recognised.

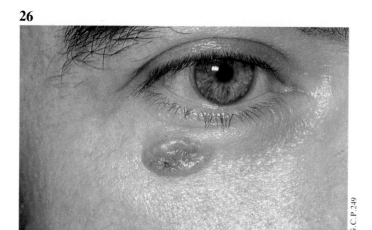

26 A typical basal cell carcinoma with a pearly, rolled edge and central ulceration.

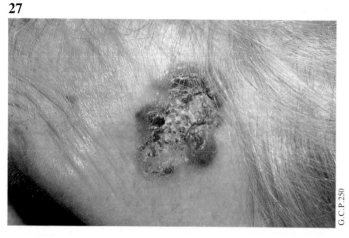

27 This basal cell carcinoma shows irregular pigmentation and focal ulceration.

Aetiology

Aetiological factors are principally those of cumulative ultra-violet light exposure, perhaps coupled with innate ageing, and the factors previously described 'as of importance in the development of squamous carcinomas, e.g. occurrence in scars and previous arsenical ingestion. The rare, autosomal dominantly inherited, basal cell naevus syndrome is associated with numerous basal cell carcinomas developing at an early age with associated abnormalities of the ecto-skeleton, eyes and reproductive system. Patients with xeroderma pigmentosum are also at increased risk for basal cell carcinoma development. Basal cell carcinoma may occur in association with hamartomatous lesions arising from epidermis and glandular tissue.

Pathology

The malignancy of the lesion is expressed by local invasion. Despite this infiltrative capacity metastases are rare, though without adequate treatment considerable local tissue destruction may occur.

In the nodulo-ulcerative variety the small darkly-staining basal cells arise from the overlying epidermis and associated hair follicles often in a multifocal manner, and grow in well-defined aggregates in the dermis. The delineation is accentuated by peripheral aligning or palisading of the outer layer of cells. Numerous mitoses and associated individual cell death are seen. In the cicatricial (morphoeic) type the cellular tumour islands appear entrapped and squeezed by dense fibroblastic tissue.

Histology

Basal cell carcinomas exhibit variable growth patterns, often showing differentiation towards hair follicles, sebaceous units, sweat gland structures etc. Basal cell carcinomas of skin appendage type may show a slower growth potential but are nevertheless best regarded as lesions with local infiltrative capacity. In basal cell carcinomas, where the rate of cell proliferation and cell death is high, the stroma-tumour interaction is probably of importance in determining the growth pattern.

28

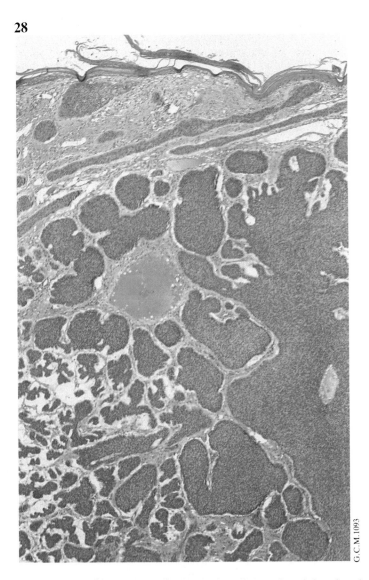

29

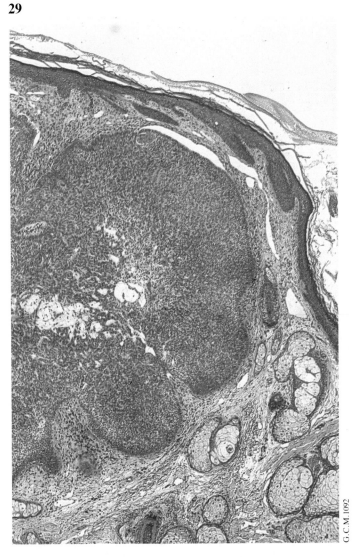

28   A nodular basal cell carcinoma showing islands of neoplastic basal cells growing in well-defined nests. *(H&E × 60)*

29   Basal cell papilloma. The peripheral palisading of basal cells is well illustrated; centrally these islands may undergo cystic degeneration. *(H&E × 60)*

Epidermal tumours *(Continued)*

Epidermoid and pilar (sebaceous) cysts

The term 'sebaceous cyst' is applied to a wide variety of cystic and non-cystic epidermal lesions. Most of these cystic lesions are of follicular origin.

'Sebaceous cysts' contain degenerate, cellular material, not sebum. When the cysts are incised the keratin content of the epidermoid variety is generally soft and compressible whereas that of the pilar cyst is hard.

Histology

The classification of these cysts is based on the character of the lining epithelium. Histologically, epidermoid cysts exhibit a true squamous epithelial lining, the cells of which show intercellular bridges and maturation through a keratohyaline granular layer to laminated keratin formation. The pilar cyst has a lining whose cells exhibit peripheral palisading, lack obvious intercellular bridges and show a gradual homogenization and fusion of cells as they merge with the amorphous and eosinophilic intracystic or luminal content. In both instances previous cyst rupture may excite a foreign body giant cell reaction with associated scarring in the surrounding dermis.

Pathology

Both epidermoid and pilar cysts present as firm, slowly growing, dermal or subcutaneous nodules which may have a surface punctum and may be multiple. Most are epidermoid, but pilar cysts are the commonest type found on the scalp.

31

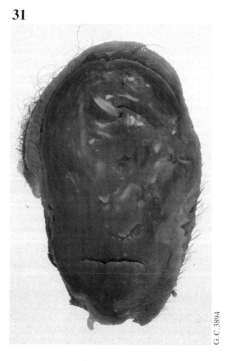

30

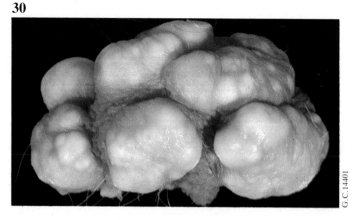

30 Multiple cysts of follicular origin on the scrotum. Histological examination is required in order to classify these.

31 This pilar (sebaceous) cyst of scalp is filled with inspissated, lipid-rich material.

Histology

32

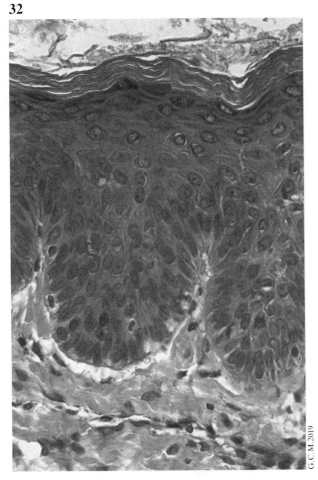

33

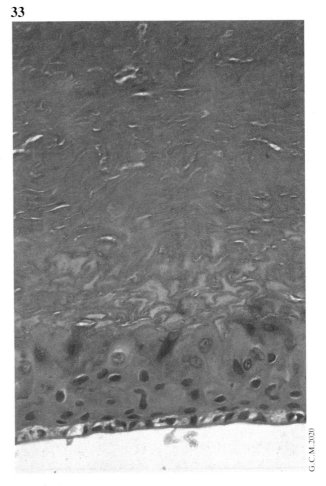

32 In this epidermoid cyst, the wall comprises maturing squamous epithelium with keratinisation (top of picture). *(H&E × 416)*

33 This pilar cyst shows a gradual loss of cell outline, the cellular degeneration contributing to the cyst content (top of picture). *(H&E × 416)*

Many solitary, circumscribed lesions thought clinically to be follicular cysts are in fact benign skin appendage tumours of a variety of histogenetic types.

Epidermal tumours *(Continued)*

Appendageal tumours

Numerous and varied benign tumours of skin appendage origin are recognised. Their classification is a largely histopathological one, based on the presumed cell of origin. They may be either solid or cystic and their importance lies in their differential diagnosis from basal cell carcinoma and epidermoid and pilar cysts. They are all usually benign with only very rare instances of malignant transformation being described. The tumours arise from presumed eccrine and apocrine sweat glands and ducts at varying depths of the appendageal unit and they include the syringoma, eccrine spiradenoma, hidrocystoma and cylindroma. The latter with their multiple dermal nodules and predominant origin in skin of the scalp are occasionally referred to as 'turban' tumours. An interesting benign appendage tumour, the calcifying epithelioma of Malherbe is thought to be of hair shaft derivation and is now termed a pilomatrixoma. It is dermal in site and is formed by proliferating strands of basal and squamous epithelium whose cells die by nuclear loss producing shadow cells. It matures by progressive cell loss, inflammatory reaction and calcification.

Similar appendageal neoplasms which exhibit hair follicle differentiation are termed tricholemmoma, trichofolliculoma and trichoepithelioma, the terminology based loosely on the hair follicle cell of origin and its degree of maturation towards hair structure.

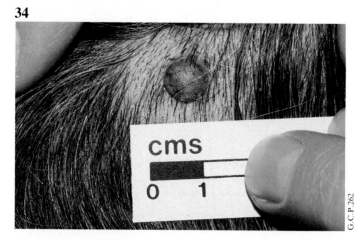

34 This eccrine spiradenoma, dermal in site, is difficult to differentiate from other adnexal cystic lesions on clinical grounds.

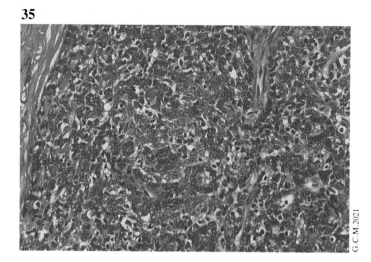

35 Eccrine spiradenoma is a circumscribed benign tumour of eccrine origin, comprising strands and occasional glands of basophilic cells with an intimate vascular component. *(H&E ×250)*

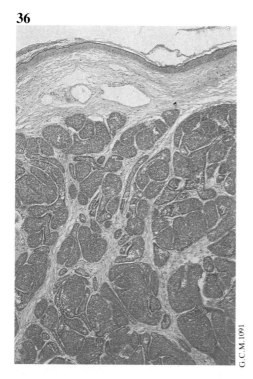

36 Cylindroma. Islands of basophilic cells lie in the dermis. This benign appendage tumour is of probable apocrine origin. *(H&E ×50)*

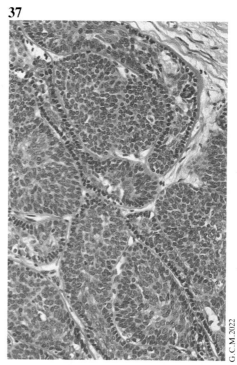

37 The basaloid islands in a cylindroma are closely apposed and defined by a thick hyaline condensation of collagen (top right). *(H&E ×250)*

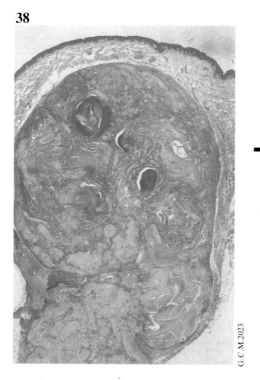

38 Pilomatrixoma (calcifying epithelioma of Malherbe) an unusual benign tumour of hair follicle origin shows basaloid cells, viable and degenerate (shadow), with extensive keratin production. *(H&E ×10)*

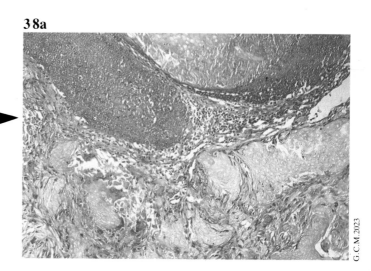

38a Pilomatrixoma showing basaloid islands, shadow cells and giant cell reaction. The necrotic areas calcify with time. *(H&E ×100)*

Benign pigmented lesions

There are about 2000 million melanocytes in the human skin, the number being similar irrespective of race or colour. Hyperplasias and tumours of skin melanocytes occur mainly in the light-skinned races.

Freckles (ephelides)

Freckles are so well known that their clinical description is almost unnecessary. They are common in red haired and blond individuals and are seen as sharply demarcated light brown-gold macules of usually less than 5mm in diameter often in profuse numbers. They are especially obvious on the face, upper trunk and upper limbs. They increase in number and become darker with sun exposure. This is of special significance in relation to caucasoids who migrate to tropical countries.

Histology

Increased melanin pigment is seen in the basal layer of the epidermis without increase in the number of melanocytes and without elongation of the rete ridges.

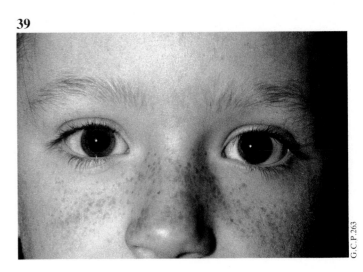

39 Characteristic facial freckling.

Lentigo

Both simple and senile lentigines appear clinically similar. They vary in colour from light to dark brown, are impalpable and vary in size from 1mm to 1cm. They often have an irregular outline. Simple lentigines arise most frequently in childhood and appear as a few scattered lesions without predilection to areas of sun exposure.

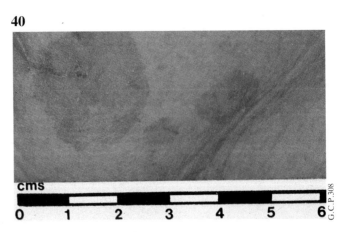

40 Simple lentigines in an elderly person.

398

Histology

41

The rete ridges are elongated and there is an increased number of melanocytes and considerable hyper-pigmentation in the basal layer. Occasionally a small area of junctional activity of melanocytes (*see* melano-cytic naevi) may be seen.

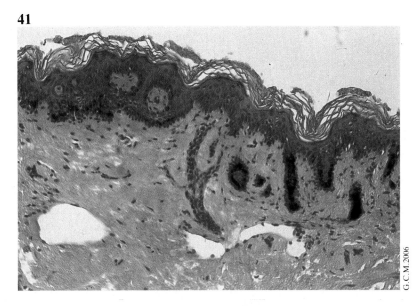

Simple lentigo. *(H&E ×180)*

Conditions associated with multiple lentigines

a   Peutz–Jeghers' Syndrome. Profuse lentigines are seen on and around the lips in this autosomal dominantly inherited condition. Scattered lentigines also occur on the buccal mucosa, gums and hard palate. The syndrome is of some surgical importance because of associated gastro-intestinal polyposis involving especially the small intestine. Complications include recurrent intussusception and rarely malignant transformation of polyps. (*See* Vol. 1. p. 326)

b   Cronkhite–Canada Syndrome. Multiple lentigines on the backs of the hand and diffuse pigmentation of the palms and volar aspects of the fingers. May also be associated with gastro-intestinal polyposis. Alopecia and deformity of the nails complete the rare but characteristic clinical picture. (*See* Vol. 1. p. 327.)

c   'Leopard' Syndrome. An acronym for generalised lentiginosis associated with cardiac abnormalities demonstrated by E.C.G., ocular hypertelorism, pulmonary stenosis, abnormal genitalia, retardation of growth and deafness.

Melanocytic naevi

Naevi are birth marks comprising a local excess of one or several normal constitutents of the skin. Melanocytic naevi (moles) are localised benign proliferations of melanocytes, sometimes associated with hyperplasia of other skin components. They therefore conform to the definition of a hamartoma.

Origin of melanocyte and naevus cell

The normal melanocyte, found in the basal layer of the epidermis, is a neuroectodermal derivative. Its stem cell, the melanoblast, arises from the neural crest (a strip of specialised ectoderm flanking the neural plate) and migrates as early as the fourteenth week in utero to the epidermis. Similar cells also migrate to the choroid – meninges. Once in the epidermis melanocytes form a self-replicating population of cells, which retain their ability to migrate even in adult epidermis. So called 'mongolian spots' are formed by dermal melanocytes and may be due to incomplete migration of melanoblasts from neural crest to epidermis.

Naevus cells, modified melanocytes, may originate from melanoblasts which have failed to reach the epidermis, from Schwann cells of cutaneous nerves or from melanocytes which have migrated from the epidermis to dermis.

Neurofibromatosis, where pigmentary abnormalities are associated with tumours of nerve and adrenal is a reminder of the pluripotentiality of neural crest cells.

Classification of melanocytic naevi

Congenital melanocytic naevus

Dysplastic naevus

Acquired: Junctional naevus
         Compound naevus
         Intradermal naevus
         Blue naevus
         Spitz naevus (Juvenile melanoma)
         Halo naevus

A convenient way of classifying common acquired melanocytic naevi depends on the predominant site of the aggregates of naevus cells.

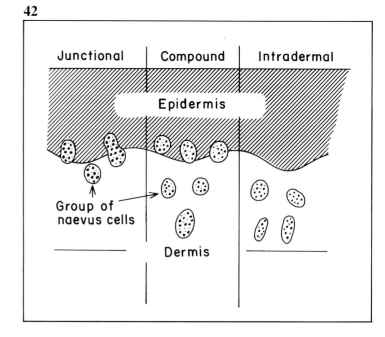

42　Histological types of melanocytic naevi.

Congenital melanocytic naevus

These naevi are present at birth, seldom less than 1cm in diameter and may be very large as in the so-called 'bathing trunk naevus'. They vary from brown to blue-black and may become protuberant and hairy, developing a cerebriform surface. Congenital naevi represent a rare potential origin of malignant melanoma.

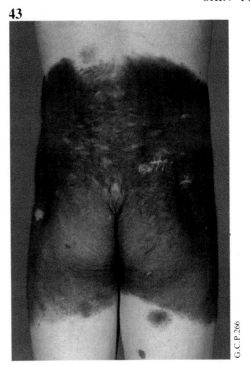

43 Giant congenital melanocytic naevus.

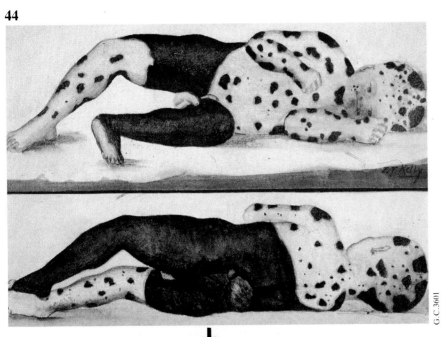

44 An extensive giant bathing trunk type of naevus surrounded by large but discrete congenital melanocytic naevi. The tumour seen on the right mid-back is probably a malignant melanoma.

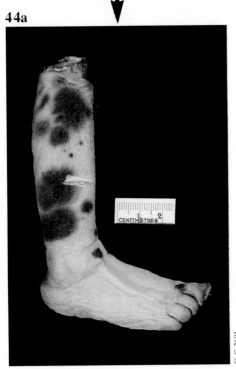

44a Lower leg and foot of child depicted in (**44**).

44b Specimen taken from lower leg. In this instance the histology is that of a heavily pigmented intradermal naevus. *(H&E ×50)*

Dysplastic naevus

Recently a syndrome has been described in which clinically and histologically atypical naevi are associated with familial and sporadic cases of malignant melanoma. There seems to be little virtue in retaining the names of 'B–K mole syndrome' and 'familial atypical multiple mole-melanoma syndrome' for familial examples: 'dysplastic naevus syndrome' seems more appropriate. This syndrome is characterised by the following features.

Clinical

Multiple irregularly pigmented melanocytic naevi. Most profuse on trunk and may be present in scalp. There is irregularity of the edge and a wide variation in size of naevi. Inflammatory halo around some lesions.

Histological

Junctional nests exhibiting epithelioid or lentiginous melanocytic dysplasia (nuclear pleomorphism and hyperchromatism). Fibroplasia of papillary dermis. Lymphocytic inflammatory response.

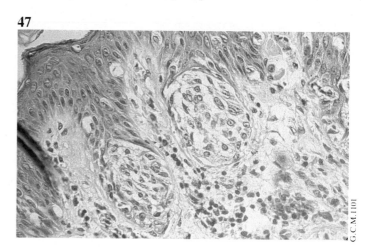

47 Dysplastic naevus. Histology reveals junctional proliferation of atypical melanocytes, with subjacent fibrosis and lymphocytic infiltration. (×250)

Dysplastic naevus syndrome

45 Multiple irregularly pigmented naevi on the back of a young man who has already had a malignant melanoma overlying the left scapula removed.

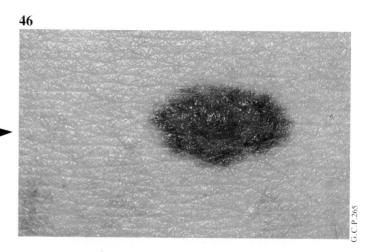

46 Dysplastic naevus (1.5 × 0.9cm). Note irregular pigmentation.

Acquired melanocytic naevus

Clinically it is not easy to predict the histological appearance of melanocytic naevi, but discrete macular or barely palpable pigmented lesions are most likely junctional naevi, whereas dome-shaped papules and papilliferous, even pedunculated lesions are usually compound or intradermal naevi.

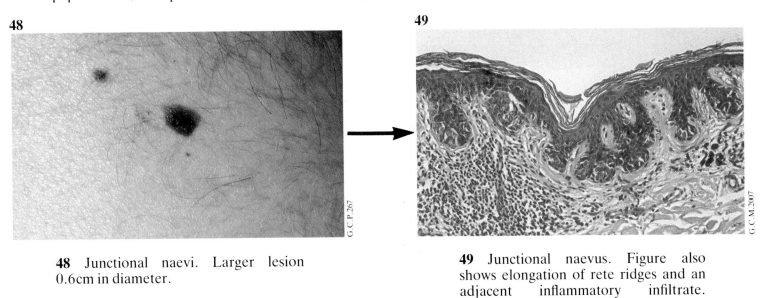

48 Junctional naevi. Larger lesion 0.6cm in diameter.

49 Junctional naevus. Figure also shows elongation of rete ridges and an adjacent inflammatory infiltrate. *(H&E ×150)*

50 Compound melanocytic naevus. Note long-standing symmetrical halo of even light brown pigmentation surrounding the lesion which does not suggest malignancy.

51 Compound hyperkeratotic melanocytic naevus. Occasional foci of junctional activity are apparent but most naevus cells lie in the upper dermis. *(H&E ×40)*

403

Acquired melanocytic naevus *(Continued)*

52

52 Intradermal melanocytic naevus.

53

53 Intradermal melanocytic naevus. Clusters of naevus cells in superficial and mid dermis. No junctional activity. *(H&E ×100)*

Benign clinico-pathological variants include Blue naevus and Spitz naevus (juvenile melanoma), the latter presenting subtle histological features which distinguish it from malignant melanoma.

Blue naevus

54

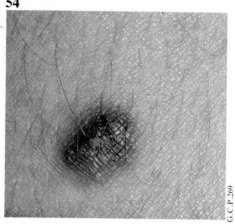

54 Blue naevus on back of wrist.

Spitz naevus

55

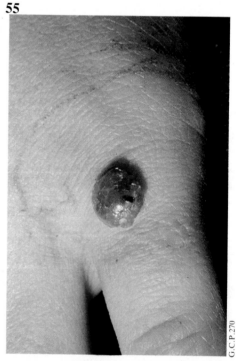

55 Spitz naevus. Solitary pink dome-shaped nodule overlying metacarpophalangeal joint.

56

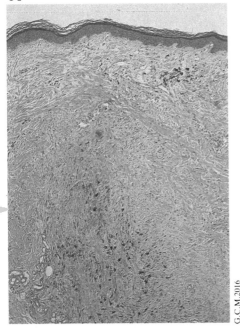

G.C.M.2016

56a

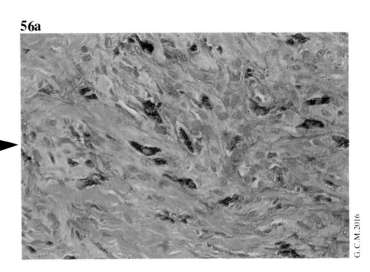

G.C.M.2016

56 Blue naevus. There is no junctional activity and the lesion is seen primarily in the mid and deep dermis. At low power melanophages are especially obvious. *(H&E ×50)*

56a Blue naevus. High power view of (**56**). The elongated dendrites of melano-cytes are now easily seen. In addition there are melanophages, without dendritic processes, filled with coarse melanin granules. *(H&E ×250)*

57

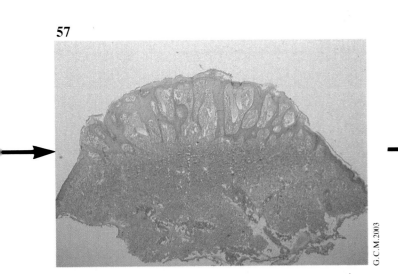

G.C.M.2003

58

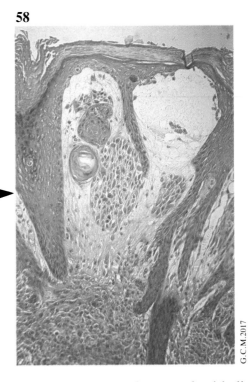

G.C.M.2017

57 Spitz naevus. Scanning view to demonstrate symmetry of lesion. Dermal oedema and dilated capillaries are obvious in the subepidermal zone. *(H&E ×10)*

58 Spitz naevus. Groups of epithelioid naevus cells are seen within and deep to a grossly oedematous superficial dermis. Giant naevus cells and scattered mitoses are also apparent. *(H&E ×100)*

Malignant melanoma

Malignant melanoma is a malignant melanocytic tumour which, although rare, attracts much attention from both the profession and the public because of the potentially tragic sequence of events triggered off by the appearance or change of an apparently trivial black spot.

Incidence

Skin colour

The tumour is rare in negroids except on their less pigmented palms and soles.

Sex

The higher the incidence of the tumour the nearer the F:M ratio approximates 1. In areas of low incidence the F:M ratio may reach 2.

Latitude

There is a significant increase in incidence of cutaneous malignant melanoma in those with white skin living in sunny climates near the equator compared with those living in more temperate zones. The incidence of ocular melanoma appears independent of latitude.

Age

The tumour is very rare before puberty. In the South-east of Scotland the incidence between the ages of 30 and 70 years is about 5/100 000 p.a. but increases in those over 70.

Incidence of malignant melanoma (/100 000 population/year).

Scotland   5
Arizona, USA   27
Queensland, Australia   35

Figures from many parts of the world indicate that the incidence of this tumour is increasing rapidly.

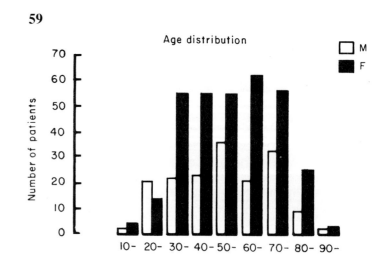

59

59 Histogram of age and sex of 477 patients presenting with primary malignant melanoma in South-east Scotland, 1961–1976.

Site

Few sites are exempt. In areas of low incidence the tumour is most commonly seen on the female lower leg. As the incidence increases more tumours are seen on the trunk, especially of males. Primary malignant melanomas occur occasionally on mucous membranes and rarely at other sites where a few melanocytes are found such as the nail matrix, leptomeninges and gastro-intestinal tract. Ocular melanomas, although rare, are the commonest primary intraocular tumour in adults. About 5% of patients present with metastatic melanoma with no primary lesion detectable ('occult primary melanoma').

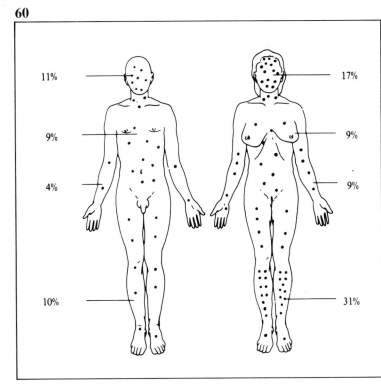

60   Primary site of 477 cutaneous malignant melanomas (66% of tumours in females and 34% in males). South-east Scotland series 1961–1976.

Aetiology

Causative Factor	Evidence
Genetic	Occurs in both white and black races. Increased incidence in whites with blond hair, fair skin which tans poorly, severe freckling. Persons of Celtic origin may be more susceptible. Familial occurrence reported (some related to dysplastic naevi).
Sunlight	Incidence and mortality increases with decreasing latitude. Higher incidence on exposed skin.
Pre-existing pigmented lesion	Increased incidence in people with congenital melanocytic naevi, dysplastic melanocytic naevi. Pre-existing naevus seen histologically in about 30% of malignant melanomas.
Trauma	Increased incidence on feet of barefoot African Bantu.
Virus	RNA tumour viruses have been noted in metastatic deposits of human melanoma and in some animal melanomas.

Malignant melanoma *(Continued)*

Early recognition

About two-thirds of all malignant melanomas, including those developing in melanocytic naevi, have a radial (horizontal) growth phase within the epidermis before dermal invasion takes place. Early recognition of this superficial growth phase is critical because prognosis is directly proportional to the thickness of the tumour removed. Malignant change should be excluded by *excision biopsy* in all pigmented lesions in which the following changes occur:

    itch
    enlargement
    increased or decreased pigmentation
    irregularity of surface or edge
    ulceration
    bleeding

61 Development of invasive melanoma within expanding radial (horizontal) *in situ* area of growth. The reniform projections and notches at the edge of the radial growth phase and the varying colour hues within it are characteristic signs of *in situ* malignancy.

The current classification is based on site and distinctive histological appearances.

In situ malignant melanoma	Invasive malignant melanoma
Lentigo Maligna (Hutchinson's melanotic freckle, Mélanose circonscrite précancéreuse) ⟶	Lentigo Maligna Melanoma
Superficial spreading melanoma *in situ* ⟶	Superficial spreading melanoma
No *in situ* phase	Nodular melanoma
Acral lentiginous melanoma *in situ* ⟶	Acral lentiginous melanoma
Mucosal lentiginous melanoma *in situ* ⟶	Mucosal lentiginous melanoma

62

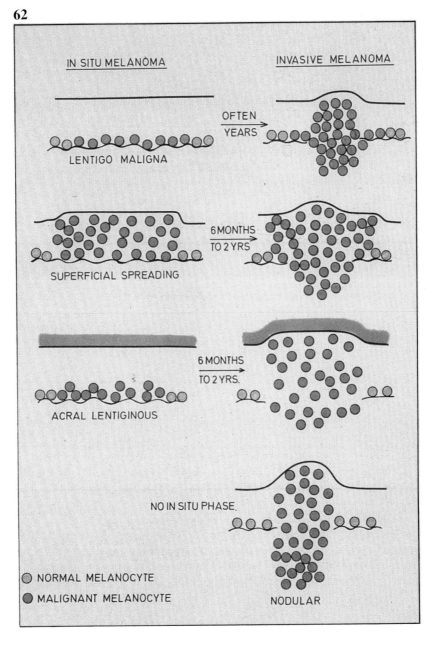

62 Histogenetic classification of malignant melanoma.

Malignant melanoma *(Continued)*

Lentigo maligna

Usually develops on the sun exposed skin of the elderly. It appears as a slowly increasing patch of irregular pigmentation. It is seldom palpable and comprises all shades of light brown to black. Spontaneous regression in some areas causes patches of relative depigmentation.

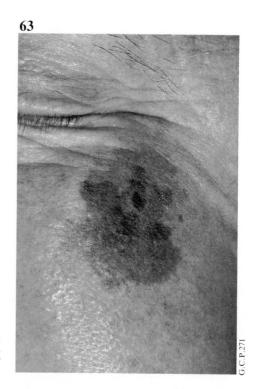

63

63 Lentigo maligna. Lesion on cheek of an elderly patient. Slowly expanding over a period of 5 years.

Lentigo maligna melanoma

A patch of lentigo maligna may expand slowly for years before dermal invasion develops. This is seen as an indurated area of nodule, often dark brown or bluish-black indicating transition to lentigo maligna.

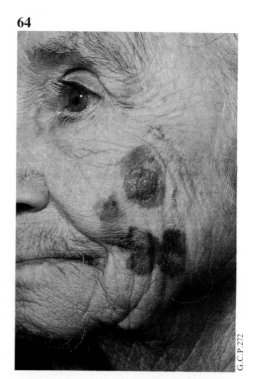

64

64 Lentigo maligna and lentigo maligna melanoma. This old lady had four very slowly expanding pigmented patches on her left cheek (lentigo maligna). Treatment was not sought until the nodule developed within the upper lesion (lentigo maligna melanoma).

Lentigo maligna has a characteristic histology. In the early stages there is hyperpigmentation of the basal layers in the epidermis and marked hyperplasia of atypical melanocytes. These malignant cells are often spindle shaped and contain large pleomorphic angulated hyperchromatic nuclei. A band of chronic inflammatory cells and scattered pigment within macrophages is seen in the adjacent superficial dermis. Prior to dermal invasion the atypical melanocytes aggregate in clusters. Helpful clues in diagnosing this histogenetic pattern are the frequent involvement of melanocytes in the external root sheath of hair follicles and signs of solar damage to the collagen in the adjacent dermis (elastotic degeneration).

65

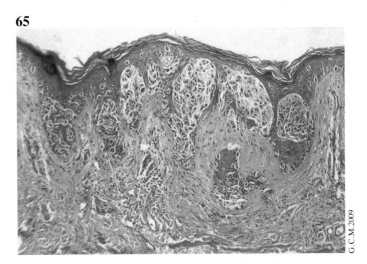

65 Lentigo maligna. Atypical melanocytes, many in large groups are seen along the entire length of the section and in the wall of the hair follicle (centre). No clear cut sign of dermal invasion. *(Masson trichrome ×100)*

Epidermal attenuation and dermal invasion by the atypical cells signifies transition to lentigo maligna melanoma. There is downward streaming of the tumour cells from the epidermis and the tumour nodule is usually composed of spindle shaped melanoma cells. Pigmentation within the tumour may be minimal, but there is often considerable melanin uptake by surrounding melanophages.

66

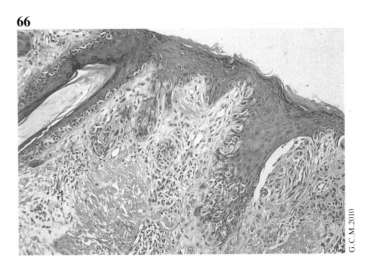

66 Lentigo maligna melanoma. Early dermal invasion has occurred in two areas. Note atypical melanocytes in wall of hair follicle and elastotic degeneration in the dermis. *(H&E ×100)*

Malignant melanoma (*Continued*)

Superficial spreading melanoma *in situ* and superficial spreading melanoma

Superficial spreading melanoma *in situ* appears initially as a slightly elevated, often arciform lesion with prominent indentations and reniform projections at the margins. The colour variations are similar to those of lentigo maligna but more shades of pink and blue are seen. In contrast to lentigo maligna invasion occurs earlier (within one to two years), usually before the lesion is larger than 2–3cm in diameter. Induration, nodule formation, ulceration and bleeding are all signs of transition to an invasive superficial spreading melanoma.

67

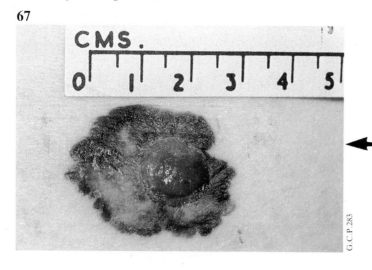

67 Superficial spreading melanoma. Radial growth phase was present for about three years before the amelanotic invasive nodule developed within it. Note different hues including depigmented areas signifying spontaneous regression, in radial area of growth. Protrusions and notches at edge of lesion suggest malignancy.

Histologically the malignant melanocytes of superficial spreading melanoma *in situ* are seen invading the epidermis in a manner reminiscent of that seen in Paget's disease of the breast. From the beginning a few similar cells may also be seen in the papillary dermis. Again the atypical cells have a distinctive appearance, they are uniform in shape and size, often contain abundant finely granular cytoplasm and large nuclei with prominent nucleoli. When dermal invasion, i.e. transition to superficial spreading melanoma occurs, the tumour nodule may comprise epithelial cells, spindle cells, naevus-like cells or combinations of each. Pigmentation within and around the tumour cells is variable. A chronic inflammatory infiltrate is usually present in the subjacent dermis.

68

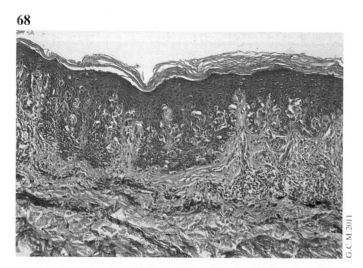

68 Superficial spreading melanoma *in situ*. Note proliferation of atypical melanocytes throughout epidermis. (*H&E ×100*)

69

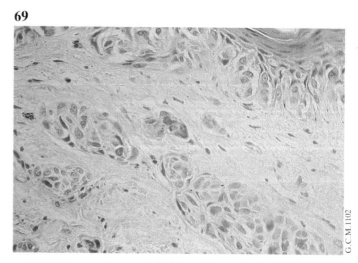

69 Superficial spreading malignant melanoma. Melanocytes invade the papillary dermis. (*×250*)

Nodular melanoma

This type of melanoma starts as an elevated, often deeply pigmented nodule which grows rapidly and frequently ulcerates. Although relatively amelanotic variants occur careful examination (with a lens) usually reveals flecks of pigment.

Histologically no preceding intraepidermal phase is evident. In most cases, including when malignancy develops in a melanocytic naevus, malignant melanocytes proliferate at the dermo-epidermal junction and invade the dermis. The tumour nodule may be indistinguishable from that of lentigo maligna melanoma and superficial spreading melanoma but the absence of an intraepidermal component is an important clue in diagnosing the histogenetic pattern.

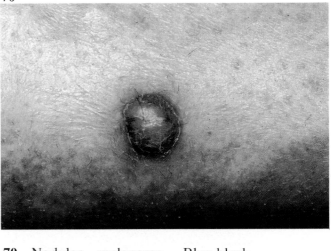

70

70 Nodular melanoma. Blue-black nodule appeared three months before this photo was taken. No radial growth phase apparent.

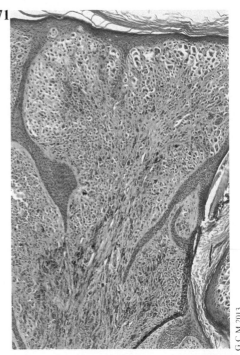

71

71 Nodular melanoma. Field shows epithelioid and spindle tumour cells containing pigment. The latter is also present in melanophages. *(H&E ×62)*

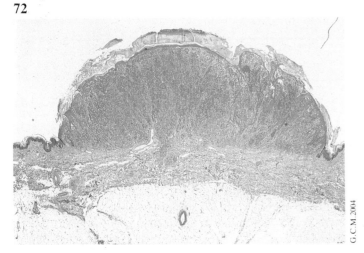

72

72 Nodular melanoma. No *in situ* abnormalities seen within the epidermis adjacent to the tumour nodule. *(H&E ×7.5)*

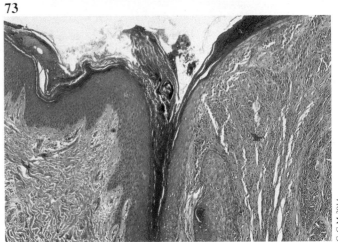

73

73 Nodular melanoma. No *in situ* changes evident at margin (left) or tumour nodule (right). *(Masson's trichrome ×50)*

413

Malignant melanoma (*Continued*)

Acral lentiginous and mucosal lentiginous melanoma

Acral and mucosal melanomas are clinically and histologically similar in many ways. Both types are preceded by an *in situ* radial growth phase similar to that seen in lentigo maligna. Histologically their *in situ* appearance has features of both lentigo maligna and superficial spreading melanoma *in situ* though abnormal melanocytes with long dendrites may be demonstrated by special stains.

74

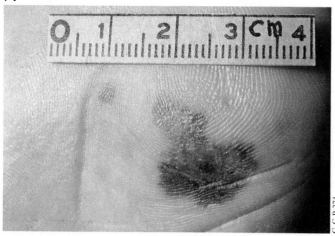

74 Acral lentiginous melanoma *in situ*. Barely palpable irregular patch of pigmentation on the foot – slowly expanding and present for three years. Excision, not observation, essential.

75

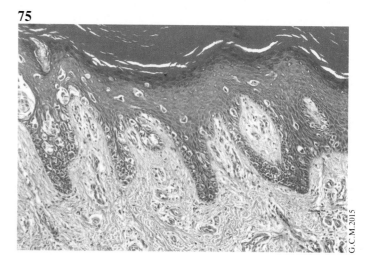

75 Acral lentiginous melanoma *in situ*. Note thick horny layer of sole. Atypical melanocytes are seen in base of epidermis and permeating mid epidermis. (*Masson's trichrome ×100*)

76

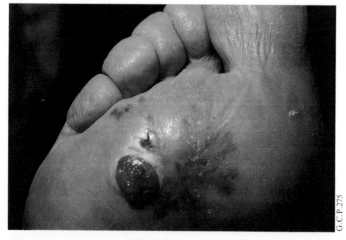

76 Acral lentiginous melanoma. The *in situ* phase was neglected; invasive, relatively amelanotic tumour is now obvious. Prognosis, even after extensive surgery, will be poor.

77

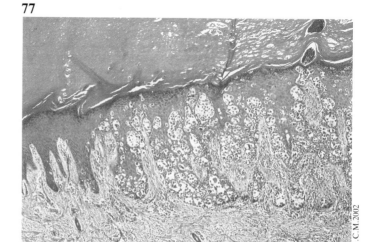

77 Acral lentiginous melanoma. Thick horny layer of sole again evident. Early invasion of malignant melanocytes into superficial dermis is present. (*H&E ×40*)

Subungual melanoma

First described as 'melanotic whitlow' by Sir Jonathan Hutchinson in 1886 because, except for the pigmentation, it resembled ordinary whitlow infections. This presentation is rare in Caucasoids accounting for only 3% of melanomas, but is relatively more common in negroids where it accounts for 15–20% of melanomas.

About half occur under fingernails and half under toenails, by far the most common sites being the nails of big toes and thumbs. The majority of patients who develop subungual melanomas are over 50 years old. Most produce little discomfort, and usually begin as brown to black discoloration in the nail bed. Thickening, splitting, distortion or destruction of the nail plate may occur. The nail bed, proximal and lateral nail folds may then show variable degrees of pigmentation, inflammation and purulent discharge. Approximately one fifth of subungual melanomas are amelanotic.

The differential diagnosis includes ingrowing toenail, chronic paronychia, subungual exostosis, or haematoma.

Diagnosis

Removal of the nail and excision biopsy of the lesion should be carried out if possible. If this is not feasible, biopsy of a portion of the lesion is reasonable at this site though, if the histology is inconclusive, repeat biopsies should be performed.

78

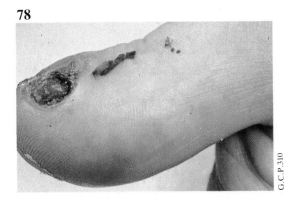

78 Subungual malignant melanoma. The pigmented tumour nodule of the nail bed has destroyed the nail plate. There are tumour satellites proximally.

79

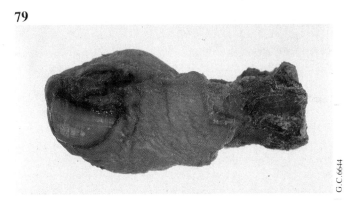

79 Melanoma of nail bed with partial destruction of the nail. Duration – 1 year. Histologically a highly pigmented tumour with fusiform cell formation.

Malignant melanoma *(Continued)*

Clinical staging

The generally accepted tumour – node – metastases (TNM) system of classifying tumours is not found to be satisfactory when assessing the melanomas. An alternative classification is:

Stage I
Local disease
    Stage IA   Primary lesion alone.
          IB   Primary and satellites within 5cm.
          IC   Local recurrence within 5cm of primary site.
          ID   Spread more than 5cm from primary site but within primary lymphatic drainage area.

Stage II
Nodal disease
  (regional draining nodes)
    Stage IIA Regional lymph nodes; clinically positive, histology not done.
          IIB Regional lymph nodes; clinically negative, histology positive.
          IIC Regional lymph nodes; clinically positive, histology positive.

Stage III
Disseminated disease
    Stage IIIA Remote cutaneous/subcutaneous melanoma.
          IIIB Remote nodal involvement only.
          IIIC Both of above.
          IIID Visceral spread.

(New York University Melanoma Co-operative Group)

Microstaging

Microstaging depends on the measurement of the thickness of the invasive nodule. This indicates the prognosis. Breslow's method, using an ocular micrometer, measures the depth of the invasion from the granular cell layer. Clark's method assesses the invasion of the tumour by relating it to the micro-anatomical layers of the skin penetrated. As the latter method does not require the use of an ocular micrometer both are illustrated below.

80

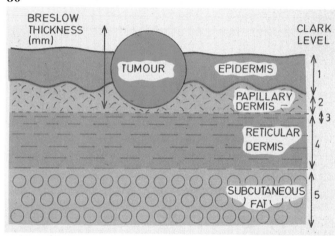

80 Schematic representation of Breslow's and Clark's method of microstaging of malignant melanoma.

81

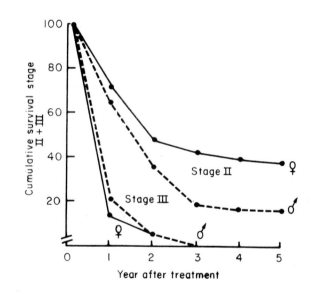

81 South-east Scotland series 1961–1976. Survival curves for 100 patients with stage II and 32 patients with stage III malignant melanoma.

Prognosis

Indicator	Prognostic significance
Depth of primary tumour	Breslow < 1.5mm Good Breslow > 3.5mm Bad
Sex	Females fare significantly better than males.
Age	Prognosis worsens after the age of 50 years, especially in males.
Site	Poorer prognosis with tumours on trunk, upper arms, neck and scalp.
Ulceration of primary tumour	Signifies poorer prognosis.
Clinical stage	Stage I – 5 year survival 75% Stage II – 5 year survival 25% Stage III – 5 year survival 0–5%

Spread

In approximately 75% of patients in whom the tumour recurs the first recurrence is at the primary site, in the local lymph node or in the intransit area. Blood borne spread to the liver, lungs or a distant subcutaneous site occurs in the remaining quarter. In general the nearer the recurrence to the site of the primary lesion, the sooner it is diagnosed. In the South-east Scotland series it was found that 35% of all cases recurring within 10 years of treatment did so within the first year, 65% within three years and 81% within five years. Recurrences can even occur up to 20 years after treatment. It has been calculated that spontaneous regression in metastatic melanoma occurs in one patient per 400 with metastatic disease.

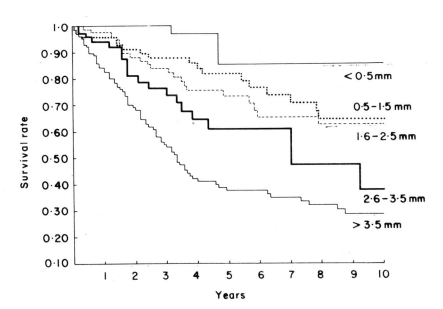

82 Survival curves illustrating the predictive value of tumour thickness (measured by Breslow's method) on prognosis. Curves based on a series of 477 patients with malignant melanoma treated in Edinburgh between 1961 and 1976.

Malignant melanoma *(Continued)*

Differential diagnosis

All brown-black tumours should be considered in the differential diagnosis. Those most often confused with malignant melanoma include seborrhoeic wart, pigmented basal cell carcinoma, sclerosing haemangioma, haematoma and so-called 'Talon noir' (black heel). Rarely malignant melanoma presents as a truly amelanotic tumour with no hint of pigment visible even with the help of a lens. Excision biopsy, if possible, should be carried out to settle the issue histologically. Occasionally electron microscopy is helpful in defining the nature of an amelanotic tumour.

83

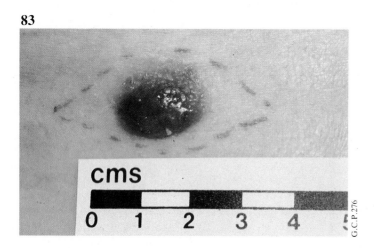

83 Inflamed seborrhoeic wart.

84

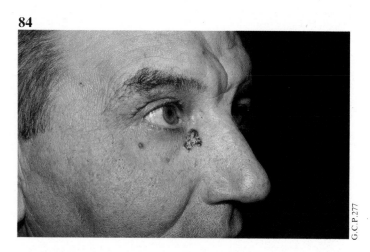

84 Pigmented basal cell carcinoma. Site and opalescent nature of lesion should arouse diagnostic suspicion.

85

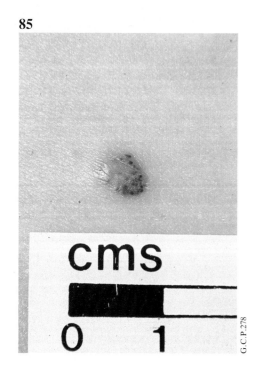

85 Sclerosing haemangioma. Thrombosed capillary heads and frosted glass-like surface are useful pointers to the diagnosis.

86

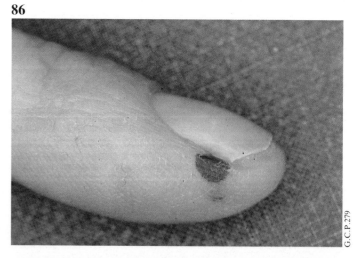

86 Periungual haematoma. Appearance and history of trauma allow paring to be carried out and the avoidance of an unnecessary operation.

87

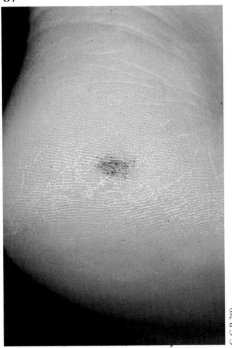

87 'Talon noir'. Squash player with new shoes. Once the peppery appearance of the capillary heads is seen and recognised it is never forgotten. Paring satisfies everybody.

88

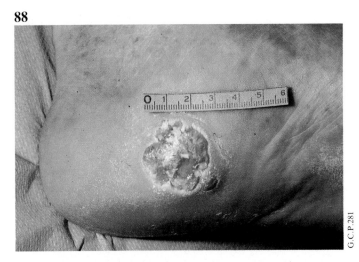

88 Amelanotic melanoma. Beware of the slowly growing atypical 'corn'. Appearance may be altered by self treatment with wart paints etc.

89

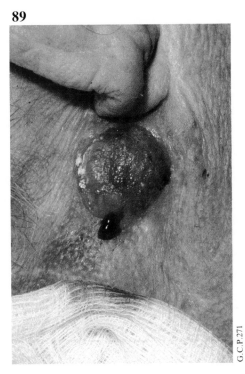

89 Amelanotic melanoma. Rapidly growing skin coloured tumour. Appearance not specific and could be due to an anaplastic squamous cell carcinoma or to another malignant tumour.

90

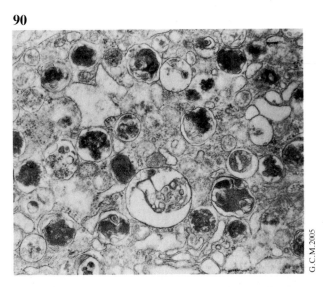

90 Electron micrograph of part of a melanoma cell. The presence of grossly abnormal melanosomes (pigment granules) may allow a definitive diagnosis to be made in undifferentiated malignant tumours.

Ocular malignant melanoma

Though an unusual site for its development, primary malignant melanoma is the commonest primary intra-ocular neoplasm in adults. It may arise from any area of the uveal tract though the choroid and ciliary bodies are involved more often than the retina. Since uveal tract melanomas may arise from pre-existing naevi, early diagnosis is clearly beneficial; in the case of choroidal melanomas, however, presentation may not be until the tumour has attained considerable size.

As with skin melanomas, the size of the lesion is a factor in determining outcome though less attention is paid to the depth, the overall size of the tumour being a useful prognostic factor. In the past, the degree of pigmentation was used as a prognostic indicator, heavily pigmented lesions having a worse outlook than sparsely pigmented variants. It is now thought that this component has little if any independent role in predicting outcome.

Illustrative case

From an adult female.
42 years   Patient noticed reduced right visual acuity (6/18) and went to optician, then general practitioner, then hospital clinic.
Clinic diagnosis: malignant melanomas of choroid.
43 years   Right enucleation.

91

91a

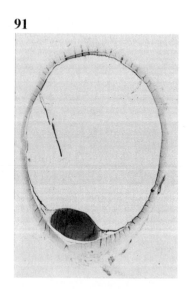 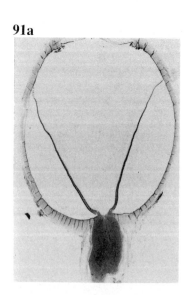

Right globe (without cornea) 23mm AP × 24mm × 24mm + 5mm of optic nerve. Externally normal. Section shows a small, sessile nodule 6mm in diameter × 3mm in thickness arising in the choroid near the optic nerve head.

Histology

The histological classification into spindle A, spindle B and epithelioid seems to be valuable in predicting the growth potential of the lesion. The spindle A are small spindle-shaped cells with fusiform nuclei often exhibiting a central groove. Lesions formed entirely of these cells conform to a melanocytic naevus. The spindle B cells are larger and show varying pleomorphism with large nuclei, prominent nucleoli and increasing mitotic activity. The epithelioid cells are not a distinct cell type but are probably an intralesional transformation of spindle B into cells of varying size, some giant, with abundant eosinophilic rather granular cytoplasm. Mixed cell variants occur. The proportion of these varying cell types in the lesion is useful in assessing prognosis; thus lesions with spindle A and B or pure B show a 70% five-year survival whereas those with an epithelioid component have a five-year survival of only 50%.

91b

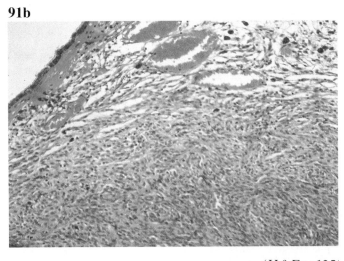

(H&E ×125)

91c

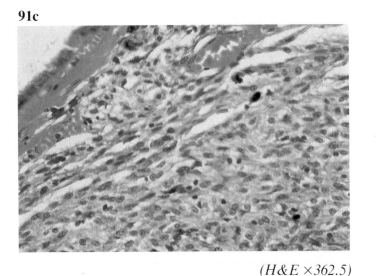

(H&E ×362.5)

91d

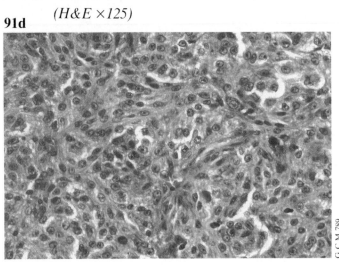

(H&E ×362.5)

The tumour is a poorly pigmented melanoma of the choroid. It forms a very discrete lenticular mass limited externally by sclera and internally by the pigmented epithelial layer of the retina. The tumour is of the mixed cell type (spindle B and epithelioid). The tumour does not involve the optic nerve; the optic cup is slightly excavated. No other abnormalities are seen.

Dermal tumours

Vascular tumours of skin

These lesions, dermal in site, may be either hamartomatous or acquired. The former usually represent disordered proliferation of endothelial-lined spaces of varying calibre and are termed haemangiomas. Haemangiomas usually occur sporadically without genetic predisposition. Their classification is confusing as there is no true clinico-histological correlation. They may be macular (capillary haemangioma, naevus flammeus or 'port-wine' stain) or elevated (capillary-cavernous haemangioma or 'strawberry' naevus). Macular haemangiomas are present at birth and are usually permanent. Elevated haemangiomas become obvious and grow in the first few months of life and involute spontaneously after a variable period.

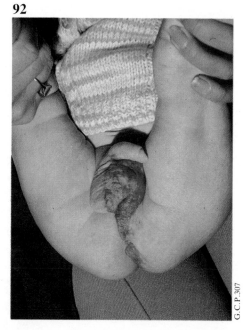

92 Capillary cavernous haemangioma (strawberry naevus). Appeared soon after birth, rapidly enlarged, and is now beginning to fibrose. Spontaneous involution anticipated and no surgical treatment necessary.

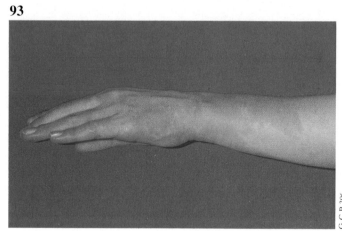

93 Capillary haemangioma (port-wine stain) left hand and wrist. Present since birth and no sign of resolution.

Pathology

Haemangiomas may be classified according to their histological pattern as capillary, cavernous or mixed. The capillary haemangioma comprises a fine network of capillary channels located in the upper and mid dermis. The cavernous haemangioma consists of multiple ectatic channels of varying calibre located in upper, mid and lower dermis and sometimes involving subcutaneous fat. The channels contain blood and have a flat endothelial lining.

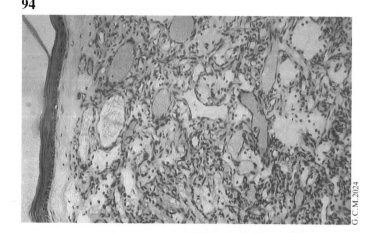

94 Capillary haemangioma. Multiple thin-walled channels of small to medium calibre lie in the dermis. (*H&E ×150*)

95

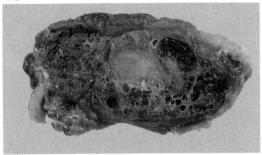

95 Cavernous haemangioma. Large blood-filled vascular spaces are seen on the cut surface.

95a

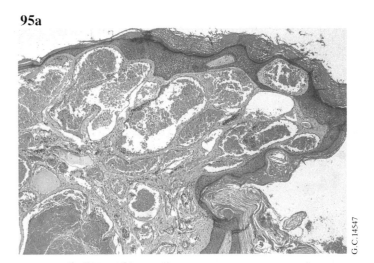

95a Cavernous haemangioma. Dilated blood-filled vascular channels lie in upper, mid and deep dermis. *(H&E ×40)*

Lymphangioma

Lymphangiomas are also hamartomatous. In the superficial form, lymphangioma circumscriptum, the dilated lymphatic channels, containing pale-staining lymph and occasional erythrocytes, lie in upper dermis, closely applied to the overlying epidermis which may show variable acanthosis and hyperkeratosis.

96

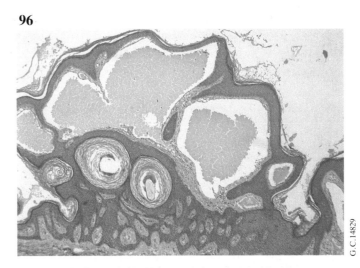

96 Lymphangioma circumscriptum. Dilated thin-walled channels containing lymph lie closely opposed to a papillomatous epidermis. *(H&E ×44)*

Dermal tumours *(Continued)*

Glomus tumour

This is probably a true neoplasm derived from small arteriovenous shunts, most often in the skin of the fingertips or under the nails. When solitary, the lesion is often painful. Multiple lesions are less often symptomatic. They may be red or bluish in colour.

Histology

Histologically the tumour contains vascular channels but the cellular element is seen to comprise polygonal, regular, eosinophilic cells with dark staining centrally placed nuclei, located between the vascular lumina beneath a flat endothelium.

The glomus tumour has a very rich supply of nerve fibres.

97

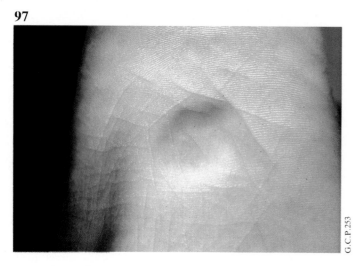

97 Glomus tumour. This dermal lesion has a bluish colour visualised through the intact epidermis.

98

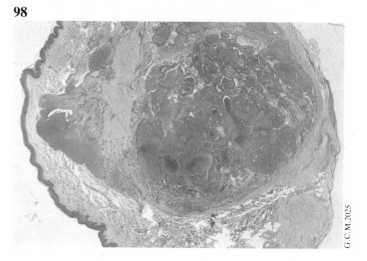

98 Glomus tumour. This cellular and highly vascular tumour lies in the dermis and subcutaneous tissue. A well defined capsule encloses its deeper aspect. *(H&E ×12.5)*

99

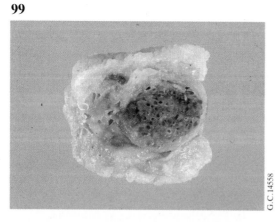

99 Glomus tumour. A transection of the lesion shows numerous vascular channels with intervening cellular walls.

100

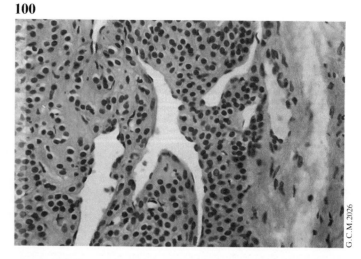

100 Glomus tumour. At higher magnification the small cuboidal eosinophilic constituent cells lie between vascular channels, beneath a flat endothelium. *(H&E ×312)*

424

Pyogenic granuloma

These benign usually solitary vascular proliferative lesions are often associated with a history of trauma and may cause concern due to rapid growth, surface ulceration, bleeding and pain.

Histology reflects the clinical appearance, the lesion comprising proliferating capillary channels arising from moderate calibre arteriolar vessels at the base and forming a dome-shaped nodule. The epidermis at the margins shows reactive acanthosis but is usually ulcerated over the surface where an intense fibrinous and inflammatory exudate is found. The inflammatory component extends throughout the stroma of the lesion. Healing may occur by surface epithelialisation at which time it may be difficult to distinguish these healed lesions from pre-existing hamartomatous haemangiomas. The tumour is therefore inappropriately named as it is neither pyogenic nor granulomatous.

101

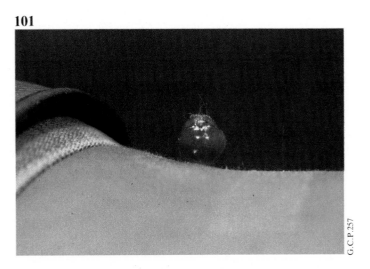

101 Pyogenic granuloma is an elevated, often ulcerated and bleeding lesion which may grow rapidly.

102

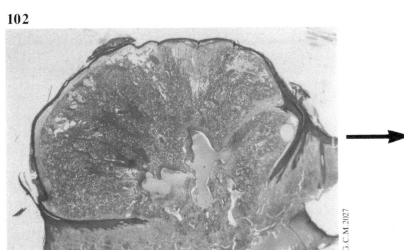

102 Histologically the pyogenic granuloma comprises leashes of varying calibre vessels invested by a thinned epidermis. The epidermis is usually ulcerated but on this section is intact. *(H&E ×15)*

102a

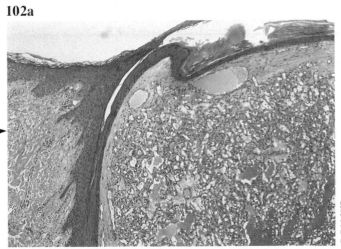

102a Same section – the bottom left-hand edge of the lesion seen at a higher magnification. The surface capillary network is embedded in a stroma which may be inflamed. The epidermis at the margin shows reactive hyperplasia. *(H&E ×50)*

Dermal tumours *(Continued)*

Dermatofibroma

These benign dermal lesions are subject to a wide range of confusing nomenclature: fibrous histiocytoma; sclerosing haemangioma; nodular subepidermal/dermal fibrosis. They occur as firm, discrete, usually solitary dermal nodules often on the extremities of young adults. The lesions are frequently endophytic, giving an 'iceberg' effect on palpation. There may be associated overlying pigmentation. A history of trauma or an insect bite is occasionally elicited.

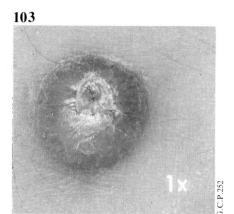

103 Dermatofibroma. The lesion is 1cm in diameter and circumscribed, and in this case, is pigmented.

Histology

Histologically the lesion is a poorly circumscribed nodule comprising a proliferation of fibroblasts with associated collagen synthesis and an admixture of macrophages, the whole merging gradually with mature and sparsely cellular collagen at the edges of and deep to the lesion.

On occasion the vascular component is particularly prominent and the stromal deposition of haemosiderin suggests an original vascular aetiology. Such an appearance may merit the term 'sclerosing haemangioma', but in most instances there is no clinical or histological evidence that the lesions arise from pre-existing haemangiomas. The overlying epidermis characteristically exhibits acanthosis, hyperkeratosis and increased basal melanin synthesis; this may reflect local growth factor production within the lesion.

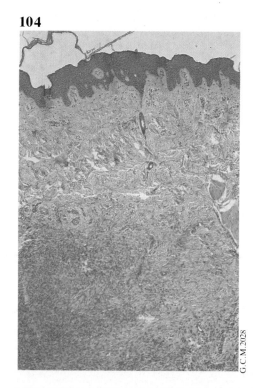

104 The proliferating fibroblasts of the dermatofibroma merge into the sparsely cellular dermis at the margins. The overlying epidermal hyperplasia and hyperpigmentation is seen. *(H&E ×50)*

104a

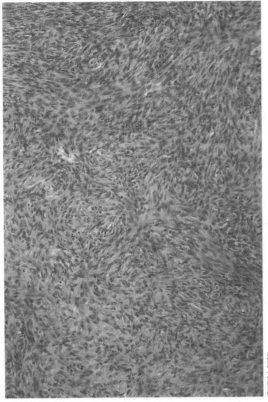

104a The cellular constituents of the dermatofibroma are fibroblasts, often proliferating in a whorled pattern, and an admixture of macrophages. *(H&E × 150)*

These lesions are almost certainly reactive rather than neoplastic, reflecting proliferation of both macrophage and fibroblast elements, the former probably releasing a growth factor for the latter. Thus nodular subepidermal or dermal fibrosis may be preferable terms.

Differential diagnosis

This lesion has to be differentiated from neurofibroma and leiomyoma, both of which may present as solitary dermal nodules, without clinically distinct features, though the latter may be painful. The diagnosis thus relies on histological evaluation.

Lymphoma

Skin infiltration may occur during the course of any malignant lymphoma, but certain types are characterised from the beginning by skin involvement. The majority of these will result eventually in extracutaneous disease spread. At present the simplest classification of skin lymphomas is into those of T and B cell types.

T cell lymphoma

105

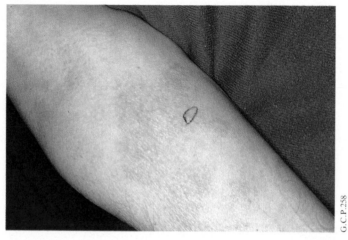

105 The premycotic stage of mycosis fungoides shows scattered barely palpable erythematous scaly patches.

Malignant lymphoma of skin-associated T lymphocytes, known as mycosis fungoides, is a disease of slow evolution with clinical phases of premycotic, infiltrative or plaque and tumour stages with eventual spread to lymph nodes and other tissues late in the disease. The premycotic stage may last for years. Most commonly it comprises scattered barely palpable, erythematous scaly patches; these may resemble psoriasis but they are much more recalcitrant to treatment. On close inspection epidermal atrophy with surface wrinkling is usually evident and such plaques are often slightly pigmented. Widespread poikiloderma is a rarer premycotic phase. As the lymphoma develops the scanty patches become indurated and obviously palpable. This phase is succeeded by the development of frank tumours which often ulcerate, usually within three years.

106

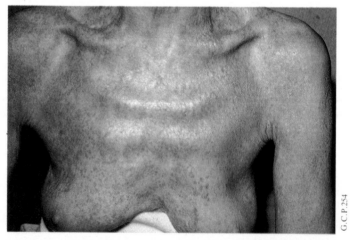

106 Less commonly, the premycotic phase is that of poikiloderma with atrophy, pigmentation and telangiectasiae.

107

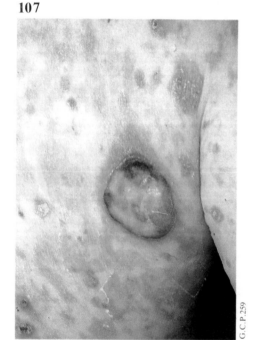

107 With evolution into mycosis fungoides the patches become palpable plaques with frank tumour formation and ulceration.

Histology

In the premycotic stage, a dense upper dermal infiltrate of lymphocytes hugs the basal layer of the epidermis and may show focal emigration or infiltration into the overlying epidermis. This epidermotropism is characteristic of T cell lymphomas. With time the cellularity of the infiltrate, its cytological atypia and its propensity for epidermal invasion increases and in the plaque stage there may be considerable invasion by groups of neoplastic cells forming so-called Pautrier's micro abscesses. In the tumour stage, the epidermal and upper dermal infiltrate is associated with extensive necrosis and involvement of deeper layers of the dermis.

Throughout the disease progression, the atypia of the cells and the number of atypical cells increases. The cells characteristically have irregular, deeply-convoluted or cerebriform nuclei but early in the disease these may be infrequent. Other appearances include larger cells with multilobulated nuclei and prominent nucleoli, a variation on the cerebriform cell. The use of monoclonal antibodies to lymphocyte subsets has allowed delineation of the identity of these cells; in mycosis fungoides the majority are T helper cells.

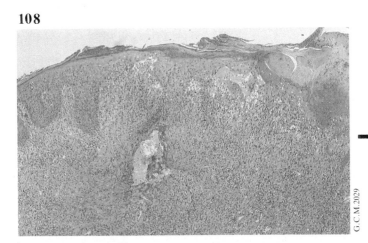

108 Mycosis fungoides. A heavy infiltrate of pleomorphic lymphoid cells invades the upper dermis and infiltrates the overlying epidermis causing ulceration. *(H&E ×50)*

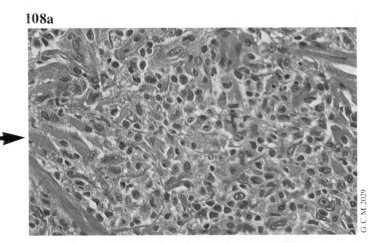

108a In the upper dermis pleomorphic lymphocytes often with cerebriform nuclei invade between collagen bundles *(H&E ×375)*

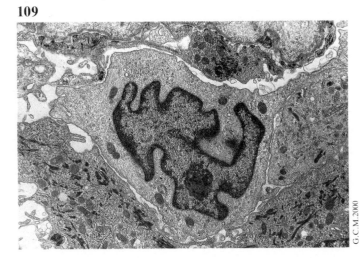

109 Electronmicrograph of a neoplastic T cell in mycosis fungoides. Note the deeply convoluted nuclear outline.

Lymphoma (*Continued*)

B cell malignant lymphoma

B cell malignant lymphomas most often present *ab initio* as scattered plum-coloured skin nodules. Histologically they are usually of follicle centre cell origin and show a perivascular distribution in mid and deep dermis, with frequent extension into subcutaneous tissues. The cells may be of centrocytic and/or centroblastic type and may be diffuse or nodular in pattern, though the former is more common. The majority of B cell lymphomas of skin develop disease at other sites (lymph nodes, liver, marrow and blood) within 5 years.

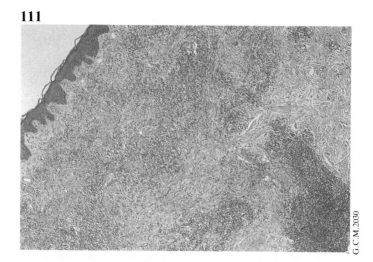

111 Histologically the B cell lymphoma typically infiltrates mid and lower dermis in a nodular or diffuse manner. (*H&E ×40*)

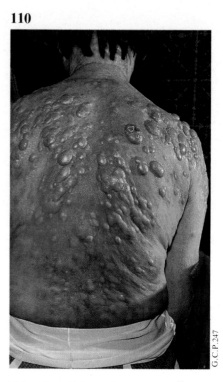

110 B cell lymphoma of skin. Multiple plum-coloured nodules cover most of the back of this patient.

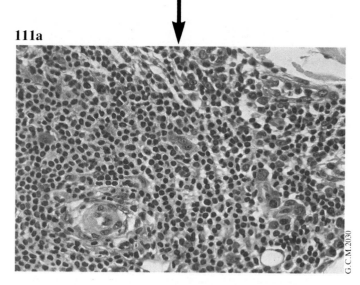

111a B cell lymphoma of skin. In this case the majority of cells are centrocytes. (*H&E ×375*)

The entity *lymphocytoma cutis* or pseudolymphoma of Spiegler–Feldt manifests itself as solitary or multiple small coloured or translucent nodules often on the face. Histologically there is lymphoid infiltration of the mid and deep dermis, the lymphocytes exhibiting germinal-centre formation or a well-organised lymphoid delineation by macrophages. These lesions may be difficult to distinguish from malignant lymphoma of nodular pattern and indeed it is now thought that a proportion of these pseudolymphomas will progress to malignant lymphoma.

In the interpretation of all lymphoid infiltration of skin the pattern, cytological appearances, delineation of lymphocyte subsets, epidermal involvement etc., must be closely correlated with the clinical features such as site, number and distribution of lesions, their duration and evolution before a diagnosis of malignant lymphoma of skin is made. The use of immunohistochemistry aids in the identification of the lymphocyte population.

Immunohistochemistry

T cell

Immunohistochemistry using monoclonal antibodies to T cell subsets demonstrates that the majority of infiltrating cells in mycosis fungoides are of T helper type.

B cell

Immunohistochemistry using antisera to immunoglobulin heavy and light chains confirms that this lymphoma shows a monoclonal expansion of B cells (in this case with IgM, Kappa expression).

112

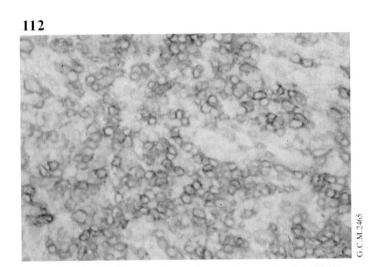

112 Cutaneous T cell lymphoma. The lymphocytic infiltrate in upper dermis is stained with a monoclonal antibody to T helper cells using an immunoperoxidase method. The brown staining product reflects antibody binding and shows that most of the neoplastic cells are of T helper type. *(×500)*

113

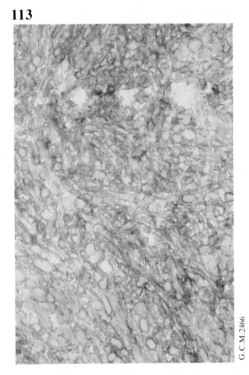

113 B cell lymphoma involving skin. This immunoperoxidase technique employs various antisera to B cell surface markers or products. Brown staining reflects a positive reaction. In this case, neoplastic cells show a predominant Kappa light chain production. *(×500)*

Kathryn McLaren

J. A. A. Hunter

Kaposi's sarcoma

This tumour was described by Moricz Kaposi in 1872 and is generally called by his name. The alternative term idiopathic multiple haemorrhagic sarcoma is also used.

The condition usually starts as small red nodules in the skin of the extremities. The nodules grow, multiply, and may coalesce forming larger, sometimes ulcerated, tumours. There is often swelling of the part and massive oedema may dominate the clinical picture. Most nodules remain small and some disappear spontaneously. The disease progresses and may involve any of the body tissues.

Kaposi's sarcoma, though widely reported, remained a curiosity of dermatology until it was recognised with remarkable frequency in the African negro after 1950. It has been reported throughout sub-Saharan Africa with a maximum incidence in north-eastern Zaire.

114

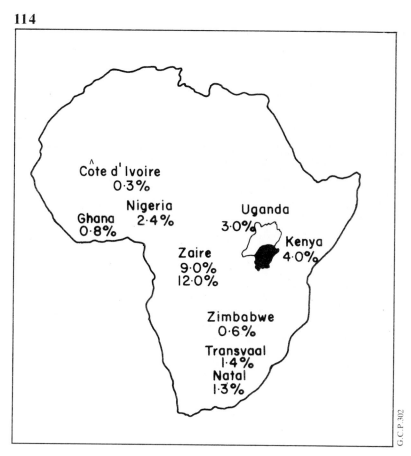

114 The figures demonstrate the incidence of Kaposi sarcoma as a percentage of all malignant tumours.

Epidemiology

Epidemiological studies of the large body of material now available shows some of the following unusual features:

1 A tendency to spontaneous regression,
2 A strong affinity for males,
3 A statistical association (outside Africa) with the reticuloses,
4 The generalised lymphadenopathic form of the disease in children.

Clinical features and length of survival

Abundant clinical studies in Africa suggest that three main patterns can be discerned:
Nodular – superficial plaques and small nodules.

Locally aggressive – including large and ulcerated lesions.

Generalised – including in children a syndrome of scanty nodules and generalised lymphadenopathy and in adults the appearance of lesions in lymph nodes, gastro-intestinal tract, heart, lungs, and skeleton.

	%	% alive at 3 years
Nodular	68	91
Locally aggressive	20	64
Generalised	12	0

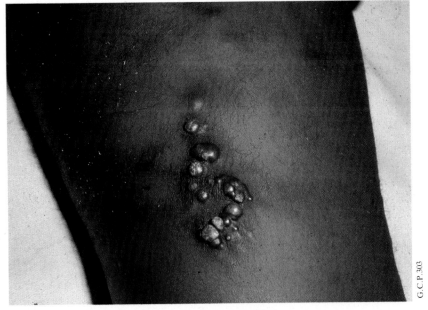

115 Volar aspect of forearm showing typical nodules, and some pigmented patches.

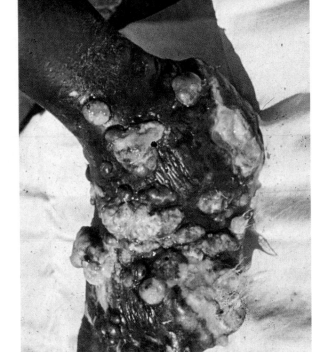

116 Foot showing locally aggressive disease.

Kaposi's sarcoma (Continued)

117

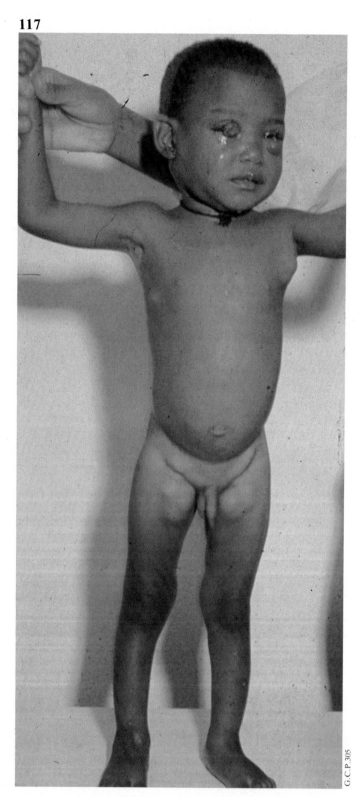

In recent years Kaposi's sarcoma has been reported in circumstances which may throw light on its aetiology. Organ transplant recipients show an increased incidence of malignant tumours of which Kaposi's sarcoma accounts for about 4%, eight times its expected incidence in the general population. Immunosuppressive agents may play a part in the development of these tumours as one example of the 'Acquired Immune Deficiency Syndrome'. Two main hypotheses have been advanced to explain these tumours, namely:

1 That Kaposi's sarcoma is a response to an 'angiogenesis factor' released in a graft-versus-host reaction between transformed and normal lymphocytes.

2 Oncogenic viruses are either activated during an immunological reaction or, more plausibly, facilitated by immune suppression.

Kaposi's sarcoma has also appeared unduly frequently in association with various rare opportunistic infections in previously healthy male homosexuals. The linking factor here may be the wide dissemination among this group of cytomegalovirus, which has been shown to have strong serological and electronmicroscopical links with Kaposi's sarcoma. The association begins to resemble that between another Herpes virus, Epstein–Barr, and Burkitt's lymphoma.

117 Kaposi's sarcoma in childhood. Lymphadenopathy and conjunctival nodules.

Histology

The microscopic appearances are of angiomatous areas of new blood vessels growing in dermis and often subcutaneous fat, set in a matrix of large spindle cells showing a moderate mitotic index. These cells sometimes part into vascular slits. There are many interstitial red cells, numerous widely scattered histiocytes, and a sparse infiltrate of small round cells. Brown granules of haemosiderin are a variable feature. The vascularity of the lesion is only appreciated on high power examination when the irregular clefts and their red-cell content reflect the attempted vascular differentiation.

The histological appearances have been classified into mixed cell, monocell and anaplastic pattern indicating aggression. The spindle cells have been regarded as the essential tumour cells and their origin is still uncertain although evidence from tissue culture and electron microscopy suggests that they are malignant fibroblasts. This fits the general view that the tumour is a multifocal angiosarcoma arising from undifferentiated mesenchymal cells in the adventitia of small blood vessels. It is probably not related to other angiosarcomas or to the lymphangiosarcoma.

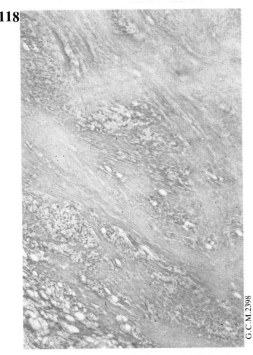

118 Field illustrating monocell appearance. *(Masson trichrome)*

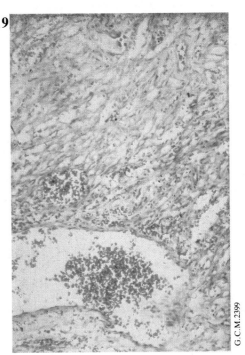

119 Low power photomicrograph of tumour showing typical features of mixed cell type. *(Phloxine – tartrazine)*

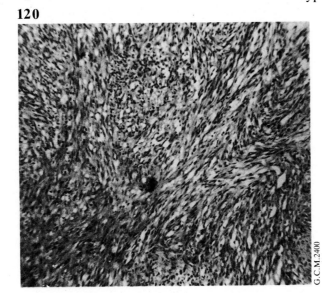

120 Field showing 'anaplastic' characteristics.

J. Cook

Index

438

Forthcoming volumes in the series

Volume 3
Genitourinary system

Congenital and acquired lesions including tumours of the renal tract. This covers the surgical pathology of the kidney, ureters and bladder. Lesions of the male genital tract including diseases of the prostate and testis. Female genital tract. The major lesions of the uterus, ovaries and fallopian tubes.

Volume 4
Cardiovascular system

This includes a study of lesions of the heart both congenital and acquired, and the vascular and lymphatic systems.
Respiratory system. The major lesions of the bronchus, lungs and pleura. Lesions of the mediastinum.

Volume 5
Orthopaedic lesions

This covers the major lesions both congenital and acquired of bones and joints.